Extracorporeal Shock V

Springer
Berlin
Heidelberg
New York
Barcelona
Budapest
Hong Kong
London
Milan
Paris
Santa Clara
Singapore
Tokyo

W. Siebert M. Buch (Eds.)

Extracorporeal Shock Waves in Orthopaedics

With 95 Figures and 51 Tables

Springer

Prof. Dr. med. WERNER SIEBERT
Dr. med. MATTHIAS BUCH
Orthopädische Klinik Kassel
Wilhelmshöher Allee 345
34131 Kassel, Germany

Translated by:
John Chinnery, Apartado 1053, 08080 Barcelona, Spain
Angie Faust, Gerberstr. 6, 30169 Hannover, Germany

ISBN-13:978-3-540-63092-0 e-ISBN-13:978-3-642-80427-4
DOI:10.1007/978-3-642-80427-4

Die Deutsche Bibliothek - CIP-Einheitsaufnahme
Extracorporeal shock waves in orthopaedics / W. Siebert; M. Buch (eds.). [Transl. by: John Chinnery]. - Berlin; Heidelberg; New York; Barcelona; Budapest; Hong Kong; London; Milan; Paris; Santa Clara; Singapore; Tokyo: Springer, 1997

Cover-Design: Design & Production GmbH, Heidelberg

Typesetting: K+V Fotosatz, Beerfelden

SPIN 10630700 24/3137-5 4 3 2 1 0 - Printed on acid-free paper

Preface

Over the past 12 years extracorporeal shock wave therapy has been successfully applied to the treatment of renal calculi. The advances in technology have lead to simplification of the technical apparatus.

In recent years, extracorporeal shock wave therapy has also been introduced in orthopaedic specialities, more and more so by physicians in private practice. The aim of this book is to review the current state of research and give an overview of the various extracorporeal shock wave applications in orthopaedics. We therefore present the literature and results from the First and the Second Shock Wave Symposium in Kassel, Germany. Furthermore, results of experiments on animals by the work group headed by Delius and Draenert (LMU Munich), some of which are published here for the first time, and results and experience gathered over years in hospitals and private practices in Germany and other countries and by the DGST/IGESTO.

Indications that have as yet not been the focus of great attention, such as treatment of spastic children with extracorporeal shock waves, are also given attention.

Taking into account that medicine is a continuously evolving science, this book can only present the current state of scientific research. Our intention is to provide the numerous colleagues who make use of this application with an overview of the various methods in extracorporeal shock wave therapy in orthopaedics. We also attempt to define goals for further research.

W. Siebert
M. Buch

Kassel, June 1997

Contents

List of Contributors

Andretta, D., Dr.
Universita degli Studi di Napoli, Frederico II, Via Sergio Pansini 5, I-80131 Napoli

Baumann, Jürg, Prof. Dr. med.
Baumann, Joyce B., Ph. D.
Orthopädische Chirurgie FMH, Felix Platter-Spital, Pavillon E, Burgfeldstraße 101, CH-4012 Basel

Beer, M.
Johanniter-Krankenhaus, Siepenstraße 33, D-42477 Radevormwald

Börner, M., Dr.
BG Unfallklinik Frankfurt, Friedberger Landstraße 430, D-60389 Frankfurt

Breitenfelder, J., Prof. Dr. med. Dr. med. habil.
St. Vincent Hospital, Danziger Straße 17, D-33029 Brakel

Buntrock, Walter, Dr.
Johanniter-Krankenhaus, Siepenstraße 33, D-42477 Radevormwald

Canero, R., Dr.
Universita degli Studi di Napoli, Frederico II, Via Sergio Pansini 5, I-80131 Napoli

Corrado, B., Dr.
Universita degli Studi di Napoli, Frederico II, Via Sergio Pansini 5, I-80131 Napoli

Delius, Michael, Dr.
Klinikum Großhadern, Institut für Chirurgische Forschung, Marchioninistraße 15, D-81366 München

Diesch, Rupert, Dr. med.
Eckener Straße 3, D-88046 Friedrichshafen

DRAENERT, K., Prof. Dr.
Zentrum für Orthopädische Wissenschaften München und Bern,
Gabriel-Max-Straße 3, D-81545 München

DRAENERT, Y., Dr.
Zentrum für Orthopädische Wissenschaften München und Bern,
Gabriel-Max-Straße 3, D-81545 München

DE DURANTE, C., Dr.
Universita degli Studi di Napoli, Frederico II, Via Sergio Pansini 5,
I-80131 Napoli

GIGLIOTTI, S., Dr.
Universita degli Studi di Napoli, Frederico II, Via Sergio Pansini 5,
I-80131 Napoli

HAHN, MICHAEL, Dipl. Ing.
Universitätsklinik Hamburg-Eppendorf, Abt. Osteopathologie,
Martinistraße 52, D-20246 Hamburg

HAIST, JOACHIM, Dr. med.
Zum Oberfeld 4, D-55286 Wörrstadt

HASSELBACH, VON, CHRISTOPH, Dr. med.
ACE Arthro-Clinic GmbH Essen, Giradetstraße 2–38, D-45131 Essen

HAUPT, GERALD, Dr. med.
Urologische Klinik der Ruhr-Universität Bochum, Widumer Straße 8,
D-44627 Herne

JAKOBEIT, C., PD Dr. med.
Johanniter-Krankenhaus, Siepenstraße 33, D-42477 Radevormwald

KEITZ-STEEGER, VON, DAG, Dr. med.
Borggrafenlacherweg 10, D-65428 Rüsselsheim

KRAEMER, M., Dr. med.
Theresienklinik, Herbert Hellmann Allee 11, D-79189 Bad Krozingen

KROLL, ULRIKE
Johanniter-Krankenhaus, Siepenstraße 33, D-42477 Radevormwald

LOHSE-BUSCH, HENNING, Dr. med.
Theresienklinik, Herbert Hellmann Allee 11, D-79189 Bad Krozingen

LÜSSENHOP, S., Dr. med.
Rehberg-Klinik, Braunlager Straße 25, D-37444 St. Andreasberg

MEISS, L., Prof.
Orthopädische Universitätsklinik Hamburg-Eppendorf,
Martinistraße 52, D-20246 Hamburg

MISSULIS, ULRICH
Johanniter-Krankenhaus, Siepenstraße 33, D-42477 Radevormwald

MOHR, GERALD, Dr. med.
Bourger-Platz 4, D-55543 Bad Kreuznach

OSENBERG, THOMAS
Johanniter-Krankenhaus, Siepenstraße 33, D-42477 Radevormwald

REIME, U., Dr. med.
Theresienklinik, Herbert Hellmann Allee 11, D-79189 Bad Krozingen

RUSSO, SERGIO, Dr. med.
Universita degli Studi di Napoli, Frederico II, Via Sergio Pansini 5,
I-80131 Napoli

SCHADEN, WOLFGANG, Dr.
Landstr. Hauptstr. 83, A-1030 Wien

SCHMEISER, ANDREA
Johanniter-Krankenhaus, Siepenstraße 33, D-42477 Radevormwald

SCHUMACHER, RALPH, Dr. med.
Johanniter-Krankenhaus, Siepenstraße 33, D-42477 Radevormwald

SCHULZE, GERHARD, Dr. med.
Bourger-Platz 4, D-55543 Bad Kreuznach

SEEMANN, D., Dr. med.
Orthopädische Universitätsklinik Hamburg-Eppendorf,
Martinistraße 52, D-20246 Hamburg

SPELSBERG, GUSTAV, Dr.
Johanniter-Krankenhaus, Siepenstraße 33, D-42477 Radevormwald

SPLITTGERBER, THOMAS
Johanniter-Krankenhaus, Siepenstraße 33, D-42477 Radevormwald

THIELE, R., Dr. med.
Deutsche Gesellschaft für Extrakorporale Stoßwellentherapie,
Kurfürstendamm 61, D-10707 Berlin

UEBERLE, FRIEDRICH, Dr. Ing.
Dornier Medizintechnik GmbH, Industriestraße 15,
D-82110 Germering

WEBER, FRED, Dr. med.
Bourger-Platz 4, D-55543 Bad Kreuznach

WELP, LARS
Johanniter-Krankenhaus, Siepenstraße 33, D-42477 Radevormwald

WINARSKI, BARBARA
Johanniter-Krankenhaus, Siepenstraße 33, D-42477 Radevormwald

WINIARSKI, BARBARA
Johanniter-Krankenhaus, Siepenstraße 33, D-42477 Radevormwald

WOLF, THOMAS, Dr. med.
St. Vincenz Hospital, Danziger Straße 7, D-33034 Brakel

PART I

General Overview

CHAPTER 1

Review

M. Buch

1.1
Effects and Side Effects of Shock Wave Therapy

In this chapter, currently known effects and side effects are presented. We first present a lecture held by Dr. Pia Steinbach at the First Shock Wave Symposium in Kassel in April 1996. It especially features the results she achieved with regard to a dosis-effect relationship at the endothelium of the blood vessels, as well as the influence of shock waves on the membrane potential of the neuron.

1.1.1
Summary of the Lecture of Dr. Steinbach

As is widely known, shock wave therapy has been employed longest for the crushing of kidney stones. However, in the meantime it is also employed to crush other calculi, such as gallstones, pancreatic and salivary calculi.

High energies are required to crush such stones. The mode of action concerning the destruction of stones is believed to be known. Interaction occurs at the interface of the liquid medium and the kidney stone, because the acoustic resistance or difference in impedance between the two materials is very high. This interaction leads to changes at the surface of the renal calculus. Pressure and shear loads occur at the transition from the liquid to the stone due to a jump in the acoustic impedance (water 1.49×10^5 g/cm^2; kidney stone $5.6–14.4 \times 10^5$ g/cm^2; Sucul et al. 1993). Water infiltrates the cracks which have been created on the surface of the stone. A further effect comes to bear, namely cavitation, i.e. gas bubbles develop in the water due to the rapid interaction between pressure and shear. The collapse of the gas bubbles also leads to the development of very fast flows, the so-called jet streams, whose impact on the stone surface leads to its further disintegration.

There are other indications for employing high-energy pressures: tumour therapy, albeit as yet only in an experimental framework. It is presumed that the destructive effect on the tumour bears on both the vascular system of the tumour and directly on the tumour cells. The effect can be enhanced by also administering cytostatic drugs. The side effects on soft tissue occuring in lithotripsy of renal calculi are employed in tumour therapy. However, the mode of action is not as clear in tumour therapy. In the literature, the preferred explanation is cavitation, whereby the development of radicals is especially believed to play an important role. The mechanical effects of cavitation, such as the jet streams, can however also contribute to the destruction, especially of the vascular system. The influence of the direct impact of the pressure wave, which plays a decisive role in the destruction of stones, may be less important, as the the differences in impedance in tissue are small.

In the following, I should like to consider two indications more thoroughly, in which the modes of action are as yet unknown: namely, the effect of shock wave therapy in the healing of bone fractures, where high pressures are also employed, and secondly, the effect in palliative therapy.

Beforehand, however, I should like to elucidate the difference between the shock waves used in lithotripsy and the waves employed in diagnostic ultrasound. Shock waves are characterized by high positive pressures up to 80 MPa and negative pressures of 5–10 MPa. Furthermore, they have a short rise time of 30–120 ns and a shorter pulse duration (5 μs). In contrast to ultrasound, shock waves have low frequencies. Just in this respect, there is less absorption by the tissue. Moreover, the shock waves are applied with a lower repetition frequency of 1–2 Hz, maximum 4 Hz, which means that they have a low time-averaged intensity. The only thing that can be said for sure is that the shock wave does not cause tissue warming. None of the known shock wave effects are due to thermal effects.

Effects of Shock Waves on Bones

There is as yet not much literature that deals with this topic. I should like to refer to two works, one of which is by Sukul and Johannes (1993). They treated formalin-fixed rabbit bones, i.e. femur and tibia, in vitro with the Lithostar Plus. The macroscopic defects found were a decortication, occurrence of bone fragments, a complete cortical bone defect and the occurrence of fractures. These effects occured after application of 1000–2000 pulses of 0.6 mJ/mm^2 (which corresponds to the upper limit in the treatment of renal calculi). No further defects were found after 5000 pulses. The lower the energy density was, the later effects occurred. The severity of damage correlated with the energy density; however, no correlation was found with the number of pulses applied.

As a reservation, it should be noted that the tests were carried out on formalin-fixed bones. It remains unclear as to whether the acoustic properties of the bones were altered due to the fixation process. The mode of action presumed and discussed is the same as in the treatment of kidney stones, i.e. that microfissures develop and cavitation bubbles occur. This is per se logical, as the acoustic impedance of a kidney stone roughly corresponds to that of bone.

The second study I should like to refer to is that by Delius and coworkers (1995), in which they studied the effects on the rabbit femur In vivo using the experimental device (XL 1) by Dornier.

Here, 1500 pulses with a voltage of 27.5 kV at a frequency of 1 Hz were applied. Ulcerations of the skin at the point of entry of the shock wave, soft-tissue swelling in the lower third of the femur, microscopic changes of the bone (detachment of the periostium, subperiosteal haemorrhages and escape of bone marrow) were encountered. Furthermore, diffuse haemorrhages at a distance of 10 mm from the focus and haematomae close to the focus in the medullary space in association with fractured trabeculae were found. At follow-up, a cortical swelling was noted, which was caused by the organization of the extensive periosteal changes. The hypotheses that similar direct effects on bone to those in lithotripsy (impedance of cortical bones 7.38 × 105 g/ cm^2) and induction of fractures occur was not confirmed by this study.

The fracture of trabeculae with displacement of the splinters and the escape of marrow rather point to cavitation effects arising from the propagation of cavities. The study does not confirm the hypothesis that the healing of pseudo-arthroses occurs due to the generation of microfractures and the breakup of sclerotic bone ends. The authors postulate that, due to pressing of the marrow from the medullary cavity, marrow hypoxia and subperiostal haemorrhages, new growth of bone is stimulated.

Effects of Shock Waves on Blood Vessels

I should now like to consider the effect of shock waves on blood vessels.

From the treatment of kidney stones, it is known that haematomas often develop. In various studies (Cornell et al. 1995; Smits et al. 1991), it was found that at the macroscopic level a temporary reduction of the tumour blood flow with subsequent metabolic inactivation and hyperacidity of the tumour occurs. At the microscopic level, interstitial haemorrhages and haematomae, damage to the arterial walls, ruptures of arteries, thrombus formation in arcual and interlobular veins (Drach et al. 1992; Rassweiler et al. 1993; Weber et al. 1992), as well as vasoconstrictions, microhaemmorhages and an increase in vascular permeability (Brendel et al. 1987) occur. These results originate from various authors from various institutions, so that there can be no doubt about these effects on blood vessels. However, the mode of action on which they are based is less clear.

I should like now to review a study on the effect of shock waves on human umbilical vessels at the Institute of Pathology of Regensburg University, in which I carried out a determination of energy threshold values, i.e. I determined which biological effects occured at which energy levels.

In our experimental setup, we used a hanging module by Siemens with which we treated a fresh, clamped human umbilical cord still containing blood in a water bath. The focus was set within the umbilical cord. As we know that the energy density decreases continuously in the lateral direction from the focus midpoint, it was possible to set up a dosage-effect relation in the umbilical cord model.

A macroscopically arisen bleeding was observable in the focal region. We then microscopically studied this region with an H&E-stained incision, concentrating on the blood vessels. In doing so, we found the most severe damage to be ruptures of the vessel walls. The erythrocytes had partially only infiltrated to the vessel wall. The least severe form of damage possible was a rupture of the endothelial layer. In a further approach, we altered the preparation method and viewed a cut vessel from the inside. By using a confocal laser scanning microscope and a scanning electron microscope, we were able to observe changes to the endothelial layer. In the focues centre, the endothelial cells were no longer monolinearly next to each other, but were scat-

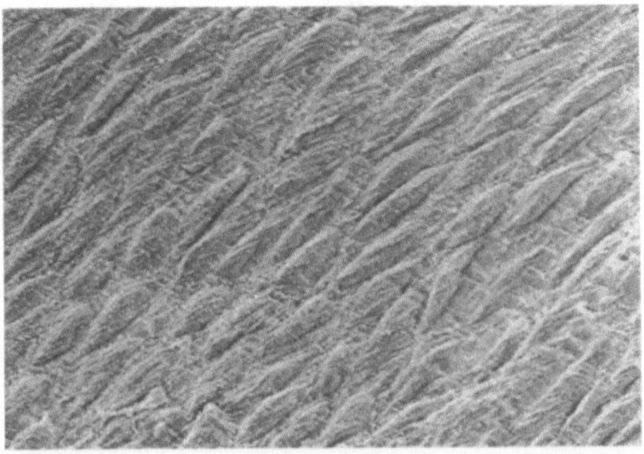

Fig. 1. Normal endothelium, × 700 magnification

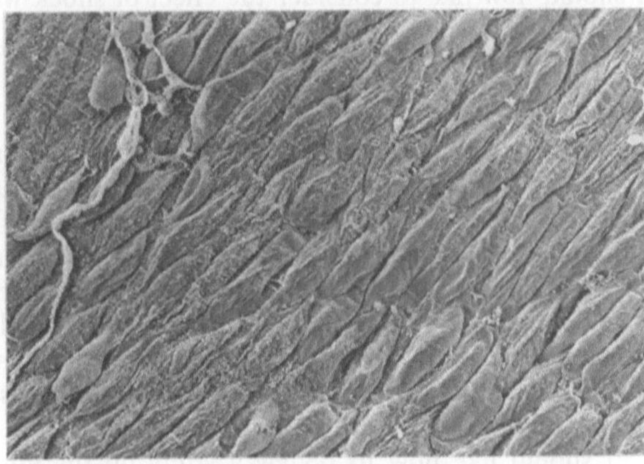

Fig. 2. Endothelium near the focus, × 700 magnification. Note the gaps between the individual cells, which point an increase in permeability of the vessel due to shock wave application

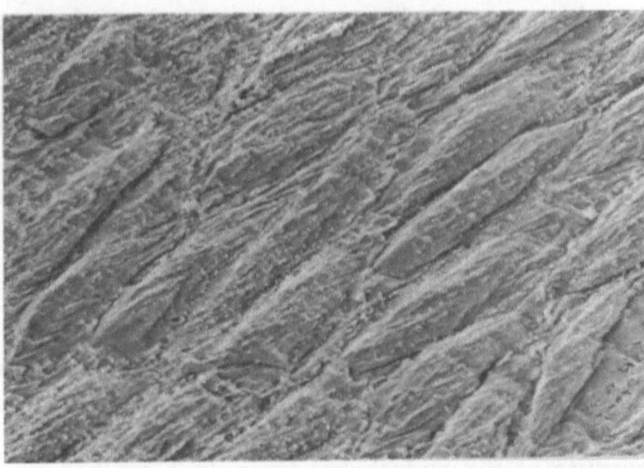

Fig. 3. As Fig. 1, × 1500 magnification

tered around, partly ripped down to the basilemma and unica muscularis. A further effect was an increase in the fibrillic actin content in the endothelial cell; the closer the cells had been to the focus, the greater the fibrillic actin

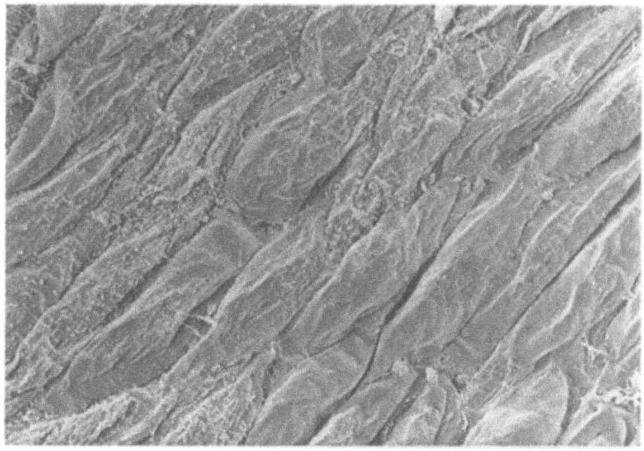

Fig. 4. As Fig. 2, × 1500 magnification

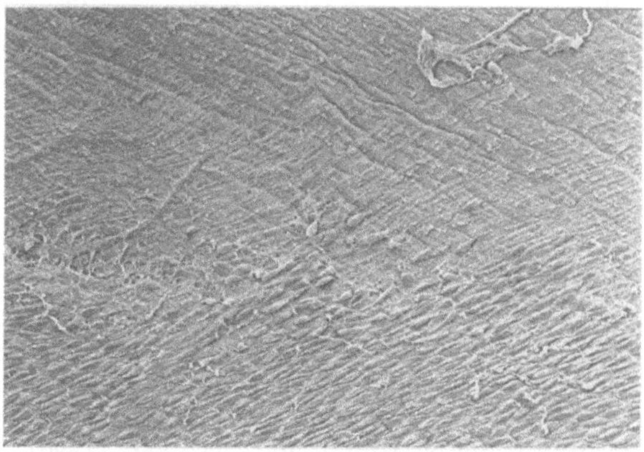

Fig. 5. Detachment of the endothelium, × 200 magnification

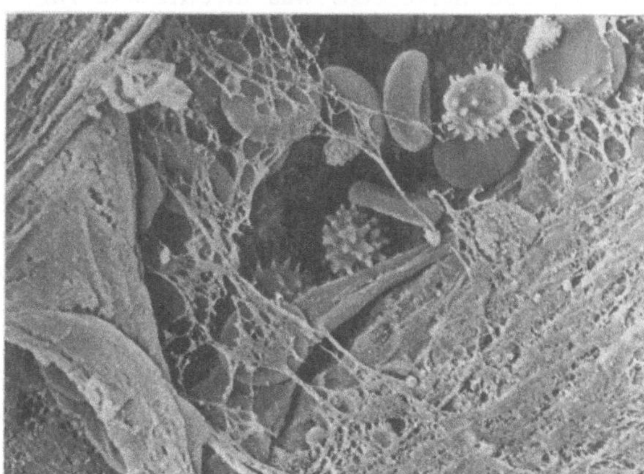

Fig. 6. Rupture of the basilemma in the focus area, × 3000 magnification

content in the cytoplasm (so-called stress fibres develop due to a variety of stimuli). Owing to the increased content of fibrillic actin in the endothelial cells, the latter retract and the intercellular distances increase, which might explain a higher vessel permeability. We then set up a energy density-effect relation. The detachment of the endothelium, being the most severe damage encountered in this experiment, occurred at an energy density of 0.3 mJ/mm^2 and the development of stress fibres already set in at 0.1 mJ/mm^2, an energies reached in palliative therapy.

Effects of Shock Waves on Nerves

I would now like to discuss the effect of shock waves on nerves and nerve cells. Schelling and coworkers (1994) carried out experiments to this effect. They treated sciatic nerves of frogs with the experimental device XL1 by Dornier set at 15 kV (50 MPa) and measured the occuring cumulative action potential. They found that 95% of all shock waves trigger a cumulative action potential, whereby the latter is characterized by a smaller amplitude but similar form compared with electrically triggered potentials. They conclude that shock waves must stimulate the same fibres as electrical stimulation.

It is important to note that the capacity to be electrically stimulated was not diminished, i.e. the neural structures were not damaged. It was hypothetically assumed that the mode of action is based on a direct mechanical effect of the shock wave on the axon membrane in the sense of an increase in permeability with consecutive depolarization and triggering of an action potential. However, it appears more probable that a cavitation-based effect plays a role in the triggering of the cumulative action potentials. After injecting gas bubbles into the medium, it was possible to trigger a cumulative action potential 8 cm from focus. If the ultrasonic therapy was however carried out in a PVA (polyvinyl alcohol) solution with high viscosity, and therefore with decreased cavitation activity, the probability of triggering action potentials decreased.

In a study by Mihran and coworkers (1990), the effect of sonic pulses on nerves and nerve cells was investigated. An axon was treated with sonic waves of differing frequency and subsequently the time interval between ultrasound and the possible electrical stimulation was studied. The result was an increase or decrease in the amplitude of the cumulative action potential, depending on the time interval between ultrasound and electrical stimulation. This effect was not frequency-dependent. The authors explain this influence on the axon by an activation of pressure-sensitive ion channels due to the radiation pressure, whereby ion flows occur at the membrane, which result in a change of the excitability due to a change in the threshold value.

Now let us consider a study I carried out in 1996 at the Institute of Pathology at the University of Regensburg. It concerned the influence of shock waves on the membrane potential of neurons. A fluorescent stain was brought into the neuron, which depending on the membrane potential changed its fluorescence intensity. In the case of hyperpolarization, the fluorescence decreased. A hyperpolarization of the neurons was achieved by means of shock wave treatment, whereby an energy dependency was discovered, i.e. the higher the energy of the emitted shock wave, the greater the polarization. These effects lasted for approximately 1 h after the shock wave. During hyperpolarization, a stimulus is necessary, which is larger than that required before shock wave treatment, to excite an action potential. Whether this effect could play a role in palliative therapy will require further study.

Finally, I would like to look into possible modes of action in tissue.

On the one hand, we have direct effects, and on the other hand, such caused by cavitation.

Direct effects. Direct effects are mechanical effects caused temporary positive pressure amplitudes during the propagation of a pressure pulse. The stability under load of the (tissue) material may be exceeded at the interface between the materials with different acoustic impedances. At such interfaces the shock waves lead to changes in the excursion, which result in tensile and shearing loads. In soft tissue, where there are no great differences in acoustic impedance, the direct effects of shock waves appear not to play a significant role.

Cavitation. The definition of cavitation is: expansion and oscillation of gas-filled cavities (pre-existing as cavitation nuclei) due to the tensile portion of a pressure wave with subsequent collapse. The cavitation results in mechanical and chemical effects.

a) Mechanical: Shearing loads develop due to the oscillation of the developed cavitation bubbles. Due to the collapse of the bubbles, there is an inflow of water (jet stream). These inflowing water masses can reach velocities between 400 and 700 m/s (Phillips et al. 1993), which correspond to the velocity of projectiles. One can surely imagine an effect of this jet stream on a mechanical basis.

b) Chemical: During the collapse of the cavitation bubbles, high temperatures develop locally inside the bubbles, which lead to the development of radicals. The induced radicals can subsequently lead to damage in the tissue.

The discussion as to which of the mentioned types of effect is responsible for the biological effects is currently still under way. In the literature, cavitation is favoured. There are numerous hints that caviatation bubbles also exist In vivo (Delius et al. 1990). Mechanical effects caused by cavitation seem to be more probable than chemical effects.

The development of intracellular radicals is a matter of controversy. Suhr et al. (1991) were able to prove the development of intracellular radicals. The results of Endl et al. (1995), however, did not confirm this. It is however, conceivable that extracellular development of radicals causes the induction of membrane damage.

Recent results of Endl and coworkers (1992) from the Institute of Pathology at the University Hospital in Regensburg are confusing, referring to direct effects without the existence large differences in impedance.

Although there are small differences here in acoustic impedance within a symplasm, the very high pressures of approximately 60 MPa might be sufficient on a mechanical basis to lead to the destruction of cells.

Finally, it should be noted that it has as yet not been clarified which mode of action is responsible for a specific effect.

Table 1. Pathophysiological effects of shock waves on human and animal kidneys (Brümmer et al. 1990)

Species	Probe	Result
Human	Renal plasma flow	No difference between treated and untreated kidney
	Renal plasma flow	5% reduced flow in 30% of treated kidneys
	Enzymuria	Change in distal tubulus epethelium
	Proximal tubulus enzymes	Perirenal soft-tissue trauma, possibly glomerular dysfunction
	Lactate dehydrogenase	Increase in blood and urine
	N-acethylglucosaminidase	Increase in urine
	Lactate dehydrogenase	Transient increase in blood and urine
	N-acethylglucosaminidase	Haemolysis
	Glutamatepyruva-transaminase	
	Creatine kinase	
	Myoglobin	
	Lysocyme in urine	Transient increase, normalization of tubulus function after 6 months
	Gamma glutamyl transferase	
	Protein in urine	Temporary increase in albumine, igG Beta-II microglobulin, Tamm-Horsfall protein; chnage in glomerular permeability
	Blood pressure	Indication of hypertension
	Fibronolytic system	Increase in fibronogen
	Activity of N-acethylglucosaminidase	Temporary renal dysfunction
Dog	Serum epinephrine	No effect on acute or chronic adrenal functions or morphology
Rat	Renal and skeletal growth	No disadvantageous effects at generator voltage of 18kV

In the following, further effects and side effects of shock waves on cell cultures, in animal experiments and in clinical trials are reviewed. Initial investigations were primarily stimulated by urologists. Preliminary experiments were carried out on cell cultures. Tables 1–3 give an overview of effects currently known.

In experiments on cells in suspension Brümmer (1990) and Smits (1994) found a cell damage pattern which is dependent on the number of shock waves and the shock wave energy applied:

- transient membrane rupture (permeability) with secondary damage (cell oedema)
- transient damage to endoplasmatic reticulum and cell nucleus
- dose-dependent vacuolization of the cytoplasma
- lesion in cytoskeleton (actin and vimentin fibres)
- complete cell rupture (e.g. haemolysis)

During their experiments in suspension, they found a clear dependency between dose and shock-wave-induced damage. The number of destroyed cells increases nearly linearly with the number of applied pulses and the energy density.

Table 2. Histopathological effects of shock waves on human and animal organs (Brümmer et al. 1990, Lingeman et al. 1988)

Species	Organ	Results
Human	Kidney	MRI: dose-dependent subcapsular accumulation of fluid. No severe renal pathological changes CT: identical results MRI: renal contusion, subcapsular haematoma (incidence 0.66%), increase of pre-existing and/or badly controlled hypertension
	Autopsy kidney	Damage to parenchyma, severe vascular damage, destruction of larger vessels
	Skin	Petechial bleeding at the point of entry of the shock wave Haemoglobininuria, decrease in kidney function, local contusion, pain, focal fibrosis
	Heart	Occurrence of ventricular arrhythmia
	Gallbladder	Vasodilation in the serosa, gallbladder wall oedema, petechial bleeding, damage to epithelium
	Bowels	Haematochezia after damage to colon
	Kidney	Haematoma (subcapsular or perirenal), increase in the occurrence of haematomae in patients with pre-existing hypertension, loss of the corticomedullary demarcation (MRI), partial to total obstruction of the ureter, delayed or total loss of diuresis of contrast agent, haematuria, enlargement of the kidney, perirenal fibrosis, maculate fibrosis of the ureter, total loss of renal function,
Dog	Kidney	Linear bleeding from cortex to medulla Haematoma and/or interstitial bleeding, fibrosis after 8000 shock waves Inner and outer perinephrial, as well as parenchymal bleeding, originating from interlobular and arciform veins venous thrombosis, tubular dilatations Light and reversible renal-tissue damage
	Lung	Bleeding after cholelithotripsy
	Gallbladder	Leucocystosis, increase in alanine and aspartataminotransferase levels, macro- and microscopic bleeding, oedema
	Lung	Bleeding
	Gallbladder/Liver	Small haematomae and haemosiderosis
Pig	Kidney	Interstitial capsular and perivascular fibrosis in small areas in approx. 70% of treated cases; some weeks after treatment: interstitial and perivascular fibrosis with chronic lymphoid infiltration

Table 2 (continued)

Species	Organ	Results
Golden hamster	Skin	Vasoconstriction of all arterial microvascular segments
	Muscle	Microhaemorrhages, escape of macromolecules
Rat	Kidney	Renal cortical necrosis, haemorrhages
		Bleeding, cortical, tubular necroses, cellular infiltrations
		Loss of the microvili and cilia at the surface of the tubulus cells, cellular vacuolation, rupture of glomerula
		Perirenal bleeding, 5000 shock waves in one session: death of animal; 5000 shock waves fractionated in two sessions: animal survives
	Liver	Hepatocellular necrosis
	Lung	Interstitial cellular intrapulmonary infiltration
		Petechial bleeding
		Bleeding
	Thorax	Massive haemoptysis
	Bowels	Intestinal bleeding
	Colon	Petechial bleeding
	Bones	Focal epiphysial growth plate dysplasia in 44% of treated tibiae
	Bone/Femur	Temporary dose-dependent haemorrhagic lesions, polymorphonuclear infiltrations, inflammation
	Epeidermis	Dose-dependent effects: focal bleeding, cellular infiltrations
	Ovary/Foetus	Rat ovaries appear to be resistant to shock waves of 20 kV generator voltage
	Bladder	Loss of epithelium due to cavitation
	Kidney	Long-term changes in MRI

Apart from the above-mentioned side effects, there has been other important preliminary research concerning the side effects of shock wave application, the results of which have been a decisive contribution to the compilation of a list of indications and contra-indications.

Newman (1987), based on neurological deficits after ureter lithotripsy in dogs investigated the influence of shock waves on the spinal cord. On fentanyl/pancuronium anaesthesia in three dogs, 2000, 4000, and 6000 shock waves were directed at the posterior part of the intervertebral space L3/4 or L4/5. During the experiment, a movement similar to the patellar tendon reflex and temporally slightly displaced from the impulses was observed. There was no change in the neurological status after shock wave application after 24 h and 48 h. The animals were not subsequently subjected to euthanasia. In accordance with the results of Delius et al. and Schelling et al. cited by Steinbach, one can currently not rule out damage to neural structures on application of shock waves.

Haupt et al. (1990) published results of research on the influence of shock waves on wound healing. Four pigs were afflicted with skin wounds (with a

Table 3. Effects of shock waves on cell cultures and tumours (Brümmer et al. 1990, Lingeman et al. 1988)

Cells	Results
Total blood	In vitro: dose-dependent haemolysis, In vivo: no increase of haemoglobin in the plasma of the rabbit
Human lymphocytes	Proliferation not influenced
Human neutrophiles	In suspension cell rupture, tumefaction of mitochondria, plasma membrane ruptures: changes in cell permeability and of the cyto-skeleton
Human melanoma	Reduction of the cellular vitality, drop in the development of colonies, selective decrease in cells in the G2 and M phases No influence on cell cycle, reinforcement of the cytostatic effect on treatment in media at 37 °C or 40 °C
Human renal carcinoma	Dose-dependent reduction of survivability in vitro, complete inhibition of cell division for 5 days
Human cervical carcinoma	No influence on cell cycle, reinforcement of the cytostatic effect on treatment in media at 37 °C and 42 °C In suspension dose-dependent cell damage, no effect on immobilized cells
Human prostate carcinoma	All cells displayed sensitivity to shock waves
Human renal carcinoma	After 2000 shock waves, reduction of survivability of cells and in cell growth
Human embryonic renal cells	In vivo: delay in growth, doxorubicin in combination with shock waves displays inhibitory effects
Normal human marrow	Reduction of 50% in cell viability after 700 shock waves, reduction in the development of colonies
Rat prostate carcinoma	Reduction of cell survivability, decrease in the number of colony-developing units, selective decrease in cells in G2 and M phases, delay in tumour growth after reimplatation, swollen mitochondria, destroyed cristae mitochondriales, In vivo there was no sign of a histopathological or ultrastructural effect after exposure to shock waves In suspension delay in growth, ultrastructural damage, In vivo delay in growth Dose-dependent reduction in cell survivability and colony growth, cells pre-treated with shock waves became more sensitive in chemotherapy and immunotherapy
Prostate tumour of rat	No effect on primary growth and frequency of metastatic spread
Bladder tumour of rat	Palpable tumours were not influenced by 800 or 1400 shock waves, 2000 shock waves lead to a significant inhibition of tumour growth
Leukemia of mouse	In suspension: dose-dependent cell damage, no effect on immobilized cells
Breast neoplasm of mouse	In suspension: dose-dependent cell damage, no effect on immobilized cells
Leukemia of mouse	In suspension: dose-dependent destruction of cells, reduced cell growth was evident in combination with adriamycin and cisplatin

keratoma; 1×1 cm, 0.3–0.5 cm deep). Some of the animals were pre-treated radiologically with a dose of 1500 rad. Subsequent shock wave application was carried out with the XL1 experimental lithotripter (Dornier, Germering, Germany) at 14 or 18 kV generator voltage. So as to achieve an even distribution of energy at the wound site, the wound was positioned 0.7 cm above

Table 4. The shock-wave-induced renal lesions were classified in four groups according to Rassweiler (1993)

Level of lesion	Morphology
Level 0	No macroscopically visible lesion, intratubular accumulations of erythrocytes, individual tubulus necroses
Level 1	Petechial bleeding in the medulla, rupture of venules, small tubulus necroses
Level 2	Focal haematoma in the renal cortex, subcapsular ecchymoses, rupture of venules and arterioles
Level 3	Perirenal and cortical haematoma, rupture of interlobular arteries and glomeruli, massive tubulus cell necroses

the F2 point. After treatment, a shock-wave-dependent influence on the healing of the wound was observed. High doses of energy (18 kV, 1000 pulses) lead to an inhibition, low doses (14 kV, 1000 pulses) to an acceleration in healing of the wounds. At morphological examination, a significantly higher number of microvessels and a significantly thicker, new epithelial layer was found in the group treated with low-energy doses.

In routine clinical treatment, this has, however, not been implemented to a greater extent.

Reproductive Organs/Pregnancy

Extracorporeal shock wave application is currently the therapy of choice with regard to distal ureter stones. Due to the proximity of the distal ureter and the female reproductive system, one focus of discussion in the past was the possibility of a mutagenic and fertility-diminishing effect. Therefore, animal experiments were carried out to investigate the possibility of damaging effects of shock waves on these organs.

Rüdiger et al. (1991) reported on experiments with rat testicles. Two thousand pulses with various energy intensities were applied to the right testis of each of 48 rats after intraperitoneal anaesthesia, using the Piezolit (Wolf). Some animals were killed after 24 h and subsequently examined. Energy-dose-dependent tubular damage with haemorrhages and tissue destruction was observed. In the group examined after 3 months, signs of repair were found and the level of damage considerably lower. Here and there, interstitial fibroses were encountered.

Mendoza et al. (1991) researched the influence of shock waves on the ovaries and pregnancy. The ovaries of 18 nonpregnant rats were treated with shock waves (Lithotripter HM 3, Dornier, Germany; 1500 shock waves, 18 kV). Another 24 rats were subjected to the same treatment on the 15th day of pregnancy. Of these, 12 were laparotomized directly after shock wave application and the remainder completed pregnancy. Of the ovaries treated, 20% displayed small extravasations, the blood vessels being intact. In the case of the animals killed directly after shock wave application, 1/3 displayed haemorrhages in the placenta. The children of the last group were of normal size and weight.

In the past, urological shock wave treatment has been administered to unconsciously pregnant women without a negative influence on the pregnancy being observed. Shock wave therapy administered to a woman with a stone trapped high in the ureter in the 22nd week of pregnancy did not result in damage to either child or mother (Chaussy et al. 1993, 1995).

The work group lead by Frankenschmidt investigated in detail the foetotoxicity and teratogeneity of shock waves in a Swiss hare rabbits (In: Chaussy et al. "Die Stoßwelle" 1995). The first group was exposed to shock waves on the 25th day of pregnancy, 24 h after which autopsy was carried out. The second group underwent exposure on the 20th day of pregnancy and autopsy was on the 29th day (the day before bringing forth the children). The shock waves were focused by ultrasound on the skull, abdomen and thorax of the foetuses of three of the animals. In a further three animals, the shock waves were focused between two foetuses at a distance of 2 cm from the uterine horn.

The application of shock waves to the foetal skull resulted in the death of all six animals (haematoma of the skull, intercranial bleeding). The application to the thorax lead to the death of five of the six animals (haemothorax, haematopericardium, bleeding of the lung, mediastinal soft-tissue haematoma). Shock wave application to the foetal heart resulted in cardiac arrest during treatment. The application to the abdomen lead to three fatal outcomes (one acute, two delayed resorptions). The surviving animals showed areas of bleeding in kidney, mesenterium and intestinal walls.

The focusing between two foetuses resulted in death due to haemorrhage of the placenta. In the remaining cases, haematoma were found at the corporeal periphery of the foetuses, which did not endanger the vitality of the foetuses.

In the group where parauterine focusing at 2 cm was applied, there was no foetal damage. In these cases, only soft-tissue haematoma in the mothers was encountered.

As regards the experiments concerning teratogeneity, shock waves were applied on the teratologically sensitive 12th day of pregnancy to the lower kidney pool (approx. 4 cm from the uterus). The mothers were killed on the 29th day of pregnancy and the children delivered by section. The number of corpora lutea, the implantation sites, the primary losses, the foetuses, the litter sizes the courses of pregnancy and the development of weight of the mothers showed no significant statistical differences to the untreated animals. This also applies to the foetal measurments of the body and vitality tests.

Nevertheless, pregnancy is still a contra-indication for shock wave therapy. However, accidental shock wave treatment during unknown pregnancy does not have to result in abortion.

1.2 The Effect of Shock Waves on Bones

In this chapter, we shall report on the effects and side effects of shock wave application to bones. Delius et al. present their in part as yet unpublished results concerning the effect of high-energy shock wave application on bones. Furthermore, the literature is reviewed with regard to experiments on animals as concerns the effect of shock waves on bones, on the healing of fractures, the benefit of shock waves in cases of bone cement loosening in revision arthroplasty and the effect of shock waves on the growing bone *(see Chapter 3).*

A publication originating from the Orthopaedic University Hospital Mainz (presented in Baden-Baden in 1996) investigates the effect of shock waves on tendinous tissue. In 48 rabbits, the Achilles tendon was treated 1 cm above the point of attachment to the calcaneum with various energies (1000 pulses each of A: 0.08 mJ/mm^2, B: 0.28 mJ/mm^2, C: 0.6 mJ/mm^2) . The animals were followed up sonographically four times (days 1, 7, 14, 28 / 7.5-MHz linear transducer, proxon lead). Liquid accumulations and thickness measurments of the tendon were documented and compared with the situation before shock wave application. The authors classified the changes in various groups:

- Level 0: Difference in diameter up to 0.5 mm
- Level 1: Difference in diameter between 0.5 mm and 1 mm
- Level 2: Difference in diameter more than 1 mm

After 28 days, no changes were sonographically detectable in any of the cases. Only in a few cases in the medium- and low-energy ranges was level-1 (3 cases of level-2) thickening observed, especially in the first days of examination.

In the higher energy ranges, 9 cases (7 high energy, 2 medium energy) showed a weak-echo paratendinous border, which was interpreted as liquid accumulation. In no cases was a change in the echo texture or an interruption of continuity of the tendon observed. Histologically, a lack of tenocytes and eosinophilia was observed as a manifestation of tendon damage in the group treated with high energy levels.

In view of the differing results concerning shock wave application to bones in the animal experiment, the question as to the mode of action arises. In the literature [18, 19], various hypotheses are proffered:

1. Microfissures at the fracture ends
2. Development of a haematoma
3. Development of small cortical/spongiosa chips
4. Transformation of local connective-tissue cells

In the literature, there are several works dealing with the question of cell activation due to shock waves.

Yang et al. (1988) observed dose-dependent necrosis of bone marrow cells after shock wave application. The bone marrow of healthy patients was treated with 400, 800 and 1500 shock waves from a lithotriptor HM3 (Dornier) at 18 kV generator voltage and at a frequency of 100 shock waves per minute. After 400 pulses, the survival rate was 57.7±3.1%, at 800 pulses it was 27.7±4.2% and at 1500 pulses it fell to 10.7±5%.

Sukul and Johannes (1994) investigated the effect of shock waves on human fibroblast cultures. They observed cell damage proportional to to the shock wave intensity and number, which occurred 24 h after application. They explain the positive effect of shock wave application on fracture healing often mentioned in the literature rather by better blood supply than by direct cytostimulation. The conclude that a small number of high-energy shock waves should be applied in clinical practice.

Notwithstanding the shock wave application to the bone/tendon interface and to the bone itself already practiced in many hospitals, fundamental studies concerning dose-effect relationship of shock waves in the bone and at the bone/tendon interface are still lacking. In both cases we have "a therapeutic effect with speculated mode of action" (Rompe 1996).

The changes after shock wave application in the area of the epiphyses reported by Yeaman (1989) and cited by Delius (herein) could theoretically be used in clinical growth manipulation. Animal experiments in this respect have been carried out in Germany by the work group lead by Lüssenhop *(see Chapter 4).*

Haist describes his experience in shock wave therapy in osteorestoration. He belongs to the users with the greatest experience in this field *(see Chapter 5).*

Diesch has implemented shock wave therapy in his private practice for many years. Thankfully, he has documented his observations for the past 3 years. His main experience is, however, in the field of shock wave application in pseudo-arthroses *(see Chapter 6).*

Shock wave therapy is also used successfully in other European countries. Schaden gives an account of his experience regarding delayed bone union and loosened cement-free endoprotheses *(see Chapter 7).*

Russo elucidates his experience in shock wave application to navicular pseudo-arthroses *(see Chapter 8).*

The following table (Table 5) gives an overview of the data published to date concerning the efficacy of shock wave therapy in delayed bone union/ pseudo-arthroses in clincial practice.

In view of these data, it becomes apparent that further animal experiments and multicentre studies concerning the application of shock wave therapy in delayed bone union/pseudo-arthroses are necessary before recommendations concerning a golden standard of shock wave number and intensity to be applied in specific forms of fracture can be made. Final proof of efficacy of shock wave therapy in the generally accepted pseudo-arthrosis model has as yet not been found in animal experiments.

Shock Wave Therapy in Tendopathies and Tendinosis Calcarea

In the following, the results from experienced clinicians and practitioners concerning the implementation of shock wave therapy in enthesiopathia and tendinosis calcarea is presented *(see Chapters 9–13).*

At the end of the 1980s, first reports of shock wave application in delayed bone union appeared in the literature (Schleberger 1992, Vachalnov 1991). In the majority of treated cases, a secondary finding was that a pronounced analgesia was observed in the area of treatment, even when low energies were applied. Dahmen and Haist belonged to the pioneers who used shock waves for analgesia in the locomotor system in cases of enthesiopathiae at the beginning of the 1990s.

Loew published results of the successful implementation of shock wave therapy in tendinosis calcarea of the shoulder in 1993, which he also presented at the First Kassel Shock Wave Symposium (Buch 1996). According to

Table 5. Overview of the data published to date

Author(s)	Year	Number of cases	Shock wave parameters	Apparatus	Success rate
Schleberger et al.	1992	7	18 kV / 2000 pulses	Dornier MFL 5000 and HM3	75% of patients displayed callus formation after 6 weeks
Valchanov et al.	1992	?	1000–4000 pulses / 1000–1700 bar	?	70 of 82 patients showed ossification
Schleberger et al.		45 pseudo-arthroses	16/18 kV/2000 pulses	MFL 5000	success in 41 of 45 patients
Haupt et al.	1995	29 pseudo-arthroses	28 kV/3000 pulses	HMT/Ossatron	20 of 29 patients displayed consolidation after one session
Rompe	1994	30 pseudo-arthroses, 31 delayed bone union	3000 pulses/ maximum intensity	?	18 of 30 pseudo-arthroses consolidated after 8.5 weeks, 25 of 31 delayed bone unions consolidated after 6 weeks
Bürger et al.	1991	10	2500 pulses/ 17.5–19 kV	Lithostar	Controls after 1–6 months showed 2 successes, in the majority scintigraphic increased enrichment
Bürger et al.	1992	30	2500 pulses/ 17.5–19 kV	Lithostar	After 2–10 months, 9 ossifications, 9 beginning ossifications and first signs of ossification after 4–8 weeks
Schultheis (HTM)	?	?	?	?	80% consolidated after 3–6 months, 60% with one session, 20% with two sessions, 20% failures

his theory, a secondary impingement between the head of the humerus and the acromion/coracoacromial ligament occurs due to large calcium deposits, which are mostly situated in the area of the supraspinatus muscle. His train of thought was to break up these calcium deposits, which often lay quite near the surface, by means of high-energy shock wave treatment, and thus to effect "via naturalis" disintegration or to convey them to the bursa subacromialis. His theory concerning the mode of action of this form of treatment contained the following strategies:

1. *Direct mode of action*: Due to the development of cavitation bubbles and implosion phenomena, an increase in pressure occurs in the calcium deposit, which leads to a rupture of the calcium masses and release into the bursa subacromialis.
2. *Indirect mode of action*: Due to a loosening of the structure, an partial fragmentation and disintegration of the calcium deposit occurs in a cell mediated mechanism.

To study the mechanical effect of a shock wave on a calcium deposit in the shoulder, a reference stone[1] was implanted in the shoulder of a freshly slaughtered Merino. Based on this model experiment, it was possible to determine a dose-effect relationship, i.e. it was determined how many pulses at which energy level lead to the disintegration of the stone. It was noted that higher energy intensities than in a water bath were required to achieve a mechanical effect on the stone, i.e. a large portion of the energy must have been absorbed on its path through the shoulder.

Based on these data, shock wave therapy was applied in a pilot study to patients with large type-1 or type-2 (according to Gärtner 1993) calcium deposits. In average, the specific complaint had had a duration of 3 years. The age of the patients was between 40 and 50 years. Females suffered from this complaint more than males. The apparatus used was a Lithotripter Compact (Dornier). The patient lying prone, the transducer was coupled to the shoulder ventrally. The arm was then rotated in such a way that no bone obstructed the path between the deposit and the transducer. Localization and fixation of the calcium deposit in the focal point of the shock wave source was controlled radiologically in two planes. The area of the focus was anaesthesized locally before treatment.

With approval of the ethics committee, 20 patients were randomly allotted to four groups. Group 1 was treated twice in intervals of 14 days with a high charging voltage of 22 kV. Group 3 was treated with the same voltage once. Group 2, as the control group, was not treated. Group 4 was treated once with a low charging voltage of 18 kV. Follow-up examinations were carried out after 6 and 12 weeks, so as to evaluate the direct effect of the shock waves on the calcium deposits and to rule out as far as possible spontaneous disintegration. Subjective information from the patient, constant score, as well as radiological and nuclear magnetic resonance tomographic control examinations were evaluated. According to the patients in the control group quasi no change had occurred (see Fig. 7).

Significant differences were observed in the four groups. The changes in constant score are shown in the following graph (Fig. 8).

Radiologically observed changes 12 weeks after treatment are presented in the graph below (Fig. 9).

As some of the patients did not state an improvement, although the calcium deposit had dissolved, the data as regards the radiological data and the subjective statements concerning the complaint were again compared. A statistically significant positive correlation between the radiologically observed

[1] Limestone is used by manufacturers of shock wave apparatuses to determine the effect of the shock wave source.

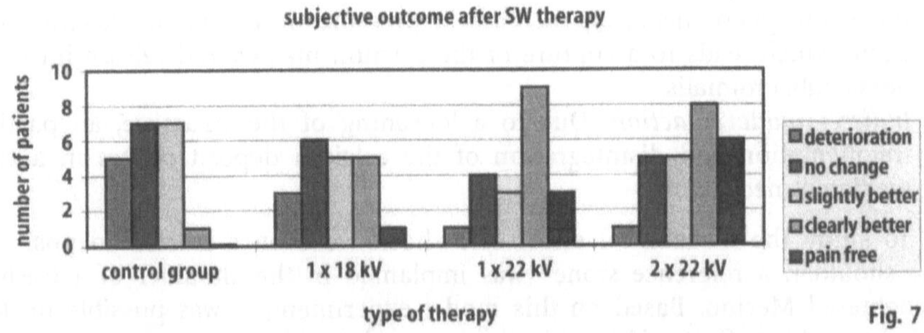

Fig. 7

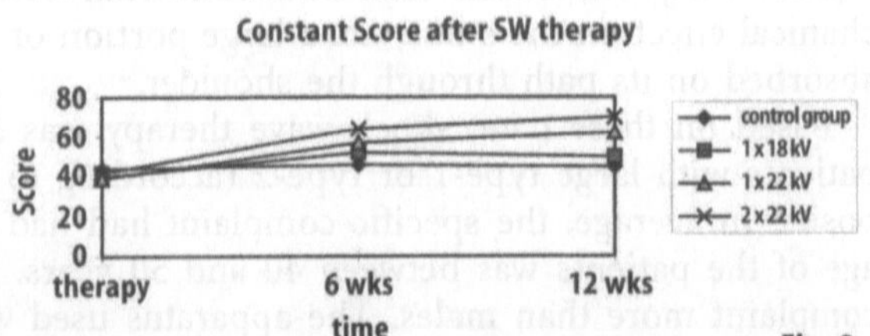

Fig. 8

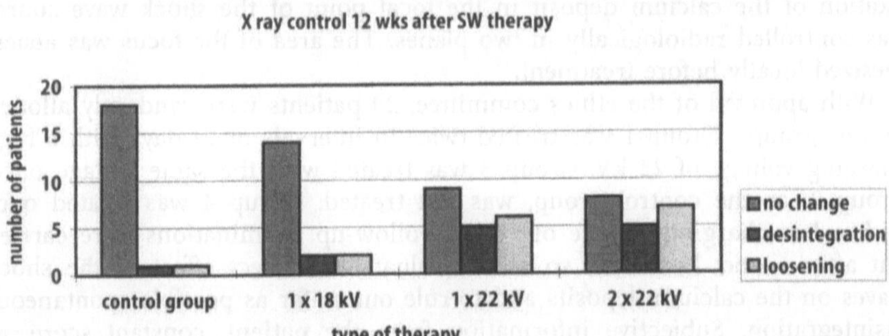

Fig. 9

success of therapy and the subjectively experienced success was found. According to the nuclear magnetic resonance tomographic control examinations, no changes occurred in the areas of the humerus head or tendons of the rotator cuff.

The following side effects were observed: the treatment is painful. Some of the patients displayed skin erosion or petechiae at the point of entry of the shock wave after therapy. In some cases a haematoma developed.

The failed patients subsequently underwent surgery. In some of these patients, biopsy samples were taken from the area of the tendinosis calcarea. A membrane-like, cell-rich layer, in which giant cells were encountered, was found around the calcium deposit. The adjacent tendon tissue had, however, not changed. In patients, where partial disintegration of the calcium had occurred, it was histologically observed that a considerable number of phagocytes had grown into the deposit. This supports the theory of cell-induced calcium disintegration.

In summary, with high charging voltages and application of shock waves once or twice, there exists a pronounced physical effect, which leads to desintegration of the calcium deposit and to subjective freedom from complaints in 60–70% of the cases.

The insights gained were put to clinical use in the Orthopaedic University Hospital in Heidelberg. In a prospective study, the results of high-energy shock waves applied once (2000 pulses/22 kV/54 patients) and twice (2 × 2000 pulses/1-week interval/22 kV/61 patients) were compared.

Inclusion criteria were: therapy-resistant pain and calcifications larger than 1 cm and corresponding to type 1 or type 2 according to the classification after Gärtner.

Exclusion criteria were: limited movability of the shoulder joint, osteoarthritis of the shoulder, pathological neurological changes or calcifications of type 3 after Gärtner.

After 3 and 6 months the subjective statements of the patients, the constant score and the radiological were followed up. At the 3-month control, 45% of the patients of Group 1 (one session) stated that they thought that therapy was successful (complaint-free or considerable improvement). In Group 2, (two sessions) approximately 50% answered thus. After 6 months, 45% of Group 1 were of the opinion that therapy had been successful and in Group 2 54%. In both groups, there was a significant increase in constant score. Group 1 had a constant score of 49 before treatment, which increased to 62 after 3 months and to 67 after 6 months. Group 2 had a constant score similar to that of Group 1 before treatment. After 3 months it had increased to 52 and to 69 after 6 months. After 6 months, dissolution or disintegration of the calcium deposit was radiologically observed in 57% of Group 1 and in 77% of Group 2.

In summary, 6 months after shock wave therapy applied in two sessions, 54% of the patients were of the opinion that therapy had been successful compared to the pretreatment situation. Radiologically, changes were found in 77% of the cases. Here, in 54% of the cases, dissolution had occurred and, in 23%, disintegration, i.e. the same number of patients in which dissolution had been radiologically observed classified therapy as successful.

Another prospective study from the Orthopaedic University Hospital in Heidelberg, which was also presented in Kassel (Buch 1996), investigated the efficacy of shock wave application to calcaneal spurs. In a pilot study, 20 patients (12 females and 8 males, average age 42 years), who had undergone complete conservative treatment and whose average duration of complaint was 8 months, were treated with shock waves.

Inclusion criteria were: typical radiological finding of calcaneal spurs, typical local pressure pain and therapy resistance to conventional treatment.

Exclusion criteria were those generally accepted. Therapy was carried out with a Lithotripter Compact (Dornier). The foot was fixed in a special fixa-

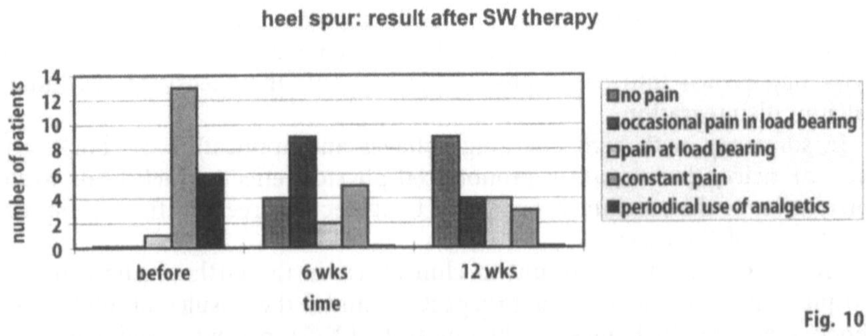

Fig. 10

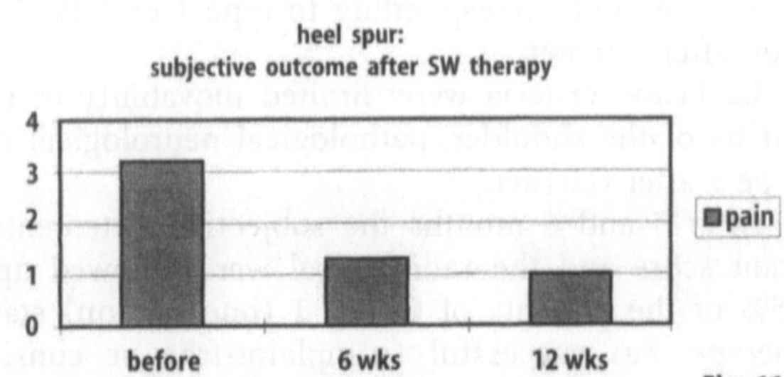

Fig. 11

tion device. The calcaneal spur was then localized radiologically in two planes and local anaesthesia administered to the target area. The transducer was coupled from the lateral side and 3000 pulses each of energy settings 4–5 applied. Follow-up was carried out after 6, 12 and 18 weeks, whereby the the patients' subjective impression of a decrease in pain was classified according to a visual analogue scale, and the local pressure pain and the use of accessories were evaluated (Fig. 10).

The subjective impression concernig pain according to the visual analogue scale is given in the following graph (Fig. 11).

In 1995 and 1996, Rompe and coworkers published the results of shock wave therapy at the Orthopaedic University Hospital in Mainz.

After a randomized prospective study on the efficacy of shock wave therapy for epicondylopathia humeri radialis had shown significant success, the study was continued with 100 patients.

Inclusion criteria were: pain at the epicondylus humeri radialis (EHR) which had persisted for more than 12 months, at least 6 months of conservative treatment, two positive provocative tests, pressure pain above the EHR, positive Thomsen's sign, positive middle-finger extension test, positive Chair test.

Exclusion criteria were: dysfunction in the shoulder/neck/thorax region, arthrosis/arthritis, rheumatoid arthritis, pathological vascular/neurological findings, age under 18 years, pregnancy, infections, tumours and limited movability in the elbow joint.

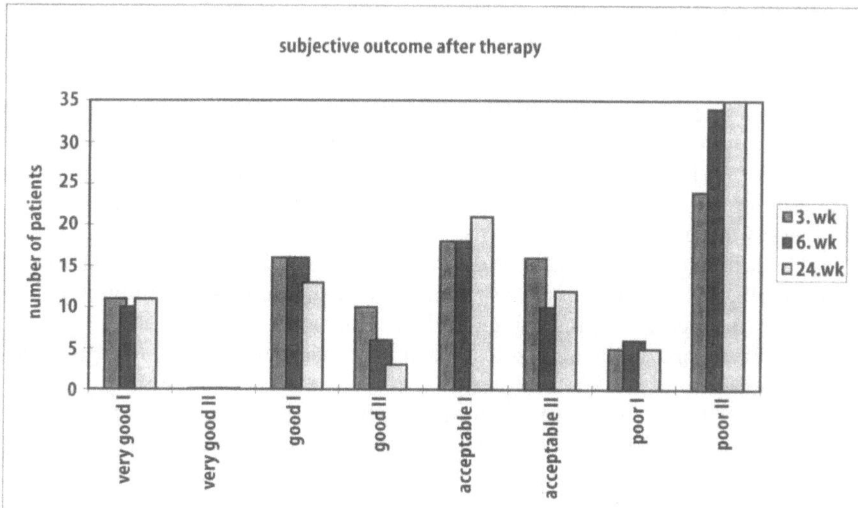

Fig. 12

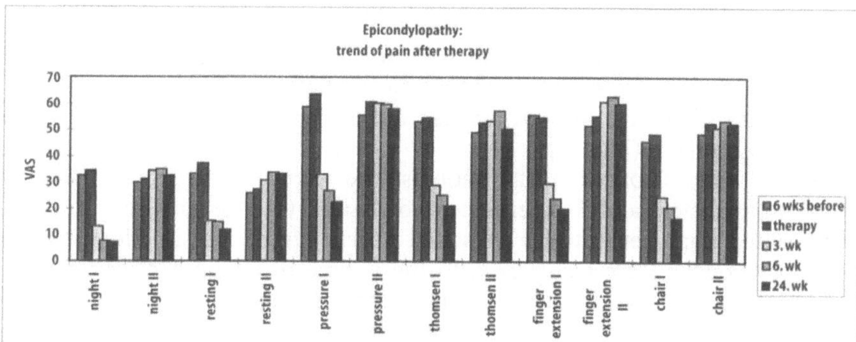

Fig. 13

A 6-week therapy-free interval was to have preceded treatment. During the control period of 6 months, no other therapies were to be carried out. The patients were randomly allotted to two therapeutic regimes:

Group 1 (50 patients, 30 females, 20 males, average age 43.9 years, average duration of complaint 24.8 months) was treated with an Osteostar (Siemens) three times in intervals of 1 week, whereby 1000 pulses of 0.08 mJ/mm^2 were applied without local anaesthesia. The EHR was positioned under radiological control in the centre of the shock wave focus, and the shock wave applied to the front part of the epicondyle and to three points within a radius of 1.5–2 cm.

Group 2 (50 patients, 28 females, 22 males, average age 41.9 years, average duration of complaint 21.9 months) were treated with only 10 pulses of 0.08 mJ/mm^2, but the same other modalities as in Group 1 applied.

Control examinations were carried out after 3, 6, 12 and 24 months with a visual analogue scale and according to the criteria of Roles and Maudsley (Fig. 12 and 13).

After these encouraging results, a prospective study of the efficacy of ESWA in calcaneal spurs was carried out (Rompe 1996).

Inclusion criteria were: a history of pain for more than 12 months under the radiologically representable heel spur, an unsuccessful conservative/surgical therapy for more than 6 months.

Exclusion criteria were: dysfunction of knee or ankle joint, local arthrosis, rheumatological primary diseases, neurological pathological findings, age under 18 years, pregnancy, infections and tumours.

Apart from provision of insoles, no other treatment was allowed 6 weeks before and 6 months after treatment.

A total of 30 patients were randomly allotted to two treatment regimes.

Group 1 (15 patients, 5 females, 10 males, average age 47 years, average duration of pain 16 months) were treated with an Osteostar (Siemens). The spur was brought into the focus of the shock wave with radiological control. One thousand pulses of 0.06 mJ/mm^2 were applied every week for 3 weeks to the spur and at three points within a radius of 1.5–2 cm from the spur.

Group 2 (15 patients, 6 females, 9 males, average age 51 years, average duration of pain 22 months) were treated as a placebo group. The coupling pillow only brought within 1 cm of the heel and no contact gel was applied, so that the shock wave energy could not be applied.

Follow-up examinations were carried out 3, 6, 12, and 24 weeks after the last therapy session (Fig. 14).

After 6 weeks Group 1 had 2 patients who were pain-free, 8 had experienced improvement and 5 experienced no change, whereas ,in Group 2, 4 patients stated improvement and 11 stated no change of the situation. All patients of Group 2 were transferred to the regime of Group 1 after 6 weeks. The graph shows the pain development over time (Fig. 15).

After 3 and 6 weeks, 3 patients of each group stated that they felt no more pain, 8 each stated improvement and 4 stated no change. After 12 and 24 weeks, 4 patients each were free of pain, 7 each experienced improvement and 4 were unchanged. Side effects were not observed.

The third published study from the Orthopaedic University Hospital in Mainz concerns shock wave therapy for tendinosis calcarea of the shoulder (Rompe 1995). The study incorporated 50 patients (27 females, 23 males, average age 47 years, average duration of pain 25 months).

Inclusion criteria were: shoulder pain with radiological proof of an at least 1-cm-large calcium deposit of type 1 after Gärtner, whereby the pain had persisted for at least the past 12 months, although conservative treatment had been carried out for 6 months.

Exclusion criteria were: subacromial impingement which was not caused by the tendinosis calcarea. Sonographic or nuclear magnetic resonance tomographic proof of a rotator cuff rupture, calcium deposits of type 2 or 3 after Gärtner, disease in the area of the throat/thorax, arthrosis, polyarthritis, neurological changes, pregnancy, infections or tumours.

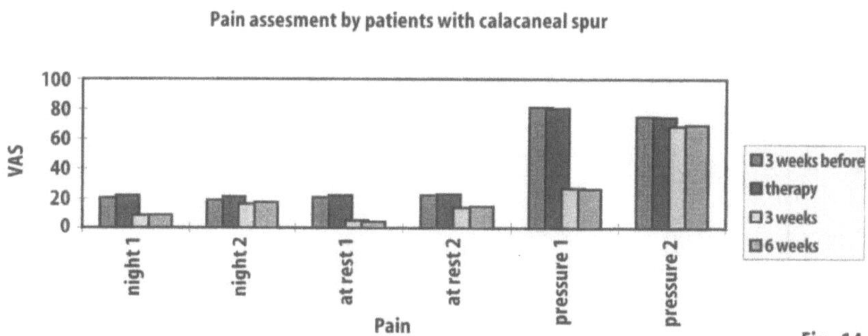

Fig. 14

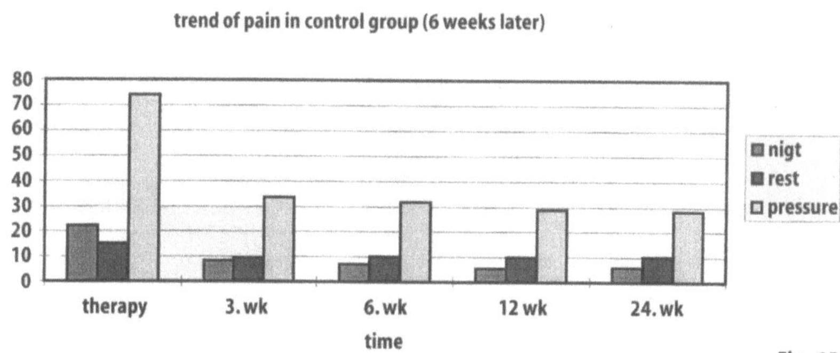

Fig. 15

Therapy was carried out with an Osteostar (Siemens) with regional anaesthesia. After positioning the calcium deposit in the focus of the shock wave source with radiological control, 1500 pulses of 0.28 mJ/mm^2 were applied in one session. In the following 3 days, the patients were kept in hospital and underwent intensive physiotherapy. They were asked to continue the exercises at home. Control examinations were carried out after 6 and 24 weeks with constant scores. Radiological changes were checked for after 3, 6 and 24 weeks. The following graph shows the changes in constant score (Figs. 16 and 17).

Before treatment the total average number of constant score points was 48.2. After only 6 weeks posttreatment it had risen to 75.4 points and after 24 weeks had reached 76.9 points. Radiologically , partial resorption had occurred in 17 cases (42.5%) after 6 weeks, dissolution in 4 cases (10%). After 24 weeks, the number of patients with partial resorption had reached 19 (47.5%). In 6 cases (15%) the deposit had dissolved.

The authors judgment any signs of radiological disintegration and achieving ≥80% of the standard values in the constant score as a success. On the basis of this judgment, 72.5% of the radiologically successfully treated patients were also subjectively successful according to the constant score.

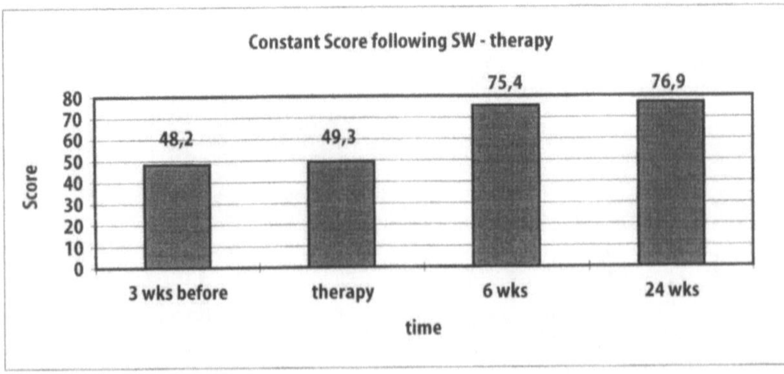

Fig. 16

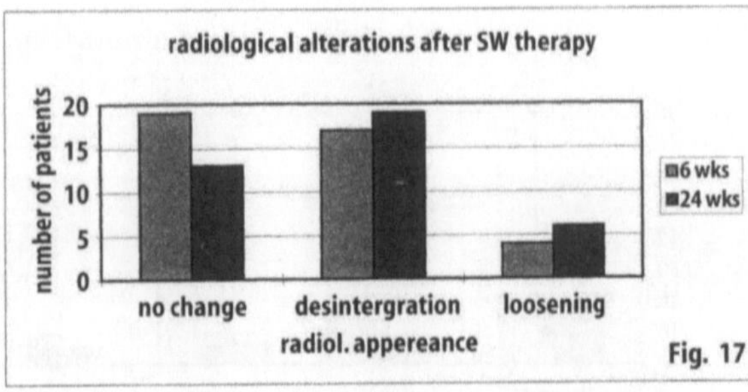

Fig. 17

1.2.1 The Influence of Shock Wave Therapy in Epicondylopathia Humeri Radialis et Ulnaris – Results from the Orthopaedic Hospital in Kassel

M. Buch · B. A. Schlangmann · D. Träger and W. E. Siebert

In the shock wave therapy of epicondylopathia humeri radialis et ulnari there are currently two different regimes:

1. low-energy treatment (Dahmen, Haist, Rompe)
2. medium-to-high-energy treatment (Schleberger, Jakobeit)

The aim of a prospective study at our institution was to differentiate between the two regimes as concerns tolerance and results.

Thirty patients each with therapy-resistant epicondylopathia were randomly allotted to one of two groups.

Inclusion criteria for our study were: pain in the epicondylus humeri radialis/ulnaris, which had persisted for more than 3 months and had been unsuccessfully treated conservatively for more than 3 months, as well as at least two provocative tests:

- pressure pain above the epicondylus humeri radialis/ulnaris,
- Thomsen's sign.

- Middle-finger extension test,
- Chair test.

Exclusion criteria were: local arthrosis, pathological neurological or vascular findings, age under 18 years, pregnancy, blood coagulation disease, infections and tumours.

No other therapy than shock wave therapy was to have been carried out 3 weeks before and during the control period after treatment.

The patients of Group 1 (30 patients, 19 females, 11 males, average age 47 years, average duration of complaint 27.8 months) were treated with a Lithotripter Compact (Dornier). Medium-/high-energy shock waves were applied under neuroleptanalgesia with Rapifen/Dormicum in two sessions 2 weeks apart. The advantage of this anaesthetic procedure is the reduced but still remaining sensitivity to pressure. This enables the patient to provide subjective information in the focusing of the pea-sized maximum-effect point of the shock wave on the epicentre of the pain in addition to the sonographic information, and also to comment on the success of therapy during treatment. We occasionally checked for Thomsen's sign to locate the point of maximum impulse of the pain anew. In each session, 2000 pulses of 0.25 mJ/mm^2 were applied.

The 30 patients of Group 2 (21 females, 9 males, average age 45.9 years, average duration of complaint 19.2 months) received 2000 pulses of 0.1 mJ/mm^2 from the Lithotripter Compact (Dornier) in each of 3–5 sessions in an interval of 2 weeks. The shock waves were applied without anaesthesia. With the help of digital examination localization the target area was localized with ultrasound. During the treatment, the patient was able to carry out localization him-/herself of the focal point on the epicentre of the pain, whereby this was sonographically checked. Here also, after about 500 pulses each, we checked for Thomsen's sign, so as to determine the point of maximum impulse of the pain.

In the follow-up examination, we used the pain intensity scale. Before and directly after therapy, 2, 6 weeks, 3, 6 months and 1 year after treatment, the patients were asked to make statements concerning pain at rest, on pressure and during the night and under go provocative tests. At the same time, they were to assess the pain experienced at the beginning and end of therapy. Furthermore, the patients assessed the success of the treatment based on the criteria of Roles and Maudsley (very good: no complaints, job and hobbies uninhibited; good: few remaining complaints, job and hobbies uninhibited; satisfactory: tolerable remaining complaints, pain considerably better, job and hobbies within limits, further conservative treatment necessary; unsatisfactory: no change in situation, pain uninfluenced).

The results are presented in the following graphs (Figs. 18, 19, 20 and 21).

The patients treated once with low energy displayed a reduction in pain at rest of 90% and Thomsen's sign test showed improvement by 64% directly after therapy. The reduction in pain lasted on average for 4.5 days and then worsened in the majority of treated patients. Only 29% of the patients in this group still had no complaints after 6 weeks. Of the patients treated in one session, 72% thought the result was very good/good directly after therapy,

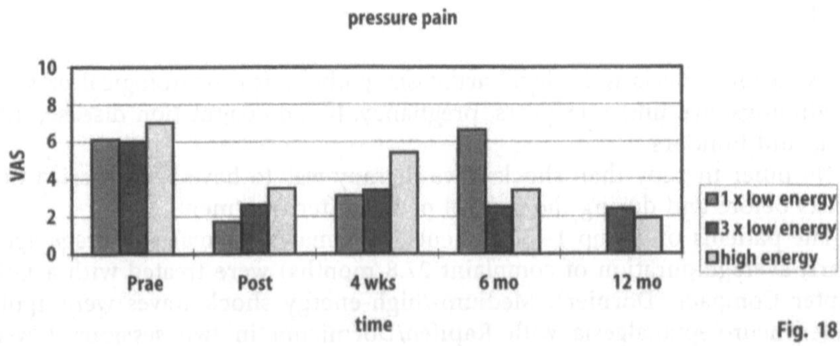

Fig. 18

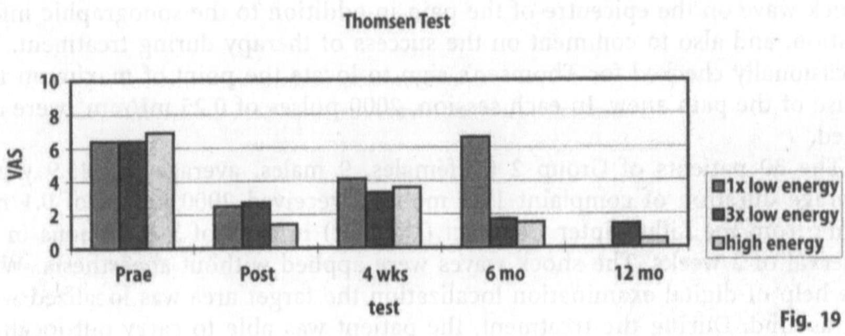

Fig. 19

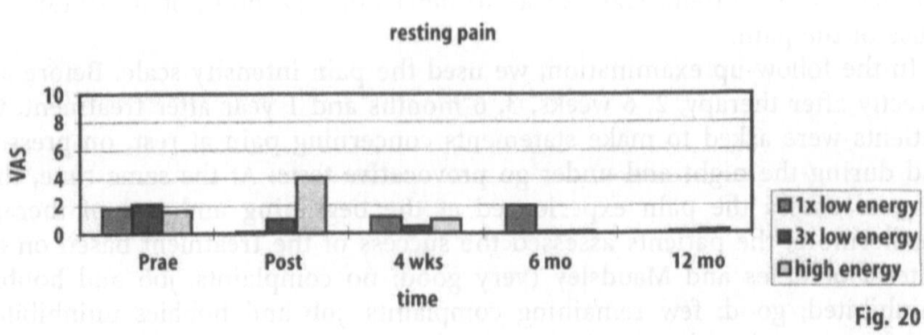

Fig. 20

based on the criteria of Roles and Maudsley. After 6 weeks, the rate had decreased to barely 30%. We subsequently abandoned the regime of the one-session low-energy-treated patients and from then on administered low-energy therapy in 3–5 sessions or high-energy therapy in 1–2 sessions.

The patients in the group treated with high energy levels showed a reduction in pain at rest directly after therapy by about 55%. In the Thomsen's sign test, they showed an improvement of about 70%. The level of pain in-

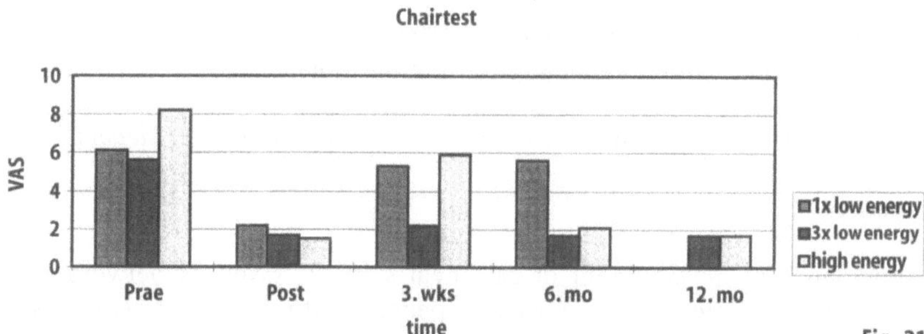

Fig. 21

creased up to the 4th week and then improvement set in. After 3 months, the pain had reached about 80% of the initial value. After 1 year, 74% of the patients treated in several sessions with low energies and 82% of the patients treated with high energies regarded the outcome of therapy as successful according to the criteria of Roles and Maudsley.

An ECG recorded during high-energy therapy was not influenced by the shock wave therapy. In some patients treated for epicondylopathia humeri radialis, a pulse-synchronous finger movement was observed during treatment. As a side effect, petechiae were observed in the skin at the entry point of the shock wave in the group treated with high energy levels. No differences were observed between the patients treated for radial or ulnar epicondylopathia concerning the tolerance or success of therapy. Patients who experienced no more pain continued not to do so. No long-term side effects have been observed to date.

In our opinion, control of the patient during treatment is essential. The experience gained with the patient-controlled positioning of the shock wave focus in the point of maximum impulse of the pain is considered good. We do not think that sonographic control of the target area is absolutely necessary. Although the epicondyle is visible songraphically, which part of the depicted area is painful is not apparent. Final conclusions as to whether treatment with or without ultrasound control leads to better results is a matter of further studies.

Conclusion

With regard to the number of applications and to the subjective long-term alleviation of pain, high-energy shock wave therapy appears to be superior to low-energy treatment, even if in the latter is administered in several sessions. Further studies concerning long-term course and treatment modalities (e.g. whether the shock wave should be coupled transosseously or tangentially) are necessary, especially however studies to clarify the mode of action.

1.2.2
Results of Shock Wave Therapy of Calcaneal Spur from the Orthopaedic Hospital in Kassel: Influence of Various Parameters on the Outcome

M. Buch · B.A. Schlangmann · C. Lübbers · D. Träger and W.E. Siebert

Introduction

The incidence of development of calcaneal spurs is given as between 9 and 20%. Mostly, middle-aged and elderly people, with a greater tendency for women, are afflicted. From an aetiological point of view, an attachment tendinosis of the small muscles of the foot at the heel bone is the focus of discussion. The symptoms (stabbing exercise-dependent pain, mostly medial in the tuberculum mediale calcanei) lead to a more or less pronounced walking impediment up to complete inability to walk. There is a high frequency of patients with general structural weakness of the connective tissue, sunken arches, obesity, as well as from jobs requiring standing (teachers, physicians, nurses). Radiologically, a pointed spur is seen, which often does not concur with the symptoms. In contrast, corresponding symptoms may occur without the spur being radiologically observable. The aim of therapy is not the removal of the spur but of the irritation. Many patients experience freedom from pain when provided with insoles. Furthermore, foot baths (hot and cold alternately), antiphlogistic ointments, ultrasound and short-wave therapy, iontophoresis, electrotherapy, X-ray stimulation and local infiltration with or without corticoids are also administered. Especially as concerns the value of the last-mentioned measures, there is little found in the literature. Surgery is indicated with caution, as scar formations or recurrence of spur formation diminish the success of surgery.

In the literature, there are several accounts of the positive effect of shock wave therapy on the calcaneal spur syndrome. There is currently no knowledge concerning the dose-effect relationship in shock wave application to the bone-tendon interface. There exist hypotheses on the possible analgesic effect mechanisms of shock wave applications:

- Gate control theory
- Local formation of pain-inhibiting substances
- Influence on the receptor potential of the nerve cell

Correspondingly, there is (as yet) no consensus concerning the form of shock wave application. In the literature, success is reported for therapies using energy flux densities of 0.06, 0.16 and 0.28 mJ/mm^2. Some authors describe frontal, others lateral coupling of the transducer. The interval between sessions ranges between 1 day and several weeks. Taking into consideration that apparatuses from different manufacturers are used, which differ in the geometry of the focus zone and in the energy of the shock wave in the focal point, confusion is complete. In view of these facts, since implementing shock wave therapy at our hospital (2.5 years), we have endeavoured to determine the value of the individual parameters by effecting long-term examination and control of the patients.

The determination of "hard values" is difficult in enthesiopathiae, as the success of treatment can only be evaluated by means of subjective statements of the patients concerning pain relief based on the visual analogue scale.

Materials and Methods

The patients reported for the first time within the framework of a shock wave consultation at our hospital. The inclusion and exclusion criteria were then checked.

Inclusion criteria:

- typical local pressure and load pain
- radiologically observable calcaneal spur
- unsuccessful conservative therapy >3 months

Exclusion criteria:

- age <18 years
- pregnancy
- pathological neurological/vascular findings
- local infections
- tumours
- blood coagulation diseases

A total of 110 patients presented fullfilling these criteria, of which 66 were females and 44 were males. The average age was 44 years (25–76 years). The left foot was concerned 67 times and the right foot 43 times. The average height of the patients was 171 cm (159–186 cm), the average weight was 84 kg (61–120 kg). Pain had persisted for an average of 13 months (4 months – 4 years) and had lead to an average of 1 week of inability to work (0–12 weeks). Of the patients, 27 believed the wrong shoes or their jobs were the cause of their complaint, others were unable to name the cause. Twelve patients had had up to 12 prior physiotherapy sessions. Electrotherapy (6–18 sessions) had been administered to 33 patients. Eighteen patients had taken nonsteroid antirheumatics for several weeks. Local infiltrations without corticoids had been carried out in 54 patients, and the same with corticoids had been undergone by 34 patients. Prior to shock wave therapy, 82 patients had received 1–3 insoles. X-ray stimulation or local preoperations had been carried out in none of the cases.

Therapy was administered with two shock wave generators from Dornier:

1. Compact S: the shock wave is generated via an electromagnetic emitter in the transducer. The technical data concernig effective energy, focal energy density and the dimension of the effective area are given in the diagram (see below). A c-arch is used for localization, which displays the focal point in 3D space by two measurments. For therapy, the area to be treated is positioned in the focus, whereby the patient must be positioned accordingly on the treatment slab.
2. Epos: the shock wave is also generated electromagnetically. The technical data are given in the diagram (see below). For therapy, the area to be

treated is positioned in the focus. Fine tuning is carried out by patient-controlled focusing. The patient senses the pinhead-sized focal point and is asked to position it exactly on the point of maximum impulse of the pain. To enhance localization, provocative tests are carried out during therapy. After every 500 pulses, the patient has to walk barefoot on a hard surface, so that he/she is able to locate the main point of pain. Therapy is very much facilitated by the transducer which can be moved in 3D space. Ultrasound gel is applied between transducer and the patient's skin.

The patients were prospectively allotted to one of the following therapy groups:

1. Treatment with the Compact S apparatus with an energy flux density of 0.28 mJ/mm^2. After local anaesthesia of the spur, the heel was coupled medially to the transducer. The spur was positioned in the focus with the help of radiological control and 2000 pulses are applied (n = 24).
2. The same situation as above, but with an energy flux density of only 0.12 mJ/mm^2 and no anaesthesia (n = 14).
3. Treatment with the Epos apparatus with an energy flux density of 0.23 mJ/mm^2 and transosseous shock wave application. With controlled focusing, the patients received 2000 pulses without anaesthesia (n = 32).
4. The same situation as above, but with an energy flux density of only 0.12 mJ/mm^2 (n = 40).

The patients were examined by the physician using the visual analogue scale, whereby the former were to provide information concerning pain at rest, during the night, at work, during sports and with regard to local pressure pain. In addition, the patients were sent a questionnaire 2 weeks, 3, 6 and 12 months after therapy asking for their impression with regard to the success of the therapy according to the criteria of Roles and Maudsley (very good: no complaints, job and hobbies uninhibited; good: few remaining complaints, job and hobbies uninhibited; satisfactory: tolerable remaining complaints, pain considerably better, job and hobbies within limits, further conservative treatment necessary; unsatisfactory: no change in situation, pain uninfluenced), as well as subjectively in percent concerning the status before the first treatment as compared with the development after therapy.

Results

The following graphs show pain relief in Groups 2 and 4 according to the visual analogue scale (Figs. 22 and 23).

In the assessment of the results before the respective next session, they were rated as very good/good by 6/17 patients (43.5%) in Groups 2 and 4 after the first session, by 8/22 patients (55%) after the second session and by 9/25 patients (63.5%) after the third session.

After each session, the patients were free from pain for an average of 3 days ("feeling as if anaesthesized"), then the pain recurred, whereby the intensity of pain had decreased as compared with before the session. A large number of patients of Group 4 stated having no pain in the point of maximum impulse of the pain, but complained of remaining symptoms at the

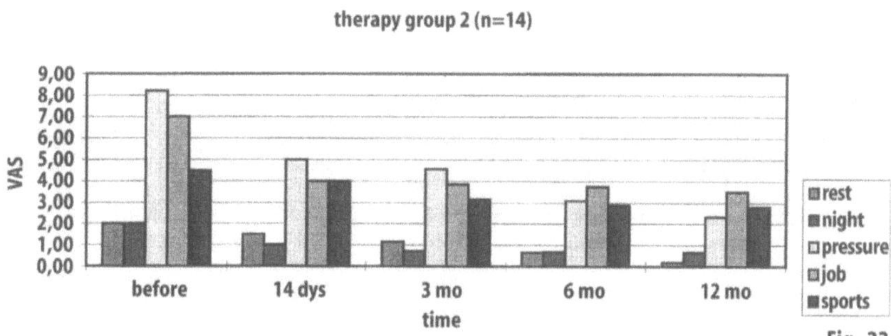

Fig. 22

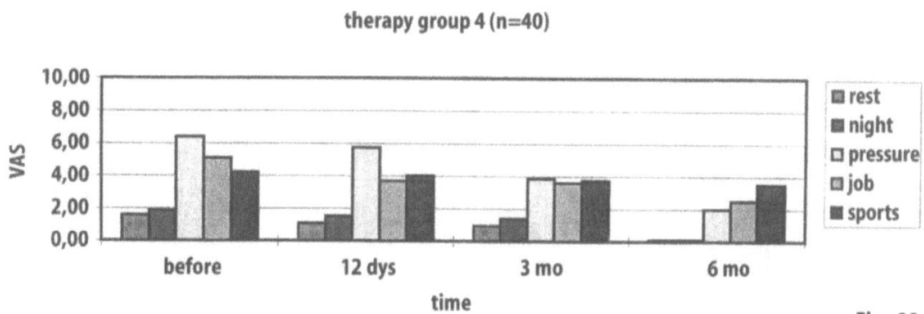

Fig. 23

medial or lateral edge of the foot. Freedom from pain was achieved by treating these areas and not the original point of maximum impulse of the pain. In the groups treated with low energies, an average of four sessions was necessary to achieve painlessness, independent of X-ray localization or patient-controlled focusing. One year after therapy 9/26 patients (65%) assessed the results as very good/good in accordance with the criteria of Roles and Maudsley. Patients who were pain-free after the last treatment remained so.

Patients treated with high energy under local anaesthesia (Group 1) reported stronger pain in the heel area up to the second week posttherapy, whereby the pain was sometimes greater than the original pain. (This phenomenon might be explained by a haematoma in the target area.) Pain receded in the following 2 weeks. Patients treated with high energy without local anaesthesia (Group 3) did not experience this phase of pain. In these two groups, an average of two sessions was necessary to achieve painlessness. At follow-up after 3 months, 9/12 patients (74%) in Groups 1 and 3 stated freedom from pain, after 6 months, the same was stated by 10/13 patients (80%). Here also, there was no recurrence of pain. The interval of between 7 and 21 days had no bearing on the result of therapy.

The low-energy shock wave treatment was repeated daily in 4 patients (Group 4). All patients of this group assessed the result after 1 year as only satisfactory.

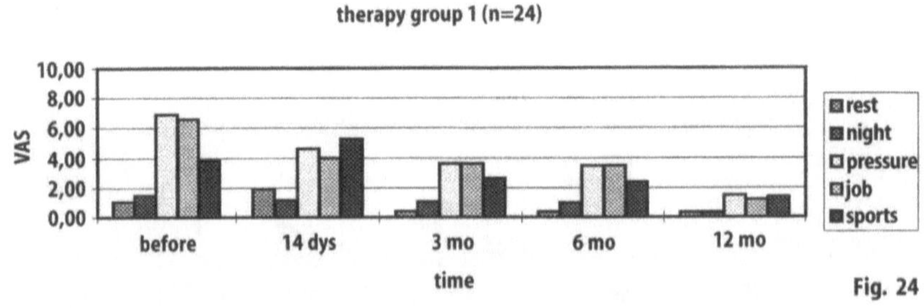

Fig. 24

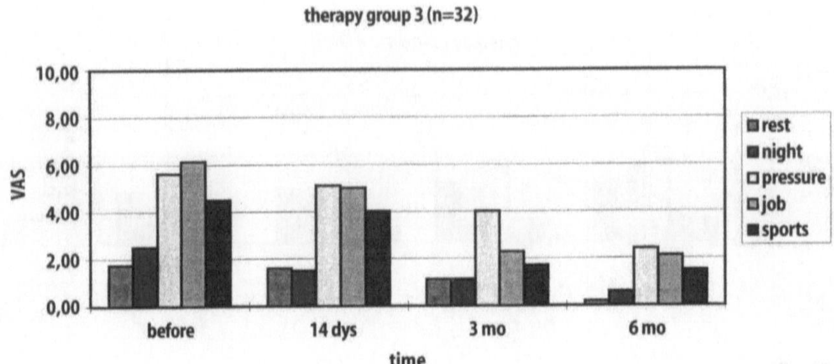

Fig. 25

There was no difference to be seen radiologically concerning the calcaneal spur 1 year after therapy, regardless of whether high or low energy had been applied. No side effects had occurred when follow-up examination was carried out 1 year (in some cases, 2.5 years) after therapy.

The following graphs show the results concerning pain relief according to the visual analogue scale for Groups 1 and 3 (Figs. 24 and 25).

Discussion

We have studied the influence of various parameters on the results of shock wave therapy of the calcaneal spur in the course of treatment. As at least six parameters (shock wave intensity, mode of coupling, type of anaesthesia, localization, interval between sessions, follow-up treatment) influence the outcome, we determined their individual value in pretrials. A controlled randomized single-blind study will be carried out based on these data. Based on the results, some conclusions can be drawn:

- High-energy shock wave therapy appears to be superior to the low-energy application with regard to the number of sessions and the rate of pain-free patients. This was also confirmed by Jakobeit et al.

- The results of the therapy does not seem to be influenced by the mode of coupling.
- Daily application appears to be less successful than application with an interval of 14 days.
- Local anaesthesia of the target area does not seem to offer an advantage. If high-energy treatment is too painful, neuroleptanalgesia can be administered. The advantage here is that the patient remains conscious but feels less pain.
- Consequent treatment of the point of maximum impulse of the pain in our patients lead to good results. Further controlled studies wil be required to determine the differences between shock wave therapy with a localization device and patient-controlled focusing. There is, however, the question as to which part of the spur/heel should be focused. Aetiologically, there are the possibilities of an irritation due to the spur, a tendopathy of the point of attachment of the plantar aponeurosis and a neural isthmus. The pain relief observed at the epicentre of the pain with remaining pain at the medial or lateral edge of the foot in our population of patients makes it highly probable that a tendopathy of the point of attachment of the plantar aponeurosis plays a role. Focusing on the spur would only in part do justice to the treatment of the entire area of attachment of the tendon.

Animal experiments are required to provide a dose-effect relationship in the area of attachment of bone and tendon and to clarify which effect mechanism is the basis of pain relief in shock wave therapy.

1.2.3 Results of Shock Wave Therapy of Tendinosis Calcarea from the Orthopaedic Hospital in Kassel: Comparison of Low- and High-Energy Shock Wave Therapy and Needling in Tendinosis Calcarea of the Shoulder

M. Buch · B.A. Schlangmann · D. Träger and W.E. Siebert

Introduction

In the literature, the frequency of tendinosis calcarea in the healthy is given as between 2.7 and 20%, and as between 6.7 and 54% in patients with shoulder complaints. It is encountered bilaterally in between 11 and 54%. Females are slightly more often afflicted (52-77%). The highest frequency of occurrence is found in the age group 30-60 years.

Aetiology and Pathogenesis

In the past decades, much has been published as to the possible cause of tendinosis calcarea – a definitive answer has, however, yet to be given. Currently, most authors take it that the calcification is to be understood as an adaptation of the cell to the insufficient blood supply. The development of a calcium deposit is initialized by the transformation of the tendocytes into chondrocytes. In living tissue mineralization occurs.

According to Uthoff, the affection has three phases:

1. precalcification phase: reversible chondroid metaplasia
2. calcification phase:
- calcium formation (hardly any complaints)
- rest period (deposits with chalk-like calcium, seen radiologically as dense and with sharp contours)
- calcium resorption (calcium consistency milky – toothpaste-like, radiologically fuzzy and without sharp contours, clinically severe pain)
3. postcalcification phase: restitution of the tendon

Corresponding to the phases, several authors describe a correlation between the radiological morphology and the clinical symptoms (Gärtner type 1–3).

Localization

The main portion of the calcium deposit is found in the points of attachment of the supraspinatus muscle (51–88%) and infraspinatus muscle (19–45%). Calcium deposits in other parts of the rotator cuff are rare.

Clinical situation. Patients often present with pain in the shoulder both at rest and following exercise, especially in rotation and abduction. Due to the pain, restriction in movability may manifest itself up to stiffness of the shoulder. Local pressure pain is mostly present in the tuberculum majus. Clinical tests such as supraspinatus test, Neer sign and painful arc are often positive. Conventional X-ray diagnosis and shoulder sonography are sufficient to determine the location and type of calcium deposit.

Therapy

As the disorder heals spontaneously, the question arises whether therapy is at all necessary. Bosworth was able to show in a patient population of more than 12,000 that over a period of 3 years spontaneous dissolution of the calcium deposit occurs in 9.3% of the cases. In this period, 34.6% of the patients became symptomatic.

We therefore believe a differentiated therapy corresponding to the kind of calcium deposit is sensible. Both in the acute and chronic phase primarily conservative therapies are applied. Randomized studies concerning the value of conservative treatment do not exist. In the following, we list some procedures and their results (Reichelt 1994).

- TENS: pain relief in 10 of 11 patients (Kaada 1984)
- Laser (infrared): comparable to placebo effect (Gusetti 1989)
- Physiotherapy: temporary effect (Harmon 1958)
- X-rays: acute phase 90% good; chronic phase 63% good (Milone 1961); no difference with or without radiation (Plenk 1952)
- Needling: 79% good in 400 patients (Harmon 1958); 61% good in 136 patients (Da Palma 1961); 70% resorption rate in type 2; 33% resorption rate in type 1 (Gärtner 1993)

The mentioned procedures are nearly all successful (spontaneous healing, dissolution of the calcium deposit and the disappearance of clinical symptoms without therapy) in the acute phase, but show weaknesses in the chronic phase.

Surgical treatment, being the last resort, is indicated when conservative therapies have failed. The aim is to remove the calcium deposit. In the literature, good results are reported for 77–96% of the cases with follow-up between 6 and 156 months.

On the background of these facts Loew developed extracorporeal shock wave therapy of large calcium deposits of type 1 or type 2. In the meantime, reports concerning high- and low-energy therapy are to be found in the literature. A mechanical effect on the calcium deposit is under discussion as concerns high-energy treatment. It is assumed that a loosening of the structure with disintegration occurs and subsequent resorption/breakthrough of the calcium masses into the bursa subacromialis. With regard to low-energy therapy, the clinical picture is that of an overstrain reaction at the point of attachment of the supraspinatus muscle, i.e. a tendinosis at the point of attachment. Here, the shock wave is focused on the tuberculum majus humeri, the point of maximum pain for the patient. The success rates vary between 54 and 89% subjective impression of improvement/pain relief and between 77 and 87% radiological observation (disintegration or dissolution of the deposit). No long-term results have been published concerning the low-energy application.

The aim of a prospective study at our institution was to determine the differences of the two above-mentioned forms of therapy and to compare them with the results of needling. Fifteen patients each with calcium deposits of type 1 or 2, who still had complaints after conservative therapy, were randomly allotted to three therapy groups:

- Two sessions of shock wave therapy at an interval of 7–10 days. The patients were in a prone position and received local anaesthesia. An energy of 0.28 mJ/mm^2 was applied and the positioning of the shock wave focus radiologically controlled (Dornier Compact S)
- Up to four sessions with low-energy (0.08–0.12 mJ/mm^2) shock waves at intervals of 5–8 days, without anaesthesia, the patient controlling the positioning of the focus in the epicentre of the pain (Compact S, EPOS)
- One session of needling (cannula with 0.9 mm diameter) of the calcium deposit with radiological control; puncturing and perforation of the deposit several times and irrigation with a 2% xylonesther (Xylonest®) solution

The patients first presented at a shock wave application consultation at our hospital. They were physically examined and the inclusion and exclusion criteria checked for.

Inclusion criteria:

- shoulder pain with tendinosis calcarea
- calcium deposit type 1 or 2 according to Gärtner
- diameter of deposit >1 cm
- unsuccessful conservative therapy for a period of at least 3 months

Table 6. Demographical data

	Age (years)	Sex	Side	Duration (months)	Calcium (months)
Needling	52.5	11 females, 4 males	10 right, 5 left	63.3	16.5
High-energy SWA	56.2	8 females, 7 males	7 right, 8 left	35.8	17.2
Low-energy SWA	49.9	9 females, 6 males	10 right, 5 left	69.1	42.9

Form and number of pretreatments are given in the following table:

	Physio-therapy	Electro-therapy	Local injections	Local injections with corticoids	X-ray stimulation
Needling	7	7	8	8	0
High-energy SWA	10	7	11	11	2
Low-energy SWA	12	7	15	15	3

Technical/clinical data are presented in the table below:

	Initial omar-throsis	AC arthrosis	Calcium type	Acromion type	Positive supraspi-natus test
Needling	0	0	13×1, 2×2	12×1, 3×2	5
High-energy SWA	5	2	12×1, 3×2	14×1, 1×2	8
Low-energy SWA	2	2	10×1, 5×2	12×1, 3×2	4

Exclusion criteria:
- calcium deposit type 3 according to Gärtner
- acromion type 3 in the y-perspective after Bigliani (thoracic outlet view)
- RM ruptures
- pathological neurological/vascular findings
- pregnancy
- omarthrosis/AC joint arthrosis
- allergic reaction to local anaesthesia
- tumour
- local infection

For evaluation, we used the visual analogue scale, the score after Roles and Maudsley, the X-ray picture 12 weeks after therapy and the statements by the patients as to the percentage by which their symptoms had evolved for the better. The patients were asked to comment on the pain experienced at rest, during the night, when pressure is applied to the tuberculum majus, at work, during exercise and at 90° abduction. This was done, using the visual analogue scale (0 = no pain, 10 = strongest conceivable pain), before treatment, once a week during the first 6 weeks after therapy and 3, 6 and 12 months after therapy.

Results

The following graphs show the development of pain during the first 6 weeks after therapy for those treated by needling and those treated with high-energy shock wave therapy (Figs. 26 and 27).

Most patients found high-energy shock wave therapy to be uncomfortable and painful. Four patients complained of more severe pain, especially at rest and during the night. In the further course, it got steadily better. Only at 90° abduction did the complaints persist up to the sixth week.

Of the patients treated by needling, 9 developed severe pain in the first 2 weeks, which caused them to visit our hospital several times. In these cases, the pain could only be subdued by administering analgesics actic on the central nervous system. Two patients developed a frozen shoulder, which were treated successfully by means of stationary balneophysical measures.

At the end of week 6 posttherapy, pain had decreased by an average of four points on the visual analogue scale in the group treated with high energy levels. In the group treated with needling, it was only by 1.5 points. In

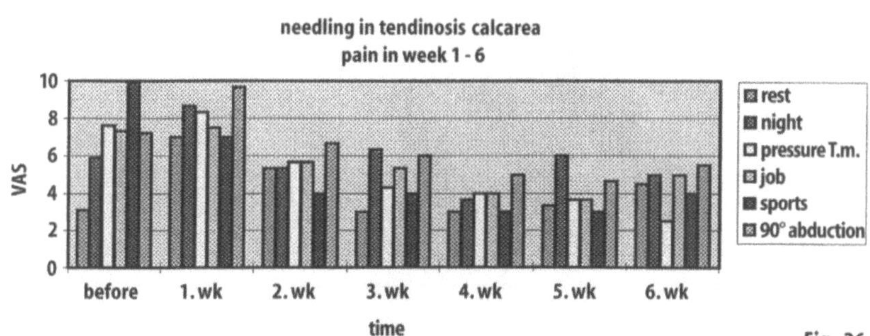

Fig. 26

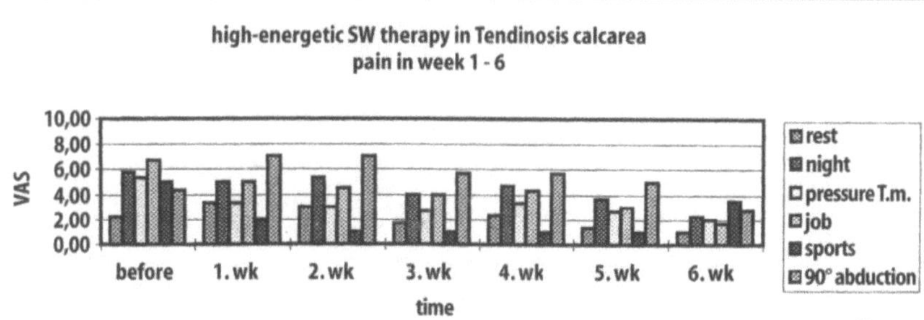

Fig. 27

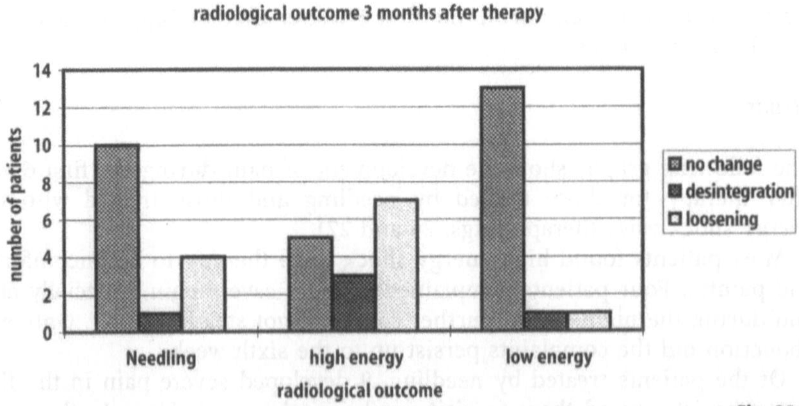

Fig. 28

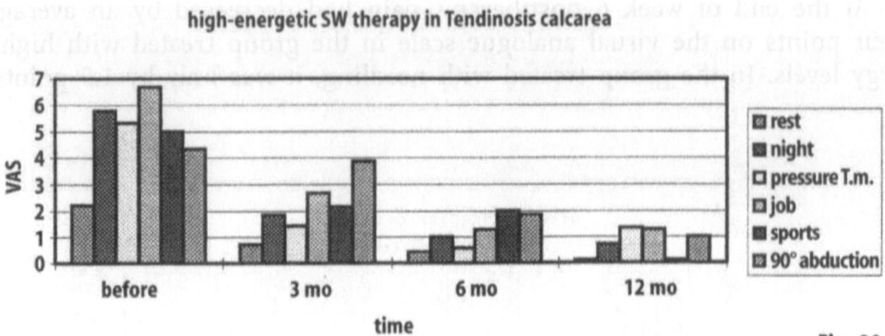

Fig. 29

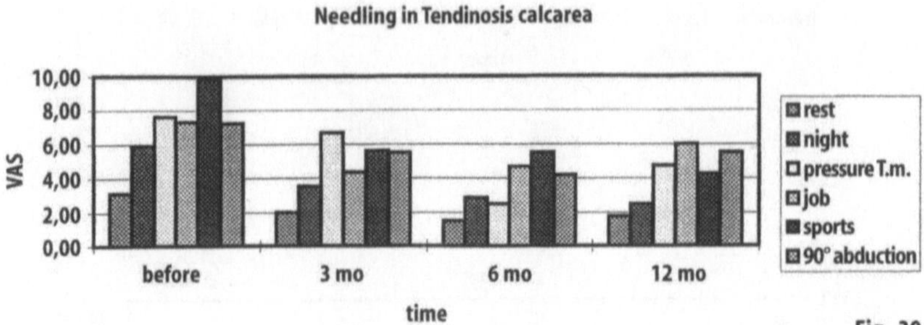

Fig. 30

the case of the patients treated with low energy levels, they stated on average an improvement of approximately 33% after the first session, 60% after the second session and 75% after the third session.

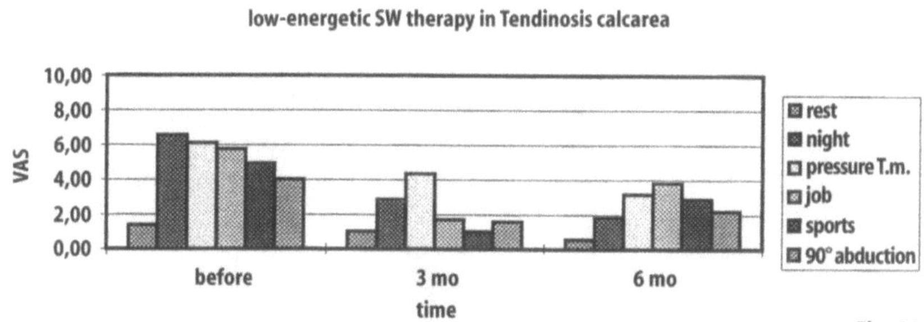

Fig. 31

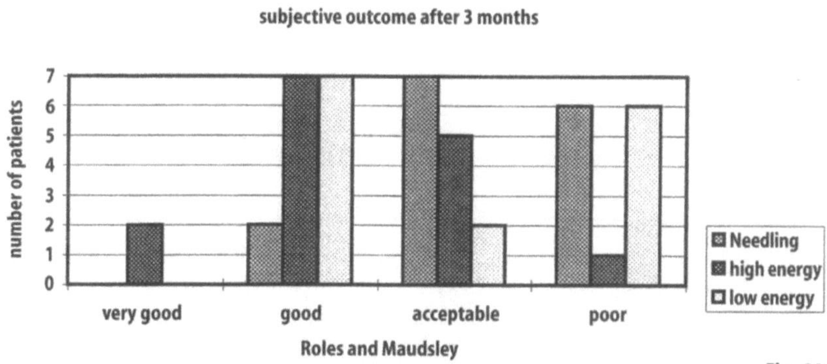

Fig. 32

All patients were followed up radiologically concerning the shoulder after 3 months. The results are shown in the following graph (Fig. 28).

If, in accordance with Loew, the dissolution and disintegration (change in the morphology of the calcium shadow, e.g. transition from type 2 to type 3) is classified as a radiological success, it is permissible to say that, after 3 months, 10 cases in the high-energy group, 5 cases in the needling group and 2 cases in the low-energy group were a success.

The development of pain according to the visual analogue scale is depicted in the following graphs (Figs. 29, 30 and 31).

These results are in parallel with the patients' comments concerning their impression concerning pain relief according to the criteria of Roles and Maudsley (see Figs. 32, 33 and 34).

- very good: no complaints, job and hobbies uninhibited
- good: few remaining complaints, job and hobbies uninhibited
- satisfactory: tolerable remaining complaints, pain considerably better, job and hobbies within limits, further conservative treatment necessary
- unsatisfactory: no change in situation, pain uninfluenced

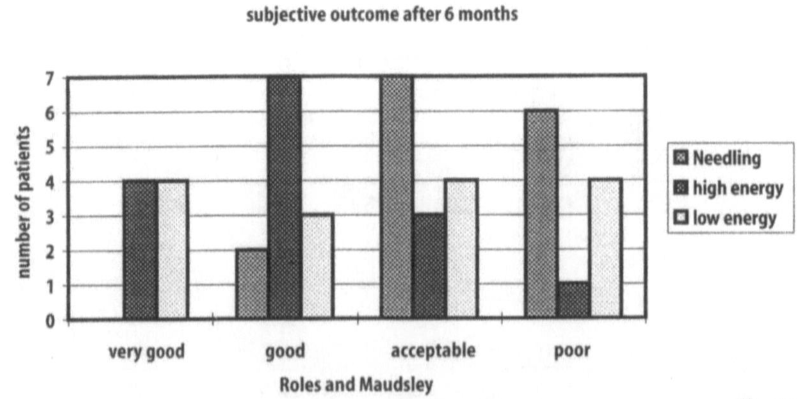

Fig. 33

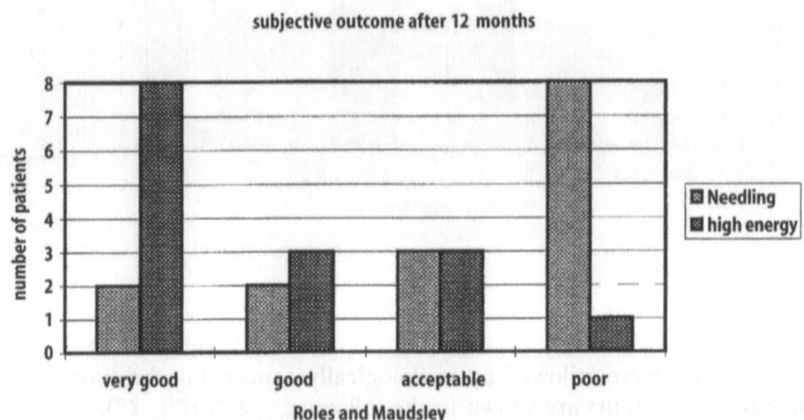

Fig. 34

Discussion

The work presented here was carried out as a field study, to gain experience of the differences in the various conservative therapies in cases of tendinosis calcarea. Statistically significant differences can as yet not be stated, as the patients were not allotted to the therapy groups according to a fixed randomization procedure and the populations are too small. Based on the data, calculations shall be made as to the population for a larger study.

Nevertheless, some trends are already observable.

With regard to the effect on the calcium deposit, the high-energy shock wave therapy appears to be superior to the other two methods, as is shown by the radiological data.

Table 7. Clinical results in cases of epicondylopathy

Author	Year	Apparatus	Therapy modalities	Number of patients	Results
Jakobeit	1996	Doli	1600 shock waves, 60% of max. energy; analogue sedation, transosseous, therapy interval 4 weeks until free of complaints, trigger zone sonographically controlled	170	86% ver good/ good, follow-up period: ?
Haist	1996	Lithostar Plus/ Minilith	10 × 150 pulses; 0.06–0.08 mJ/mm^2, no anaesthesia, transosseous, therapy interval 7–14 days, approx. 2.9 sessions/patient, region of interest sonographically controlled	1253	75.2% very good/ goo d: after 6 months (Roles/M audsley
DGST	1996	Ossatron	800–900 shock waves, 14–16 kV, local/nerve block, transosseous, therapy interval 4 weeks, 1–3 sessions/patient, shock wave application: ?	50	32% pain-free, 44% considerably better, follow-up period: ?
Wolf	1996	Minilith S	2000 shock waves; 0.08–0.12 mJ/mm^2, no anaesthesia; ?, one session/day for 5 days, 5 sessions/patient, shock wave application: ?	8	3 months: 1 × pain-free , 3 × improvement; 13 months: 0 × pain-free , 3 × improvement
Buch	1996	Compact (S)	2000 shock waves; 0.1 mJ/ mm^2, no anaesthesia, transosseous, 3–5 sessions/ patient; 2000 shock waves; 0.25 mJ/mm^2, analogue sedation, transosseous, 1–2 sessions/patient, therapy interval 2 weeks, sonographic control/patient focusing	30 each	Roles and Maudsley : after 1 year: high: 82% very good / good; low: 74% very good / good
Rompe	1996	Osteostar	1000 shock waves; 0.08 mJ/mm^2, no anaesthesia, transosseous, 3 sessions/ patient, therapy interval 1 week, radiological control: lateral epicondyle and 3 points in 2-cm radius	50	Roles and Maudsley after 24 weeks: 24/50 very good / good
Haupt	1995	Ossatron	1225 shock waves; 28 kV, anaesthesia: ?, 2.5 sessions/patient, therapy interval: ?, shock wave application: ?	10	very good/good: 70%; follow-up period: ?

The low-energy shock wave treatment leads to considerable pain relief in the treated shoulder. However, 6 months after termination of therapy, there was a new increase in pain, especially under strain (job, exercise, 90° abduction). Needling fares worst with the type of calcium we used, both as concerns the course of the pain according to the visual analogue scale and the

Table 7 (continued)

Author	Year	Apparatus	Therapy modalities	Number of patients	Results
Schleberger	1995	MFL 5000/ MPL 9000	approx. 350 shock waves; 14–16 kV, i.v. regional/local anaesthesia, sessions/patient: ?, therapy interval: ?, shock wave application: ?	36	very good / good: 65% after 9 months
Dahmen	1994	Lithostar	? shock waves, 0.08 mJ/mm^2, no anaesthesia, 1–10 sessions/week, several therapies, therapy interval: ?, shock wave application: ?	66	good: 30 patients, better: 16 patients after 1 year
Richter	1995	?	2000 shock waves, 18 kV, anaesthesia, 2 sessions/patient, therapy interval: ?, shock wave application: ?	16	very good/good: 16% after 6 months

subjective impressions of the patients as to the result of therapy. The result was classified as very good/good by 11 of 15 patients of the high-energy treatment group at follow-up 6 months after therapy. In the low-energy therapy group, the score was 7 of 15 patients and in the needling group only 2 of 15 patients.

With a larger population, it could also be undertaken to assess whether it is important to concentrate on treating the point of attachment of the tendon of the supraspinatus muscle in the sense of an tendopathy, or whether the calcium really needs to be dissolved.

In general, shock waves seem to be applicable to all point-of-attachment tendinoses. In the literature, the treatment of the following indications is reported:

- tendopathies of the thoracic girdle
- point-of-attachment tendinosis in the greater femoral trochanter
- patellar apex syndrome (jumpers knee)
- achillodynia
- adductor strain in the pelvis

However, the populations have as yet been small. Here also, there is a differentiation between high- and low-energy treatments. In view of the damage to the Achilles tendon proven in animal experiments, high-energy shock wave therapy of achillodynia with an energy flux density of 0.6 mJ/mm^2 should not be undertaken.

Furthermore, there are publications that describe a positive effect of shock wave therapy in the following indications:

- osteochondrosis (M. Osgood-Schlatter, M. Köhler, M. Perthes)
- osteochondrosis dissecans (knee and talus)
- shock wave application in cases of loosened cement-free endoprotheses
- phantom pain

Table 8. Clinical results in calcaneal spur

Author	Year	Apparatus	Therapy modalities	Number of patients	Results
Jakobeit	1996	Doli	1600 shock waves, 70% of max. energy (high energy); neuroleptanalgesia, transosseous, 2 sessions/ patient 1600 shock waves, 30% of max. energy (low energy); no anaesthesia, transosseous, up to 4 sessions/patient therapy interval 4 weeks, respectively, trigger zone sonographically controlled, respectively	113 high energy 79 low energy	pain-free/little pain 84.1% HE 79.8% LE
DGST	1996	Ossatron	800–1000 shock waves, 14–16 kV, local/nerve block, transosseous, therapy interval 4 weeks, approx. 1.53–3 sessions/ patient, shock wave application: ?	28	21% pain-free, 61% improvement
Wolf	1996	Minilith S	2000 shock waves; 0.08–0.12 mJ/mm^2, no anaesthesia; one session/day for 5 days, shock wave application: ?	10	6 months: 1 × pain-free , 2 × improvement; 13 months: 3 × pain-free
Buch	1996	Compact (S), EPOS	2000 shock waves; 0.28 mJ/mm^2 (HE1) 6000 shock waves; 0.23 mJ/mm^2 (HE2) 2000 shock waves; 0.12 mJ/mm^2 (LE1+ 2) local anaesthesia (HE1), otherwise no anaesthesia, max. 3 (HE1 + 2)–5 (LE1 + 2) sessions/patient; therapy interval 1 week, HE1: medial coupling, radiol. Localization HE2: frontal, patient focusing LE1: medial coupling, radiol. Localization LE2: frontal, patient focusing	110	Roles and Maudsle y: 3 months: 74% pain-free (HE1+2) 6 months: 80% pain-free (HE1+2) 12 months: 65% pain-free (LE1+2)
Rompe	1996	Osteostar	1000 shock waves; 0.06 mJ/mm^2, no anaesthesia, 3 sessions/patient, therapy interval 1 week, radiological control: spur and 3 points in 2-cm radius, coupling: ?	15	3+6 weeks: 3 × improvement 12+24 weeks: 4 × pain-free , 7 × improve ment

In these cases, the populations are also too small to make statements concerning the therapeutic procedure or the percentage of complete healing due to the therapy. There are also no data from animal experiments concerning

Table 8 (continued)

Author	Year	Apparatus	Therapy modalities	Number of patients	Results
Loew	1996	Compact S	3000 shock waves; 0.2 mJ/ mm^2, local anaesthesia, sessions: ?, therapy interval: ?, Radiological focus on spur, lateral coupling	20	6 weeks: 4 × pain-free , 9 × occasion al pain under strain 12 weeks: 9 × pain-free , 4 × occasion al pain under strain

the efficacy/mode of action of this form of therapy in the mentioned indications.

The following tables give an overview of the results obtained to date of shock wave therapy of tendopathies and tendinosis calcarea. Comparison is in part difficult, as the results were obtained using various lithotriptors and evaluated according to different criteria.

Nevertheless, some trends can be identified and conclusions drawn on the basis of the results.

- The high-energy treatment appears to be superior to the low-energy application with regard to long-term success rates and the number of treatments.
- A therapy interval of 2–4 weeks seems to make more sense than daily sessions. Apparently, in addition to the primary pain relief lasting only a few days directly after therapy as observed by several authors, there is another effect which plays a role in the development of pain relief/healing of the disease. It must be clarified by further studies whether it is an improvement of the blood supply in the focal area detectable by Doppler sonography or the formation of new endothelium [162].
- In all orthopaedic shock wave applications no severe side effects occurred. The limit of the energy flux density of 0.3 mJ/mm^2 calculated by Steinbach is sometimes exceeded in urological (kidney stones) and biliary (gallstones) shock wave applications. Even in high-energy shock wave therapy of pseudo-arthroses this limit is sometimes exceeded (cf. Haist). In none of these therapies did clinically detectable changes/consequences such as thromboses or embolism arise. As a reservation, it should be pointed out that Steinbach carried out the tests without precursory tissue. In clinical applications, part of the shock wave energy is lost on its path through the tissue. The portion of energy actually reaching the focal point depends on the thickness and type of tissue traversed beforehand. This may vary from case to case and is ultimately not known.
- In the treatment of tendinosis calcarea type 1–2, which causes a mechanical impingement, it appears that the high-energy shock wave therapy with sonographic control of the target area leads to the best results.
- Especially in times of professional insecurity further multicentre studies concerning the efficacy of this method of treatment should be planned by a central institution.

Table 9. Clincial results in tendinosis calcarea

Author	Year	Apparatus	Shock wave parameters	Number of patients	Results: pain-free/better	Results: Radiological success	Results: C Score
Loew	1995	Compact S MFL 5000	2 × 2000 SW/21 kV (HE1) 1 × 2000 SW/21 kV (HE2) 1 × 2000 SW/18 kV (HE3) Local anaesthesia Radiol.: focus on calcium Therapy interval: 10 days	20 20 20	14 12 6	12 11 4	13×80% 11×80% 4×80% of normal
Dählke	1996	Compact S	2 × 2000 SW/22 kV (HE1) 1 × 2000 SW/22 kV (HE2) Local anaesthesia Radiol.: focus on calcium Therapy interval: 7 days	61 54	50% 45% HE1: 45% HE2: 54%	? ? after 3 months; 57% success 77% success after 6 months	49→5 2 49→5 2 →67 →69
Jako-beit	1996	Doli	1800 SW/80% max. energy Local anaesthesia/ analogue sedation Sonogr.:focus on calcium Therapy every 4 weeks until calcium-free	78	89%	87% calcium-free/ disintegration Follow-up: 1–13 months	
Wolf	1996	Minilith S	2000 SW/ 0.08–0.12 mJ/mm^2 No anaesthesia one session/day for 5 days shock wave application: ?	6		After 6 months: 1× no improvement After 13 months: 3×no improvement	
DGST	1996	Ossatron	800–1000 SW/ 16–18 kV Local anaesthesia/nerve block therapy interval: 4 weeks 1.58 sessions/ patient Radiol.: focus on calcium	127	86%	Radiol. (59 patients): dissolution/disintegration: 73%	

Table 9 (continued)

Author	Year	Apparatus	Shock wave parameters	Number of patients	Results: pain-free/better	Radiological success	C Score
Haist	1996	Lithostar Plus/ Minilith	2000 SW/ 0.27 mJ/mm^2 Anaesthesia: ? Sonogr.: focus on calcium 2.5 sessions/ patient	68		?	
Haupt	1995	Ossatron	1225 SW/15.5 kV Local anaesthesia No. therapies: ? Radiol.: focus on calcium	29	82%		
Rompe	1995	Osteostar	1500 SW/ 0.28 mJ/mm^2 Regional anaesthesia 1 session/patient Radiol.: focus on calcium	40		dissolution/ disintegration: 52.5% (6 weeks); 62.5% (24 weeks)	49.3 (0 weeks) →75.4 (6 weeks) →76.9 (24 weeks)
Buch	1996	Compact (S) EPOS	2 × 2000 SW/ 0.28 mJ/mm^2 (HE) Local anaesthesia Radiol.: focus on calcium 5 × 3000 SW/ 0.08 mJ/mm^2 (LE) No anaesthesia Patient-orientated focusing Transosseous Therapy interval: 7–10 days, respectively	15 15		6 weeks follow-up: dissolution/ disintegration: HE: 66% LE: 6.6%; (Roles/Maudsley) HE: 54% very good/good NE: 80% subjectively unchanged	HE: 37→65 NE: 41→36

1.3 Shock Wave Technology: Energy Settings

1.3.1 Dornier Compact *S*

1.3.1.1 *Dornier Compact S: Therapy Focus*

Focus describes the area in which 50 percent of the maximal energy of the shockwave is still available. The area looks like a big rice corn.

Focus Dornier *Compact S:* approx. 6.4 mm (laterally to direction of shockwave)
approx. 70 mm (parallel to direction of shockwave)

1.3.1.2
Dornier Compact S: Effective Focus Energy of Positive Part of Wave

Following values describes the positive part of the effective focus energie in the geometrical focalpoint. It is the sum of total found or measured energy within a circle with a diameter of 12 mm (=biological sensitive area). The measurement itself was made with a Imotec PVDF Hydrophon. The effective focus energy seems to be the most important value to describe the behavior and power of a shockwave therapy system.

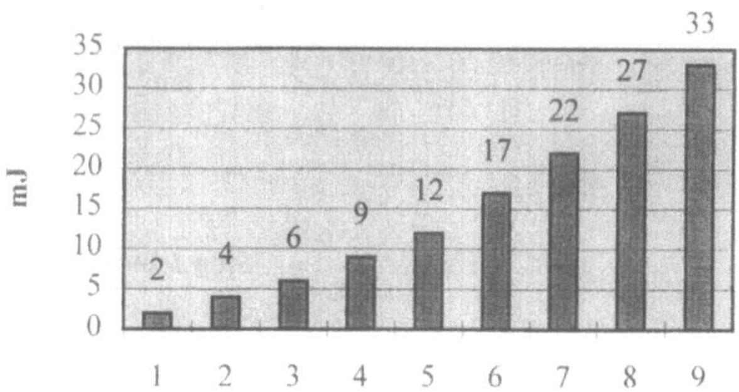

Dornier Compact S
Effective Focus Energy
[mJ]
12 mm

Step / Level

1.3.1.3
Dornier Compact S : Energy Flux Density of the Positive of the Wave

The energy flux density is measured once a time per energy level. The used sensor was a Imotec PVDF Hydrophon.

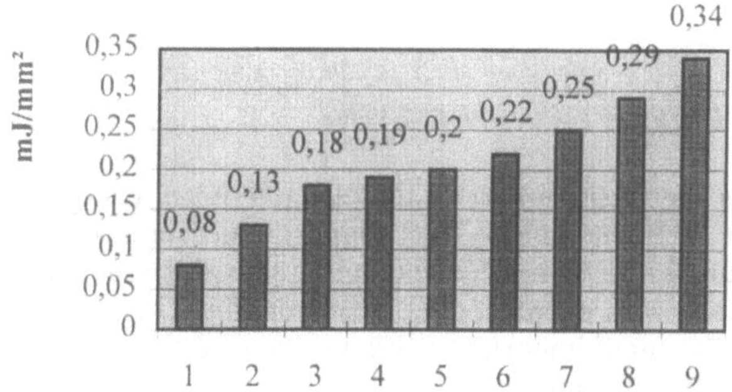

Dornier Compact S
Energy Flux Density
[mJ/mm^2]

Step / Level

1.3.1.4
Dornier Compact S: Pressure

To be complete the max. pressure of the Dornier *Compact S* is shown in the following chart. This value was measured with the use of a Imotec PVDF Hydrophon (10 bar = 1 MPa, Mega-Pascal).

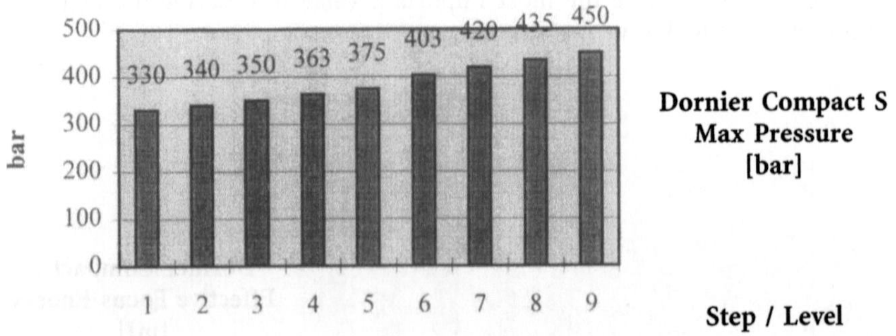

1.3.2
Dornier Epos

1.3.2.1
Dornier Epos: Therapy Focus

Focus describes the area in which 50 percent of the maximal energy of the shockwave ist still available. The area looks like a rice corn.
Focus Dornier *Epos*: approx.4 mm (laterally to direction of shockwave)
approx. 25 mm (parallel to direction of shockwave).

1.3.2.2
Dornier Epos: Effective Focus Energy of Positive Part of Wave

Following values describes the positive part of the effective focus energy in the geometrical focalpoint. It is the sum of total found or measured energy within a circle with a diameter of 12 mm (= biological sensitive area). The measurement itself was made with a Imotec PVDF Hydrophon. The effective focus energy seems to be the most important value to describe the behavior and power of a shockwave therapy system.

1.3.2.3
Dornier Epos: Energy Flux Density of the Positive of the Wave

The energy flux density is measured once a time per energy level. The used sensor was a Imotec PVDF Hydrophon.

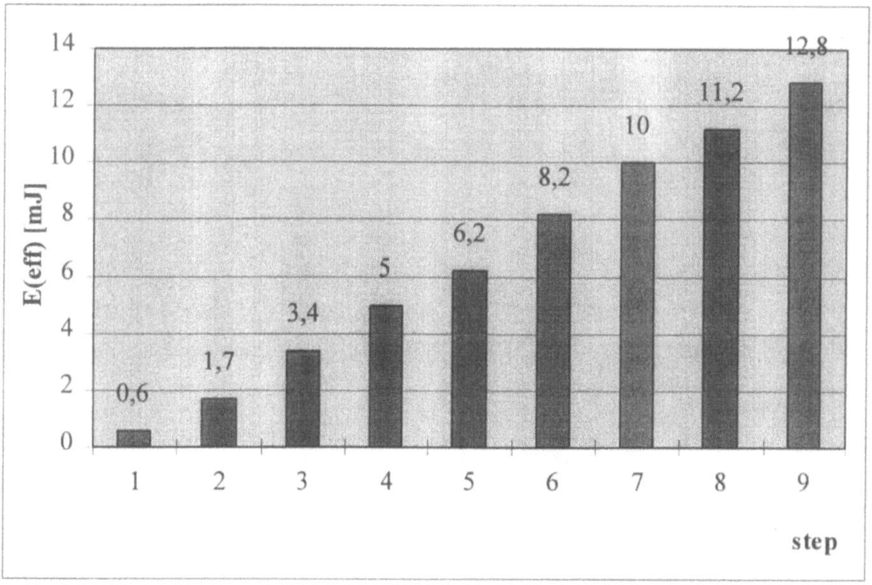

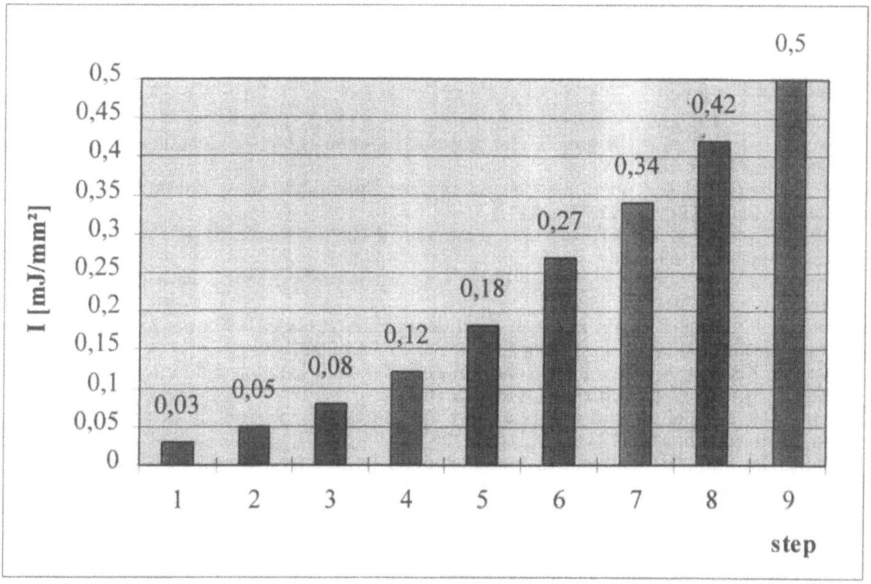

1.3.2.4
Dornier Epos: Pressure

To be complete the max. pressure of the Dornier *Epos* is shown in the following chart. Alsi this value was measured with the help of a Imotec PVDF Hydrophon. (10 bar = 1 MPa, Mega-Pascal).

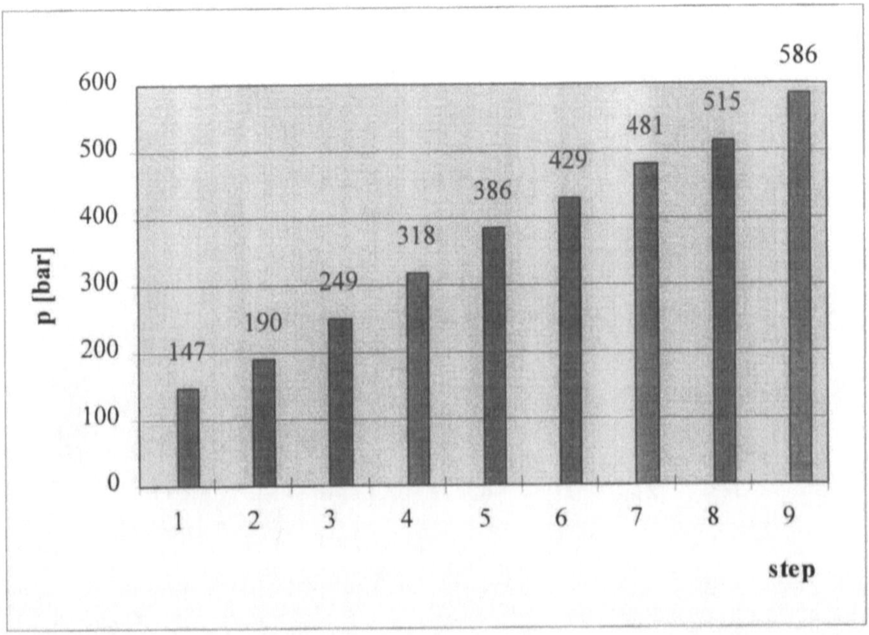

References

Aglietti P, Buzzi R et al.: Il gomito del tennisata, aspetti clinici ed anatomici. Int J Sports Traumatol 113 ff

Arcq M, Pfeiffer I., Die operative Behandlung der Epikondylopathie durch Fascia – lata – Plastik. Orthop Praxis, 12 / 92, 841 ff

Ark J W, Flock T J et al.: Arthroscopic treatment of calcific tendinitis of the shoulder. Arthroscopy 8 (2):183 – 188

Assimos DG et al.: Urinary enzyme levels after extracorporal shock wave lithotripsy (abstract). J Urol 137:45 A, 1987

Barrios R, Solchaga L et al.: Effect of high energy shock waves on bone: An experimental study on sheep. J Bone Joint Surg (Br), 1993; 75 – B; SUPP II

Biedert R, Kentsch A: Arthroskopische Revision des subakromialen Raumes bei Impingement – Syndrom.Unfallchirurg (1989) 92: 500 – 504

Bomanji J et al.: Radionuclid evaluation pre and post extracorporal shock wave lithtoripsy for renal caliculi. J Nucl Med; 28, 1284, 1987

Bosworth D.: Surgical treatment of tennis elbow. J Bone Joint Surg 47 A, No. 8, December 1965

Boyd H.: Tennis elbow. J Bone Joint Surg 55 A, No. 6, September 1973, 1183 ff

Braun, W, Claes L, Rüter A: Untersuchungen zur Wirksamkeit von Stoßwellen auf die Festigkeit des Verbundes von Knochen und Polymethyl-Metacrylat. Orthop 130 (1992) 236 – 43

Brendel W: Effect of shock waves on canine kidney. In: Gravenstein JS (ed) Extracorporal shock wave lithotripsy for renal stone disease: Technical and clinical aspects, Stoneham, Butterworth, 1986, p 141

Brümmer F, Suhr D: Standardisierte in vitro Modelle zur Charakterisierung von Stoßwellen. Biomed Tech 35, Ergänzungsband 1990, 237 ff

Brümmer F, Bräuner T, Hülser D: Biological effects of shock waves. World J Urol (1990) 8:224 ff

Buch M.: Unpublished summary of the results presented during the 1st Kasseler Shock Wave Symposium

Bürger RA, Witzsch U et al.: Extracorporal shock wave therapy of pseudo – arthrosis and aseptic osteonecrosis. Abstract

Caspari R, Raymond R: A technique for arthroscopic subacromial decompression. Arthroscopy 8 (1): 23–30
Cass AS: Colon injury with ESWL for an upper ureteral calculus. In: Newman DM (ed) Shock wave lithotripsy. New York, Plenum, 1988
Chaussy C, Eisenberger F, Jocham D, Wilbert D: Die Stoßwelle Attempto Verlag 1995
Chaussy C, Eisenberger F, Jocham D, Wilbert D: Stoßwellenlithotripsie. Attempto Verlag 1993
Chaussy C: ESWL for kidney stones: an alternative to surgery? Urol Radiol 6:80, 1984
Chaussy C: ESWL in treatment of urolithiasis. Urology 23 (Suppl), 59, 1984
Chaussy C: Extracorporal shock wave lithotripsy: Technical concept, Experimental research and clinical application. Basel S Karger, 1986
Chaussy C: The in vitro and In vivo effects of extracorporal shock waves on malignant cells. Urol Res 1988, 16, 419ff
Chaussy C, Fuchs G: ESWL: Die Evolution einer Revolution. Urologe A, 1989, 28, 126ff
Cloward RB: Cervical dicography. Ann Surg, Dec 1959 150 No 6 1052ff.
Coenen W: Über ein diagnostisches Zeichen bei der sogenannten Epikondylitis humeri radialis. Orthop, 124, (1986) 323–26.
Coleman A, Choi M: Acoustic emission and sonoluminescence due to cavitation at the beam focus of an electrohydraulic shock wave lithotripter. Ultrasound Med Biol 18, No 3, 267ff.
Coleman A, Saunders J: Acoustic cavitation generated by an extracorporal shock wave lithotripter. Ultrasound Med Biol 13, No 2, 69ff.
Constant CR.: A clinical method of functional assessment of the shoulder. Clin Orthop, No. 214, January 1987, 160ff.
Coonrad R, Hooper R: Tennis elbow: Its course, natural history, conservative and surgical management. J Bone Joint Surg 55 A, No. 6, September 1973, 1177ff.
Dahmen GP, Meiss L et. al.: Extrakorporale Stoßwellentherapie (ESWT) im knochennahen Weichteilbereich an der Schulter. Extr Orthop 15, Heft 11, 25ff..
Deam RK: Neurological damage resulting from extracorporal shock wave lithotripsy when air is used to locate the epidural space. Anaesthaesia Intensive Care 21 (4), 1993 Aug, 455ff.
Debeyre J, Patte D, Elmelik E: Repair of ruptures of the rotator cuff of the shoulder. J Bone Joint Surg 47 B, No 1; February 1965.
Delius M et al: Biological effects of shock waves: kidney damage by shock waves in dogs – dose dependence. Ultrasound Med Biol 14:177-22, 1988.
Delius M: Biologische Wirkung von Stoßwellen – mehr als "nur" Steinzertrümmerung? Zentralbl Chir 120, (1995) 259-73.
Delius M, Hofschneider P: Extracorporal shock waves for gene therapy? Lancet 345, No 8961, pp 1377.
Delius M, Weiss N: Tumor therapy with shock waves requires modified Lithotripter shock waves. Naturwissenschaften 76; 573-74; (1989).
Delius M, Denk R: Biological effects of shock waves: cavitation by shock waves in piglet liver. Ultrasound Med Biol 16, No 5, 467ff.
Delius M, Enders G: Biological effects of shock waves. Lung hemorrage by shock waves in dogs- pressure dependence. Ultrasound Med Biol 13, No 2, 61ff.
Delius M, Gambihler S: Sonographic imaging of extracorporal shock wave effects in the liver and galbladder of dogs. Digestion, 1992, 52, 55ff.
Delius M, Ueberle F: Destruction of galstones and model stones by extracorporal shock waves. Ultrasound Med Biol 20, No 3, 251ff.
Delius M, Draenert K: Biological effects of shock waves: In vivo effect of high energy pulses on rabbit bone. Ultrasound Med Biol. 21; No 9, 1219ff.
Delius M, Hoffmann E: Biological effects of shock waves: Induction of arrythmia in piglet hearts. Ultrasound Med Biol 20, No 3, 1994, 279ff.
Dellian M, Walenta S: High energy shock waves enhance hyperthermic response of tumors. J Nat Cancer Inst 86, No 4, Feb. 16, 1996.
Di Silverio F, Gallucci M: Blood cellular and biochemical changes After extracorporal shock wave lithotrypsie. Urol Res, 1990, 18, 49ff.
Doerr: Krankheiten der Sehnen – Knochen – Insertion. in: Doerr: Spezielle Pathologische Anatomie, Band 19, 203ff.
Doukas A, McAuliffe D: Biological effects of laser induced shock waves: Structural and functional cell damage in vitro. Ultrasound Med Biol 19, No 2, 137ff.
Drach GW: Report of the united states cooperative study of ESWL. J Urol., 135, 1127, 1986.

Ekkernkamp A, Haupt G et al.: Der Einfluß der extracorporalen Stoßwellen auf die Standardisierte Tibiafraktur am Schaf. in: Ittel, Siebert, Matthiaß: Aktuelle Aspekte der Osteologie. Springer Verlag 1992, 307 ff.
Ellman H: Arthroscopic Subacromial Decompression: Analysis of one to three year results. Arthroscopy: 3(3): 173-181.
Endl E, Steinbach P et al.: Flow cytometric analysis of cell suspensions exposed to shock waves in the presence of the radical sensitive dye hydroethidine. Ultrasound Med. Biol. 21:569-577, 1995
Endl E, Steinbach P et al.: Cell type specific response to shock waves of suspended or pelleted cells as analysed by flow cytometry or electricl cell volume determination. Ultrasound Med. Biol. 22 (4):515:525, 1996
Engel WJ: Hypertension due to renal compression resulting from subcapsular hematoma. J Urol, 73: 735, 1955.
Esch, J, Ozerkis L et al.: Arthroscopic subacromial decompression: Results according to dgree of rotator cuff tear. Arthroscopy 4 (4): 241–49.
Filipczynski L, Piechocki M: An attempt to reconstruct the lithotripter shock wave pulse in kidney: Possible temperature effects? Ultrasound Med Biol 18, Nos 6/7, 569 ff.
Filipczynski L, Piechocki M: Estimation of the temperature increase in the focus of a lithotripter for the case of high rate administration. Ultrasound Med Biol 16, No 2, 149 ff.
Finlayson B: A favourable commenton the practice of outpatient ESWL. Endourol Newsletter 1 (2): 1, 1986.
Finney R, Halliwell M: Measurement of lithotripsy pulses through biological media. Phys Med Biol, 1991 36, No 11, 1485 ff.
Folberth W, Köhler G et al.: Pressure distribution and energy flow in the focal region of two different electromagnetic shock wave sources. J Stone Dise 4, No1,1992, 1 ff.
Forriol F: The effect of shock waves on mature and healing cortical bone. Int Orthop (SICOT), 1994, 18: 325-29.
Gächter A, Seelig W: Arthroscopy of the shoulder. Arthroscopy 8 (1): 89–97.
Gamarra, F.; Spelsberg, F.: Complete local tumor remission after therapy with extra corporally applied high energy shock waves. Int. J Cancer: 55, 153 -56, (1993).
Gambhiler S, Delius M: In vitro interaction of lithotripter shock waves and cytotoxic drugs. Br J Cancer, 1992, 66, 69 ff.
Gambhiler S, Delius M: Influence of dissolved and free gases on iodine releasend cell killing by shock waves in vitro. Ultrasound Med Biol 18, Nos 6/7, 617 ff.
Gambihler S, Delius M: Biological effects of shock waves: cell disruption, viability, and proliferation of L1210 cells exposed to shock waves in vitro. Ultrasound Med Biol 16, No 6, 587 ff.
Gärtner J: Tendinosis calcarea – Behandlungsergebnisse mit dem Needling. Z. Orthop 131 (1993) 461 ff.
Godolias G, Pfeiffer I: Endoskopisch kontrollierte Erweiterung des subakromialen Raumes beim Impingementsyndrom. Orthp. Praxis 2 / 94; 84 ff.
Graff J, Richter KD: Wirkung von hochenergetischen Stoßwellen auf Knochengewebe. Abstract, Urol Res 16, 1988, 252 ff.
Graff Jürgen: Die Wirkung hochenergetischer Stoßwellen auf Knochen- und Weichteilgewebe. Habilitationsschrift Bochum 1989.
Gray J: Effects of strech on single myelinated nerve fibers. Journal of physiology, Band 124, 1954, 84 ff.
Haist J, Reichel W et al: Die extrakorporale Stoßwellenbehandlung der gestörten Frakturheilung – eine Alternative zu operativen Verfahren? Orthop Praxis, 12 / 93, 842 ff.
Haist J, Reichel W et al.: Einsatz der extrakorporalen Stoßwelle bei der osteosynthetisch versorgten Pseudarthrose – eine experimentelle Studie. Orthop Praxis, 5 / 93, 345 ff.
Haist J, Steeger D: Die ESWT der Epikondylopathia radialis et ulnaris. Ein neues Behandlungskonzept knochennaher Weichteilschmerzen. Orthop Mitteilungen 3/1994, 173 ff.
Harmon PH: Methods and results in the treatment of 2580 painful shoulders. (special referrence to T. C.) Am J Surg 95, April 1958.
Haucke S, Scholz J: Epikondylitis humeri radialis – ätiopathogenetische Faktoren und operative Behandlungsergebnisse. Orthop Praxis, 12 / 94, 776 ff.
Haupt G, Haupt A et al.: Influence of shock waves on fracture healing. Endourology, June 1992 XXXIX, No. 6, 529 ff.
Haupt G, Chvapil M: Effect of shock waves on the healing of partial thickness wounds in piglets. J Surg Res 49, (1990) 45 ff.
Haupt G, Haupt A et al.: Influence of shock waves on fracture healing. Urology, june 1992 34, No 6, 529 ff.

Haupt G, Haupt A et al.: Wound and fracture healing: New indication for extracorporal shock waves? Abstract.
Haupt G, Senge T: Extracorporal shock waves outside Urology-new concepts. Poster Session 38, 869.
Hedtmann A, Fett H: Die sogenannte Periarthropathia humeroskapularis. Orthop 127 (1989) 643 ff.
Hesselschwerdt H-J, Siebel T, Heisel J: Behandlungsergebnisse nach Rezidiveingriffen bei Epikondylitis Humeri. Orthop Praxis 12/92 851 ff.
Hynynen K: The threshold for thermally significant cavitation in dog's thigh muscle In vivo. Ultrasound in Med & Biol 17, No 2, 157 ff.
Janda J, Koudela K: Skelettmuskelbeteiligung bei der Enthesopathie des Epikondylus lateralis humeri. Orthop, (1988), 105 - 107.
Jansson V, Breitner S: Verlaufsbeobachtung einer aseptischen Spätlockerung eines PCA Hüftendoprothesenschaftes. Z.Orthop 131 (1993) 135 ff.
Jocham D, Liedl B: Langzeiterfahrungen nach ESWL von Harnsteinpatienten. Urologe A, 1989, 28: 134 ff.
Johannes E, Dinesh E et al.: High energy shock waves for the treatment of non-unions: an experiment on dogs. J Surg Res 57, (1994) 246 ff.
Julian F, Goldman D: The effects of mechanical stimulation on some electrical properties of axons. J General Physiol 46, 1962, 297 ff. \
Karpman R, Magee F: The lithotryptor and ist potential use in the revision of total hip arthroplasty. Orthop Rev 16, 1987, 38/81.
Kater W, Meyer WW, Wehrmann T et al.: Efficiacy, risks and limits of extracorporal shock wave lithtrypsie for salivary gland stones. Journal of endourology 8, No 1, 1994, 21 ff. \
Kenwright J, Richardson J: Effect of controlled axial micromovement on healing of tibial fractures. The Lancet: November, 22, 1986, 1185 ff.
Kim JK: Effect of shock wave treatment on femoral prothesis and cement removal. Biomed Mater Eng 4 (6), 1994, 451 ff.
Klein W, Gassen A, Laufenberg P: Endoskopische subakromiale Dekompression und Tendinitis calcarea. Arthroskopie (1992) 5: 247 - 51.
Klug W, Franke W: Tierexperimentelle szintigrafische Verlaufsbeobachtungen der sekundären Knochenbruchheilung ohne und mit Ultraschallstimulation. Z Exp Chir Transplant Künstl Organe 19, 1986 Heft 3, 185 ff.
Köster D, Schwesinger G: Operative Behandlungsergebnisse und histologische Befunde bei der Epikondylopathia humeri radialis. Orthop Praxis, 12 / 92, 849 ff.
Kroovand R, Harrison L: Extracorporal shock wave lithotrypsie in childhood. J Urol 138, october, 1987, 1106 ff.
Kuhr M, Arnold H: Langzeitergebnisse der Diszision nach G. Hohmann und ihre Wertigkeit für die Ätiopathogenese der Epikondylopathie des Ellbogens. Orthop Praxis, 12 / 92, 837 ff.
Lewis G: Effect of lithotripter treatment on the fracture toughness of acrylic bone cement. Biomaterials 1992 13 No 4 225 ff.
Liedl B, Jocham D: Prävalenz und Inzidenz der arteriellen Hypertonie bei ESWL behandelten Patienten. Urologe A, 1989, 28, 130 ff
Lingeman JE, Mcateer JE et al.: Bioeffects of extracorporal shock wave lithotrypsie. Urol Clin North Am 15, No 3, August 1988, 507 ff.
Loew M, Jurgowski W: Erste Erfahrungen mit der Extrakorporalen Stoßwellenlithotrypsie in der Behandlung der Tendinosis calcarea der Schulter. Z. Orthop, 131, (1993) 470 - 473.
Loew M, Jurgowski W, Thomsen M: Die Wirkung extracorporaler Stoßwellen auf die Tendinosis calcarea der Schulter. Urologe(A) (1995) 34: 49-53.
Mach J, Vick St: Zur Überlebenszeit von gelockerten zementierten Hüftgelenksendoprothesen. Z Orthop 131 (1993) 130 ff.
May T, Krause W: Use of high energx shock waves for bone cement removal. J Arthroplasty 5, No 1, March 1990, 19 ff.
Mendoza E, Beer M et al: ESWL during pregnancy? Abstract.
Mohr W.: Kalzifizierende Tendopathie. Tagung der DGOT 12.- 15. 10. 1994, Wiesbaden.
Morgan T, Laudone V: Free radical Production by high energy shock waves - comparison with ionizing irradiation. J Urology, 139, January, 186 ff.
Müller M: Dornier Lithotripter im Vergleich; Vermessung der Stoßwellenfelder und Fragmentationswirkung. Biomed Tech 35 (1990), 250 ff.
Neer C.: Anterior Acromioplasty for the chronic Impingement - Syndrome in the shoulder. J Bone Joint Surg 54 A, No. 1, January 1972, 41 ff.

Newman D, Coury T: Extracorporal shock wave lithotrypsie experience in children. J Urology 136, July, 238 ff.
Newman RC: ESWL Effect on canine spinal cord. Urology, Jan 1987 24, No 1, 116 ff.
Nijman R, Ackaert K: Long term results of extracorporal shock wave lithotrypsie in children. J Urology 142, August 1989, 609 ff.
Nirschl R, Pettrone F: Tennis elbow. J Bone Joint Surg 61 A, No. 6, September 1979, 832 ff.
Ohmori K, Matsuda T: Effects of shock waves on mouse fetuses. Abstract.
Okutsu I, Ninomiya S: Coracoacromial ligament release for shoulder impingement syndrome using the universal subcutaneous endoscope system. Arthroscopy 8 (1): 2-9.
Oosterhof G, Cornel, E: The influence of high energy shock waves on the development of metastases. Ultrasound Med Biol 22, No 3, pp 339-44, 1996.
Pfister J, Gerber H: Behandlung der Periarthropathia humero - scapularis calcarea mittels Schulterkalkspülung: Retrospektive Fragebogenanalyse. Z. Orthop 132 (1994) 300 ff.
Rathbun James, Macnab Ian: The mikrovascular pattern of the rotator cuff. J Bone Joint Surg 52 B No. 3, August 1970.
Rassweiler J, Kohrmann KU et al.: Experimental basis of shock wave induced renal trauma in the model of the canine kidney. World-J-Urol. 1993: 11(1):43-53
Reichelt A: Konservative versus operative Therapie der Tendinosis calcarea. Tagung der DGOT 12.-15. 10. 1994, Wiesbaden.
Richard K, Ryu R: Arthroscopic subacromial decompression: A clinical review. Arthroscopy: 8 (2): 141-47.
Richter D, Ekkernkamp A, Muhr G: Die extrakorporale Stoßwellentherapie - ein alternatives Behandlungskonzept zur Behandlung der Epikondylopathia humeri radialis? Orthopäde (1995) 24: 303-306.
Riedlinger R, Ueberle F: Die Zertrümmerung von Nierensteinen durch piezoelektrisch erzeugte Hochenergie-schallpulse. Urologe A, 1986, 25, 188 ff.
Ritzenhoff J, Knapp D: Die Langzeitergebnisse der Epikond. hum. uln. nach Behandlung analog der Hohmannschen Einkerbung bei der Epikond. hum. rad. Orthop 130 (1992) 399 ff.
Ritzenhoff J, Knapp D: Die Behandlungsergebnisse der Epikondylitis humeri ulnaris durch die Hohmannsche Einkerbung. Orthop Praxis 12/92 855 ff.
Roles N, Maudsley R: Radial Tunnel Syndrome. J Bone Joint Surg 54 B, No. 3, August 1972, 499 ff.
Rompe JD, Rumler F, Hopf C et al.: Extracorporal shock wave therapy for calcifying tendinitis of the shoulder. Clin Orthop Rel Res. 321, dec 1995 196 ff.
Rompe JD, Hopf C, Nafe B, Bürger R: Low energy extracorporal shock wave therapy for painful heel: a prospective controlled single blind study. Arch Orthop Trauma Surg (1996) 115 75-79.
Rompe JD, Hopf C, Küllmer K et al.: Low energy extracorporal shock wave therapy for persistent tennis elbow. Int ortop (SICOT) (1996) 20: 23-27.
Rompe JD, Hopf C, Küllmer K et al.: Analgesic effect of extracorporal shock wave therapy on chronic tennis elbow. J Bone Joint Surg 78 B No 2, March 1996, 233 ff.
Rompe JD, Hopf C, Küllmer K et al.: Extracorporale Stoßwellentherapie der Epikondylopathia humeri radialis - ein alternatives Behandlungskonzept. Z Orthop 134 (1996) 63 ff.
Rompe JD: Stoßwellentherapie: Therapeutische Wirkung bei spekulativem Mechanismus. Z Orthop 134, 1996 Heft 4.
Rompe JD, Hopf C, Rumler F: 2 Jahre extrakorporale Stoßwellentherapie in der Orthopädie-Indikationen und Resultate? Orthop Mitteilungen 3/1994 173 ff.
Rüdiger K, Wetterauer U et al.: Histomorphological changes of rat testicle After exposure to high energy shock wave therapy. Abstract.
Rudolph M, Hochheim B: Unsere Erfahrung mit der operativen Behandlung der Epikondylitis humeri radialis. Orthp. Praxis, 12 / 92, 844 ff.
Russo P, Stephenson A: High energy shock waves suppress tumor growth In vivo and in vitro. J Urol 135 March, 1986, 626 ff.
Sass W, Bräunlich M: The mechanism of stone desintegration by shock waves. Ultrasound Med Biol 17, No 3, 239 ff.
Schelling G, Delius M: Pain during shock wave lithrypsieis not a direct shock wave effect but results from cavitationmediated stimulation of nerve fibres. Anesthesiology 79, No 3a, Sep 1993, A824 ff.
Schelling G, Delius M, Gschwender M et al.: Extracorporal shock waves stimulate sciatic frog nerves indirectly via a cavitation mediated mechanism. Biophys J 66, Jan 1994, 133 ff.

Schelling G, Mendl G: Patient controlled analgesia for extracorporal shock wave lithotripsy of galstones. Pain, 48, 1992, 355 ff.
Schleberger R, Senge T: Non invasive treatment of long bone pseudarthrosis by shock waves. Arch Orthop Trauma Surg (1992), 111, 224-227.
Seemann O, Rassweiler J: Effect of low dose shock wave energy on fracture healing: An experimental study. J Endourol. 6, No. 3, 1992, 219 ff.
Seidl M, Steinbach P et al.: Induction of stress fibers and intercellular gaps in human vascular endothelium by shock waves. Ultrasonics 1994 32, No 5, 397 ff.
Seidl M, Steinbach P: Shock wave induced endothelial damage – in situ analysis by confocal laser scanning microscopy. Ultrasound Med Biol 20, No 6, 1994, 571 ff.
Seitz R, Seidl M, Steinbach P et al.: The effects of high energy shock waves on cell membranes and mitochondria. Ultrasonics International 93 conference proceedings, 643 ff.
Smits G, Jap P: Biological effects of high energy shock waves in mouse skeletal muscle: Correlation between ³P Magnetic resonance Spectroscopic and microscopic alterations. Ultrasound Med Biol 19, No 5, 399 ff.
Steinbach P, Hofstaedter F: Determination of energy dependent extent of vascular damage caused by high energy shock waves in an umbilical cord model. Urol Res 1993, 21, 279 ff.
Steinbach P, Hofstaedter F: In vitro investigations on cellular damage induced by high energy shock waves. Ultrasound Med Biol 18, No 8, 691 ff.
Stranne S, Callaghan J: The effect of extracorporal shock wave lithotrypsieon the prothesis interface in cementless arthroplasty. J Arthroplasty, Band 7, 1992, 173 ff.
Stranne S, Callaghan J: Would revision arthroplasty be facilitated by extracorporal shock wave lithotripsy? An evaluation including whole bone strength in dogs. Clin Orthop Related Res 287 1993 Feb, 252 ff.
Strauss JM, Rüther W: Tendinosis calcarea – Differentialdiagnose und operative Therapie. 80. Tagung der DGOT 12.-15. 10. 1994, Wiesbaden.
Sucul Kaulesa,; Johannes EJ: Extracorporal shock waves for treatment of Non unions. Hefte zu Der Unfallchirurg Heft 232, 392 ff.
Suhr D, Brümmer F: Cavitation generated free radicals during shock wave exposure: Investigations with cell free solutions and suspended cells. Ultrasound Med Biol 17, No 8, 761 ff.
Sukul K, Johannes E: The Effect of high energy shock waves focussed on cortical bone: An in vitro study. J Surg Res 54, (1993), 46 ff.
Thurner J: Deformierende Insertionstendopathie. In: Doerr: Spezielle pathologische Anatomie, Bd 18 /1, 600 ff.
Vachalnov V, Michailov et al.: Extrakorporal exposure with shock waveson bone tissue as a Factor for local osteogenesis. Abstract.
Vachalnov V, Michailov P: High energy shock waves in treatment of delayed and nonunion of fractures. Int Orthop (SICOT) 1991, 15: 181 – 184.
Vahlensieck W, Kürz H: Side effects of extracorporal piezoelectric shock wave lithotrypsie. Urol Res, 1990, 18: 53 ff.
Vakil M, Everbach E: Transient acoustic cavitation in gallstone fragmentation: A study of galstones fragmented In vivo. Ultrasound Med Biol, 19, No 4, 331 ff.
Van Arsdalen K, Kurzweil S: Effect of Lithotripsy on immature rabbit bone and kidney development. J Urol 146, July 1991, 213 ff.
Van Holsbeek E, DeRycke J: Subacromial Impingement: Open versus arthroscopic decompression. Arthroscopy: 8 (2): 173 – 78.
Van Rossum J, Buruma O: Tennis elbow – A radial tunnel syndrome. J Bone Joint Surg 60 B, No. 2, May 1978, 197 ff.
Von Hasselbach C: ESW Therapie am Bewegungsapparat. Pro Med News 1/96.
Wanivenhaus A: Differentialdiagnose der Epikondylitis humeri radialis. Z. Orthop, 124 (1986) 775 – 79.
Wehner H, Sellier K: Shockwave induced compound action potentials in the peripheral nerve. Z Rechtsmed, 1981, 86, 239 ff.
Weinstein J, Oster D et al.: The effect of the extracorporal schock wave lithotripter on the bone-cement interface in dogs. Clin Orthop Related Res (Philadelphia) 1988, No 235, oct. 1988 261 ff
Weirauch C, Skorpik G: Epikondylopathia humeri radialis – Eine Vergleichsstudie der einfachen Operation nach Hohmann mit der erweiterten Operation nach Hohmann.. Orthop Praxis, 12 / 92, 846 ff.
Weiss N, Delius M: Effect of shock waves and cisplatin on cisplatin sensitive and -resistant rodent tumors In vivo. Int J Cancer; 58, 693-99, 1994.

Weiss N, Delius M: Influence of the shock wave application mode on the growth of A-mel 3 and SSK2 tumors In vivo. Ultrasound Med Biol., 16, No 6, 595-605, 1990.
Werhan C: Biophysikalische Grundlagen der Anwendung elektromagnetischer Felder zur Beeinflussung der Osteogenese. Z Orthop, 129, 1991, 118 ff.
Williams C, Kaude J: Extracorporal shock wave lithotrypsie: Long term complications. Am J Radiol 150, Feb 1988, 311 ff.
Wolf T, Breitenfelder J: Erste Erfahrungen mit der ESWT bei Schmerzzuständen des Bewegungsapparates mit umschriebener Lokalisation. Orthop Praxis 32, 7 (1996) 480–83.
Yang C, Heston W et al.: The effect of high energy shock waves on human bone marrow. Urol Res (1988) 16: 427–429.
Yeaman LD: Effects of shock waves on the structure and growth of the immature rat epiphysis. J Urology 141, March 1989, 670 ff.
Zakharov S, Bogdanov K: The effect of acoustic cavitation on the contraction force and membrane potential of rat papillary muscle. Ultrasound Med Biol 15, No 6, 561 ff.
Zeman R, Davros W: Cavitation effects during lithotrypsie, Part 1 and 2. Radiology, october 1990, 157 ff.
Ziegler M, Kopper B: Die Zertrümmerung von Nierensteinen mit einem piezoelektrischen Gerätesystem. Urologe A, 1986, 25: 193 ff.

CHAPTER 2

Shock Wave Technology

F. Ueberle

2.1 Introduction

In 1980, the first patient with renal calculi was successfully treated with minimally invasive extracorporeal shock wave lithotripsy (ESWL). Since then the medical field of application of this form of energy has been extended. The most recent result of the medical and technical development of applications is extracorporeal shock wave application (ESWA, sometimes also ESWT) for the treatment of soft-tissue pain.

The sonic sources and systems employed in ESWL and ESWA are very similar, which is no wonder, as the first ESWA trials were undertaken with conventional kidney and gallbladder lithotriptors. One field of ESWA, i.e. the dissolution of calcific deposits, mainly tendinosis calcarea, also belongs to the domain of lithotripsy which is the crushing of concrements in the body.

Owing to this close relationship of the ESW disciplines, the terminology and knowledge stemming from ESWL can to a large extent be employed in the following technical description.

2.2 Acoustics – Sonic Waves – Shock Waves

We first need to rid ourselves of an inaccuracy in the definition of the term shock waves: not all shock waves in the medical sense are really shock waves in the physical sense. As will be shown later, shock waves are not generated at all settings of all ESWA sonic sources.

2.2.1 Definition

A shock wave is scientifically defined as an acoustic or sonic wave, at the wave front of which the pressure above atmospheric rises from ambient pressure to maximum pressure (amplitude) within a few nanoseconds (10^{-9} s). Current therapeutically used pressure amplitudes range between 10 MPa and more than 100 MPa (MegaPascal, 1 MPa = 10 bar, approximately the tenfold atmospheric pressure). As a shock wave propagates at a specific speed – as do all sonic waves – determined by the medium in which it propagates and the intensity of the shock wave itself one can calculate the shock front thickness. This is the spatial dimension between the location where ambient pressure (still) prevails and the location where the pressure amplitude has been reached. In tissue, for example, the shock front thickness is in the range of 1.5–6 μm (micrometers, 10^{-6} m)[1]. During transition of, for example, a cell wall, which has a thickness of a few molecular layers, significant forces can already come to bear on the wall, as there are immediate differences in pressure in front and behind it. The pressure gradient, i.e. the change in pressure between two locations, reaches its maximum at a given wave amplitude in the shock front as compared with other forms of sonic signals, e.g. sinusoidal ultrasound.

2.2.2 Waveforms

The simplest sonic waveform is a sinusoidal sequence of phases of positive and negative pressure (Fig. 1). As opposed to a shock wave, one can relate a definite sonic frequency to it. If the frequency is higher than about 16000 oscillations per second, this is termed ultrasound.

If only a short phase of one or a few signal periods is employed – as with diagnostic ultrasound devices – this can be termed a sonic pulse (Fig. 2).

A shock wave in the focus of an ESWA device consists typically of a single pulse of positive pressure (Fig. 3) followed within 1–5 µs after an exponential drop to ambient pressure by a phase of negative pressure of a few microseconds. After this, ambient pressure prevails again until the next wave commences after about $\frac{1}{4}$ s to 1 s.

2.3 Sonic Waves are Mechanical Waves in Media

A sonic wave is a mechanical wave which can expand in a medium, e.g. gas, liquids or solids. On wave expansion the distances between molecules change locally a little in the medium. Particularly in liquids and gases, waves propagate as longitudinal waves (Fig. 4).

In solids, other waveforms are also capable of propagation, such as transversal waves, extensional waves, surface waves, etc. These waveforms play a lesser role in ESWA and will not be discussed here.

2.4 Acoustic Properties of Media

Media are distinguished by their different mechanical properties such as elasticity and compressibility. These parameters affect sonic waves by determining the propagation speed c, as well as the acoustic impedance, $Z=\rho c$, the product of density ρ and speed of sound c. Table 1 shows some values of biological materials.

[1] Given a rise time t of 1–4 ns and a speed of sound of 1500 m/s.

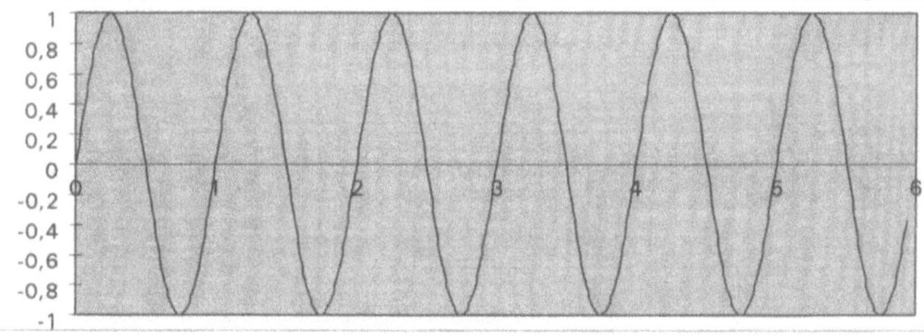

Fig. 1

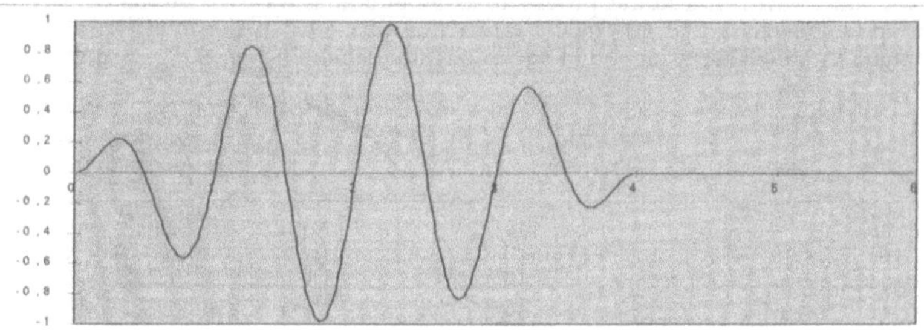

Fig. 2

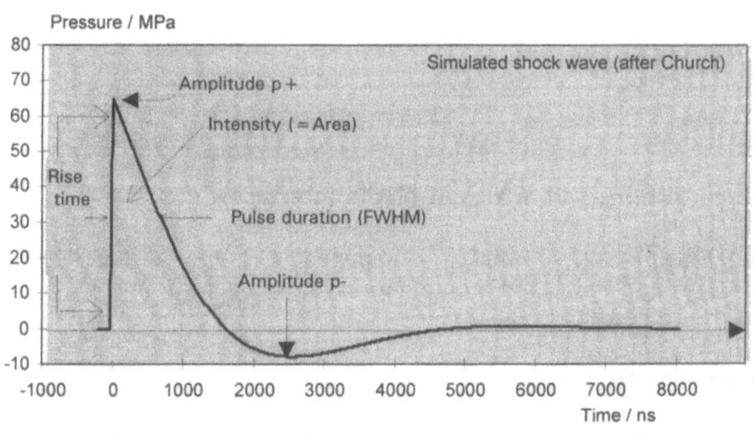

Fig. 3

Fig. 1. Sinusoidal sound wave

Fig. 2. Sound burst having a few periods of a sinusoidal wave

Fig. 3. A typical underwater shock wave is characterized by a positive pressure step having an extremely short rise time tr, followed by an exponential decay to ambient pressure. It's duration is typically some hundred nanoseconds. The following rarefaction phase has significantly less amplitude and may a duration of some microseconds

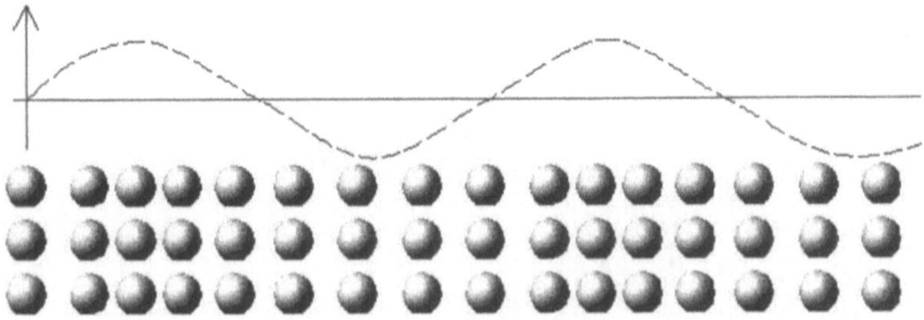

Fig. 4. Sound waves in a liquid propagate as longitudinal waves. Material density is higher in the pressure phase and less in the rarefaction phase when the wave is propagating. Accordingly, the local speed of sound varies slightly depending on the pressure of the sound wave

Table 1.

Material	Density (kg/m^3)	Sound speed (m/s)	Impedance (Ns/m^3)
Air	1.293	331	429
Water	998	1483	1.48 10^6
Fat tissue	920	1410–1479	1.33 10^6
Muscle tissue	1060	1540–1603	1.67 10^6
Bone	1380–1810	2700–4100	4.3–6.6 10^6
Kidney stone	1360–2160	1995–4659	3.2 10^6
Gallbladder stone	1100–1500	1700–2100	1.9–3.1 10^6
Model stone (gypsum)	1100	2400	2.6 10^6

2.5 Mechanical Effects of Waves at Media Interfaces

With the help of the specific acoustic impedances, one can describe the interaction of sound waves and a boundary layer between two media.

2.5.1 Reflection and Transmission

If the impedances of the media are different, e.g. at the transition from fat to muscle tissue, a part of the sound energy is reflected to Medium 1.[2] The remainder of the sound energy is transmitted to Medium 2 (Fig. 5). The examples in Table 2 show that, depending on the medium, the transmitted sound portion may already be considerably weakened.

Another, very important property of the reflected sound wave can also be derived from the reflection equation: if the impedance of Medium 2 is lower than that of Medium 1, the reflected pressure receives a negative sign. This means that the overpressure shock after reflection is reflected as an under-

[2] The specific sound amplitude reflected, p_r,is calculated according to $p_r = p_0 (Z_2 - Z_1)/(Z_2 + Z_1)$, where Z_1 and Z_2 are the impedances of Medium 1 and Medium 2, respectively. The reflected energy is calculated from the square of the amplitude.

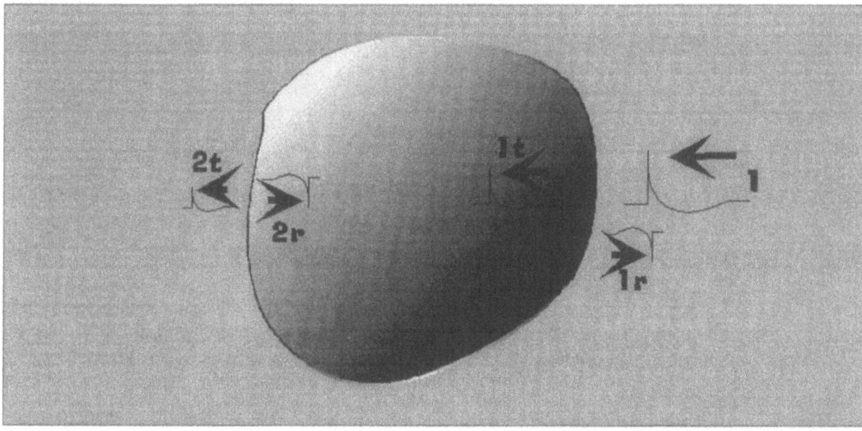

Fig. 5. At the boundary between two media the impinging sound wave is partially reflected. The portion of reflected energy is depending on the acoustic impedance mismatch between the media. If the impedance of the first medium is higher than the impedance of the second medium, the polarity of the sound wave is reversed: Positive pressure is reflected as rarefaction pressure and vice versa. This may result in high forces exerted on the surface

Table 2.

Interface	Reflected pressure	Reflected sound energy	Transmitted sound energy
Water - Fat	-5%	0.25%	99.75%
Fat - Muscle	11%	1.2%	98.8%
Muscle - Fat	-11%	1.2%	98.8%
Muscle - Bone	44–60%	19–36%	81–64%
Muscle - Model stone	22%	5%	95%
Model stone - Muscle	-22%	5%	95%
Muscle - Air	-99.9%	99.9%	0.1%

pressure shock into Medium 1. In the case of planar interfaces and complete reflection, the reflected amplitude can reach the same but negative level of the original sound pressure. The pressure gradient at the interface in this case reaches twice the height of the wave propagating in the homogeneous medium. No energy is transmitted to Medium 2. This especially occurs at interfaces between tissue and air, e.g. at the interface of lung tissue. Because nearly all the energy is reflected at this interface, from a certain wave amplitude the delicate tissue is unable to resist the forces and tears. If therefore the focus environment of a ESWA device is directed at lung tissue, severe damage can be expected. Similar results apply to gas-filled hollow bodies such as intestinal gas bubbles.

The effect of pressure reversal also comes to bear at another interface which is important in ESWA: when the sound wave transmitted into a calcific deposit leaves the latter dorsally. Here also, a portion is reflected into the calculus – this time with a negative sign, as the muscle tissue at the back of the concrement has a lower impedance than that of the calculus. This reflected wave is superim-

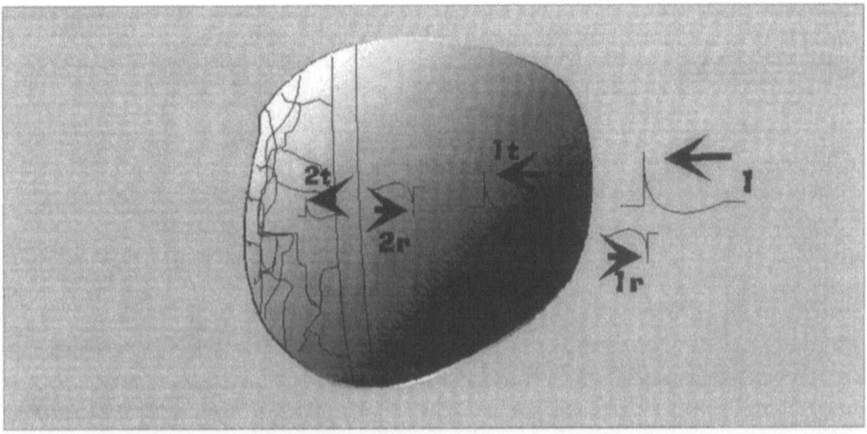

Fig. 6. If concretions are impacted in the surrounding tissue, the so-called Hopkins-effect leads to a destruction beginning at the rear side of the concretion, because the tensile strength of the material is exceeded [2]

posed with the "later" overpressure portion of the incident wave such that especially strong tensile forces act on the rear of the concrement. This so-called Hopkins effect was observed in in vitro experiments with model stones in a lamb shoulder (Fig. 6).

2.5.2 Refraction

From optics, we know that a wave entering a medium at an angle will, depending on the different propagation speeds, continue in the second medium at a different angle.[3] Analogously, this refraction effect is used for focusing sound with acoustic lenses.

2.5.3 Diffraction

Sound is – just as in optics – diffracted at an edge. A certain portion of the sound thus does not propagate linearly, but is directed around the edge.

The so-called edge diffraction wave occurs at the edge of the aperture of all sound transducers, at contours of inline scanners, etc. This wave portion which is unavoidable in transducers of finite dimension manifests itself especially on the transducer axis and in the focal region as underpressure, which follows the primarily transmitted overpressure shock.

---

[3] According to Snell's laws of refraction, the angle sines are proportional to the sound speeds: $\sin \alpha_2 / \sin \alpha_1 = c_2/c_1$. Total reflection occurs if the angle of reflection $\alpha 2$ is greater than 90°.

2.6
Mechanical Effects of Waves due to Nonlinear Phenomena

Our elucidation of the acoustic properties has up to now been based on homogeneous media whose characteristics do not change, even at large acoustic amplitudes; i.e. they are behaving linear. In the following, nonlinear effects will be discussed.

2.6.1
Steepening

High local overpressures create a strong local compression in the media, and consequently a local increase in density. At the same time, the speed of sound is also locally increased due to the elastic properties of the media, thereby enabling later portions of the sound to catch up with the front during propagation time, so that an ideally steep shock front eventually develops (Fig. 7). The location of this complete steepening depends on the pressure of the acoustic wave, the focusing, and the properties of the media.

In media with low attenuation, such as water, the steepening is reached at quite small energy settings of the ESWA devices. In tissue, however, the rapid changes in pressure, which can be described as high frequencies in the

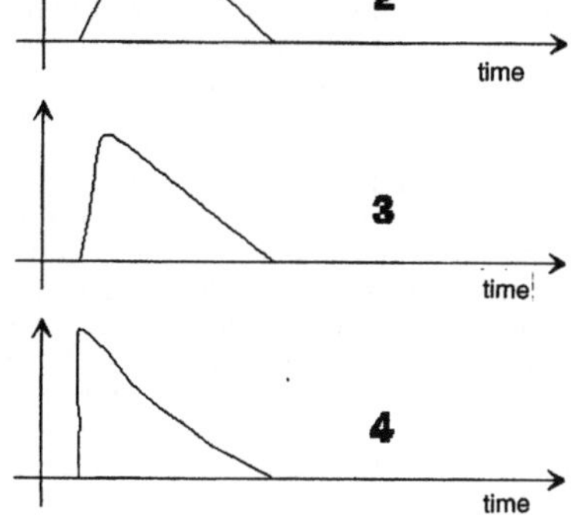

Fig. 7. Nonlinear steepening changes a propagating sinusoidal pressure wave to a shock wave on it's way from the source to the focus. The time until the wave is fully steepened depends on the pressure and the focusing parameters as well as on parameters of the propagating fluid

sound signal, are considerably attenuated.[4] Therefore, it may be assumed that, for steepening to occur in tissue, longer travel distances or higher pressures are necessary.

2.6.2
Cavitation

By cavitation we understand the occurrence of gas-filled hollow bodies in a liquid medium. Stable cavitation bubbles are in equilibrium when the vapor pressure inside the bubble is equal to the external pressure of the liquid.

When a shock wave hits a cavitation bubble, the increased external pressure causes the bubble to shrink, whereby the latter absorbs part of the sonic energy. If the excitant forces and energies are large enough, the bubble collapses, thereby releasing part of the energy stored in the bubble to the medium as a new acoustic wave.[5]

Due to the one-sided impact of the shock wave, especially near interfaces, the bubble collapses asymmetrically and sends a water jet in the direction of the surface (Fig. 8). The water jet can reach speeds of 100 to more than 800 m/s, which are sufficient to perforate aluminum membranes and plastics [3].

Due to the local effects during the collapse of a bubble, needle-shaped haemorrhages (petechiae) can be caused in tissue. On the cell level, the pitting of cell walls is attributed to cavitation [5].

For quite some years now the question whether free radicals are created by the collapse of a bubble has been investigated. They have to date only been detected in vitro in the extracellular space. There is still much controversial discussion about induction of free radicals into the cell in vivo [6].

Due to the underpressure content of the sound wave, a further cavitation effect is created: microbubbles, such as the remains of the collapsed bubble, grow during underpressure. They may reach a stable size which can be three orders of magnitude larger than the nucleus and exist for several hundred microseconds.

---

[4] According to Fourier's laws, any signal can be reduced to a series of sinusoidal components (spectral lines). It is known that in tissue sound attenuation is frequency-dependent. On average, the attenuation is 0.5–0.7 dB per cm and per Mhz sound frequency, which corresponds to a diminution by half after 8–12 cm of travel at 1 MHz. Thus, an acoustic wave loses more and more energy the farther it enters into the tissue. The energy is lost mainly in the high frequencies which result from the steepness of the shock front. Thus, a (plane) shock wave evolves into a sinusoidal impulse which finally contains only the component of the lowest frequency, i.e. the fundamental, as this is the least attenuated. The attenuation effect in focused systems counteracts the total steepening before the focus and delays it, while it causes a quicker decrease in the wave amplitude behind the focus. How strong these effects are in normal ESWAs and geometries is as yet not entirely known. However, it can be presumed that these effects are of minor importance as compared to the effects of the nonlinearity of the tissue.

[5] If the radii of the bubbles are about 500 μm (in water), in the case of collapse caused by a typical shock wave excited by a lithotriptor, most of the energy is released [3]. The bubbles collapse about 2–3 μs after being hit by the shock wave. The resulting collapse pressure is about 1/10 of the shock wave pressure and exists for typically 30 ns. Thus the sonic energy of the collapsing bubble is less by a factor of 1000 than that of the excitant shock wave. Larger bubbles do not collapse in quite such a 'hard' fashion, because they are slowed down by the rarefaction phase of the shock wave.

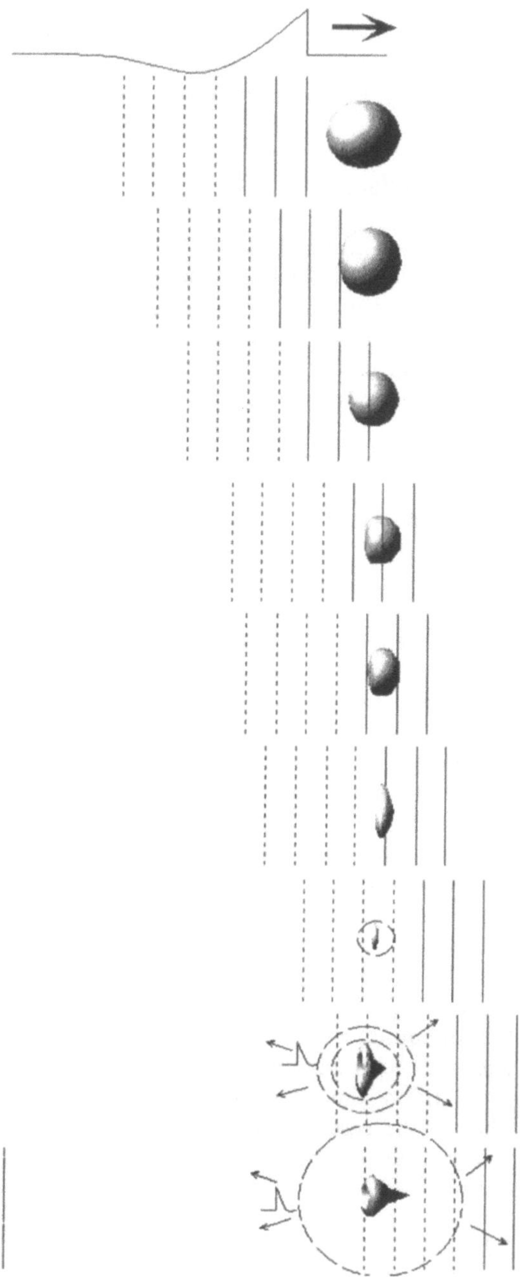

Fig. 8. A cavitation bubble hit by a shock wave may collapse, sending out a secondary shock wave and a water jet of high velocity (several hundred meters per second) preferably towards a nearby surface (plots after [3])

In the case of such stable bubbles, an oscillation phase follows until the final reduction in size. The total lifetime of the bubbles depends strongly on the ambient medium; they are at times still detectable after more than a second [7]. If these bubbles are hit by a following shock wave, this in turn leads to a collapse with the above-mentioned effects.

Thus cavitation limits the maximum pulse recurrence frequency because of the interaction with following shock waves [4].

2.7 Thermal Effects

The pulse durations of an ESWA wave are very short, usually 3–5 μs, whereby a peak sound power of more than a megawatt is reached. If one, however, calculates from this the sound energy resulting from a puls sequence of 1 to a maximum of 4 per second, the result is considerably less than one joule. This energy is not sufficient to cause a significant warming in the focus or even at a distance from it. Therefore, thermal effects can be ruled out in ESWA.

2.8 The Sound Field

In the description of the sound field, mostly those parameters encountered in practice are discussed. The biological significance of these parameters, documented by relevant metrological standards, is as yet largely unknown [18]. An important approach is the determination of energy values and energy flux density values which can be related to biological effects.

From ESWL we know that the most important variable pertaining to the crushing of stones is the acoustic energy acting on the concrement [15].

The necessary sound measurements are, in accordance with standards and because there is no adequate phantom tissue, carried out in degassed water. As water, compared to tissue, displays less attenuation and different nonlinearity parameters, the measured values are only translatable to a certain extent with regard to the individual patient. In the case of longer distances in tissue, the sound signals can be influenced by the tissue layering, the attenuation and the nonlinearity. One can generally assume a pronounced attenuation of the amplitudes, as well as a decrease in the high-frequency content of sound, which can consequently lead to longer rise times of the waves and, for each individual case, to changes in the focus geometry [8].

Common shock generators normally use water in the coupling region. Thus in the case of near-surface applications, e.g. at the elbow, the situation in the focus will be quite comparable to the metrological approaches carried out in water.

2.8.1 Signal Variations in Time

The time signal of a typical shock wave in the focus was displayed in Fig. 3.

2.8.2
Parameters: Sound Pressure, Intensity, Energy Flux Density, Pulse Duration, Rise Time

From the time signal, one extracts the amplitudes of the overpressure and underpressure phases. The rise time is measured as the time passing between 10 and 90% of the amplitude of the overpressure signal. The pulse width is defined as the signal duration between the times when 50% of the overpressure amplitude is reached. In the case of complicated signals, this may be quite misleading.

The sound intensity is a measure of the mean power transmitted by the sound pulse.[6] It is also called energy flux density per pulse, measured in Joule/m^2. Manufacturer information concerning energy flux density usually pertains to the maximum value measured in the focus.

2.8.3
Signal Position Behaviour

Only a few millimeters from the focus the pulse behaviour is drastically different. The cause is a lengthening of the signal because the pressure contents originating from different positions of the focusing system (e.g. the lense or focusing mirror) no longer reach the specific location simultaneously. Lateral to the focus the rise time of the signal increases rapidly.

The time course of the signal in front of and behind the focus depends very much on the kind of source: in the case of spark gap sources, there is always a shock front in front of the focus, whereas in the case of the less 'steep' electroacoustic shock wave emitter (EMSE) and piezoelectric sources a shock front develops only a few millimeters in front of the focus by steepening.

2.8.4
Axial and Lateral Sound Pressure Distribution, full-width half-maximum of Sound Pressure

Customarily, typical axial and lateral distributions of the overpressure in the area around the focus are represented graphically (Fig. 9). Focus dimension values which define the volume of the focus are taken from the graph. The values are so-called full-width half-maximum (FWHM) values. They characterize the distances between the locations at which half-maximum values of the curve are found.

The axial and lateral dimensions are used to calculate the volume of the focus, simplified under the assumption of an elliptical focus 'cigar' whose long axis lies in the direction of the shock wave propagation.

The medical implications of these values are, however, not yet clear. All these values are based according to norm on relative values of the positive

[6] Mathematically, the energy flux density or intensity $I = 1/Z \int p^2(t)\,dt$, integrated over the signal duration with the impedance of the medium Z. The unit is Ws/m^2 or J/m^2.

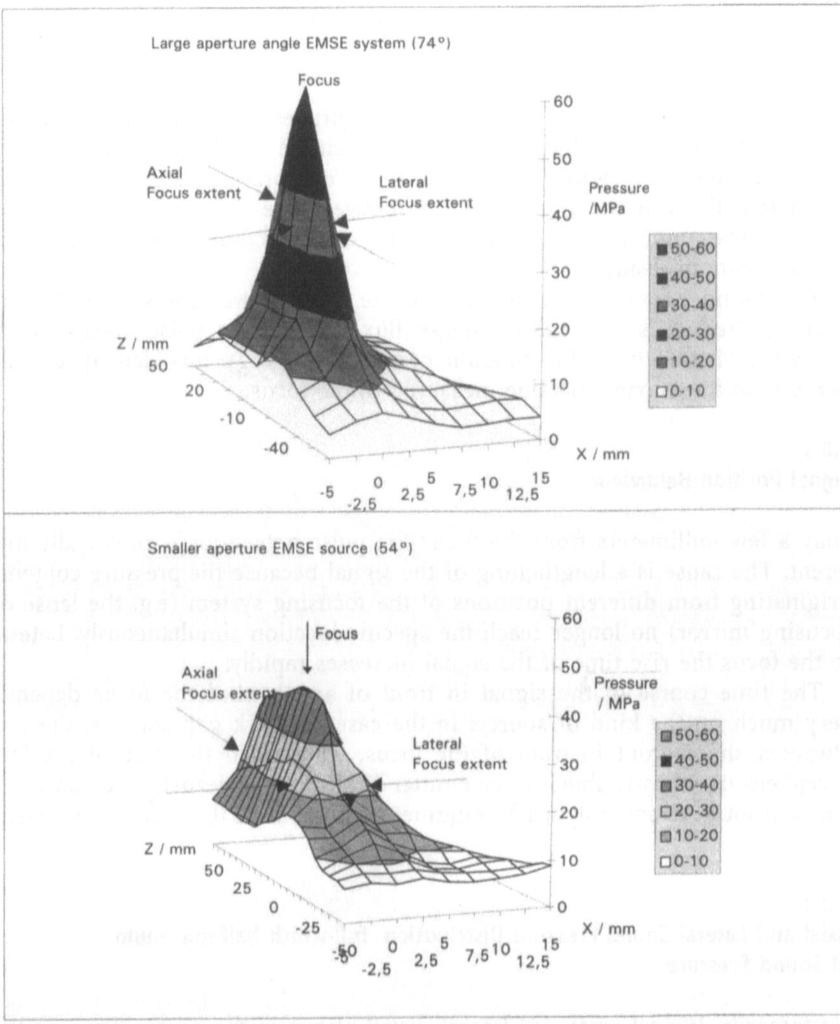

Fig. 9. The pressure distribution is characterized by axial and lateral measurements around the focus. Axial and lateral focus extent are derived from the plots at the points where the pressure amplitude has dropped to half of the maximum value at the focus

sound pressure with respect to the focal peak pressure, and therefore require suitable sensors. The peak pressure in the focus and thus the base of the FWHM values is strongly dependent on the aperture angle of the focusing system – the larger the aperture angle, the higher the focus pressure. The correlation between sound pressure and crushing effects is, however, low, as the acoustic energy is responsible for the effect on the concrements [16]. As concerns biological effects, one also does not refer to the pressure, but to the energy flux density [11], as shall be explained in the sections 2.11 and 2.15.

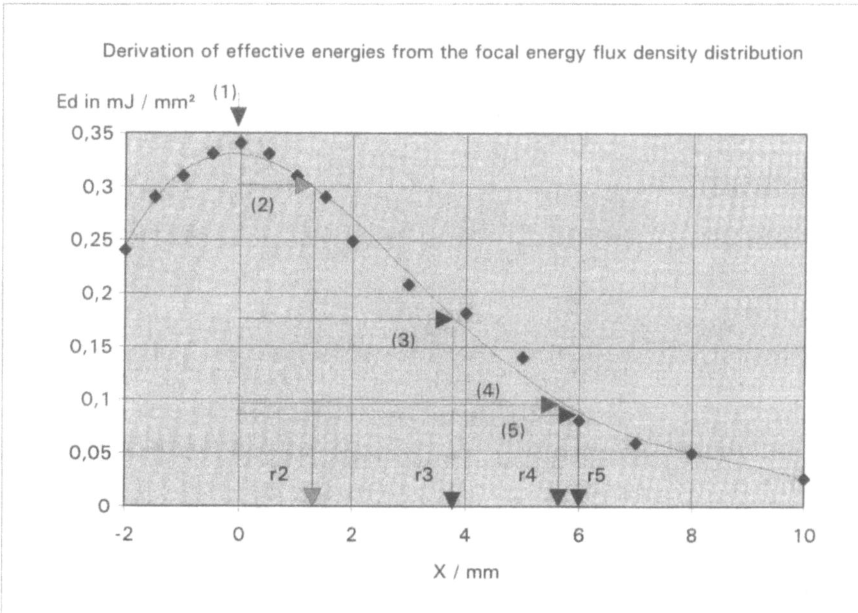

Fig. 10. Sound energies are calculated from the measured energy flux density distribution in the focal plane. Depending on the chosen area of integration several energies can be calculated. Areas of biological significance and the energy flux inside these areas may possibly derived from experiments with human umbilical cords [11]. In these experiments a stress fiber induction in cells was seen when the energy flux density exceeded 0,1 mJ/mm^2. Distraction of endothelial cells was seen for >0,3 mJ/mm^2. More threshold values for the destruction of concretions can be found.
1. Energy flux density in the focus
2. Radius r2 of the area containing energy flux densities >0,3 mJ/mm^2
3. Radius r3 of the area inside the focal lateral extent FWHM (of the pressure distribution) yields the "focal energy"
4. Radius r4 of the area containing energy flux densities >0,1 mJ/mm^2
5. Radius r5 of the area of a typical kidney stone yields an effective energy which can be used to compare several sound sources, if the radius is the same.

The area containing the whole measurable focal energy flux density distribution yields the total acoustic energy

2.8.5
Energies in the Sound Field

The spatial distribution of the energy flux density decreases at least as quickly as the distribution of the focus pressure. By means of area-weighted integration[7] of the energy flux density values in the focus plane one can calculate the energy flowing through a certain area in the focus. Mostly, the focus energy which acts within the FWHM is given (Fig. 10).

Effective energy values are characterised by the assumption of a certain effect area, e.g. a circle with a radius of 6 mm (a typical size for a stone in

[7] The energy flow through a circle symmetric area with a radius r is $E = 2\pi \iint I\,(r)\; r\; dr$; the unit is Joule.

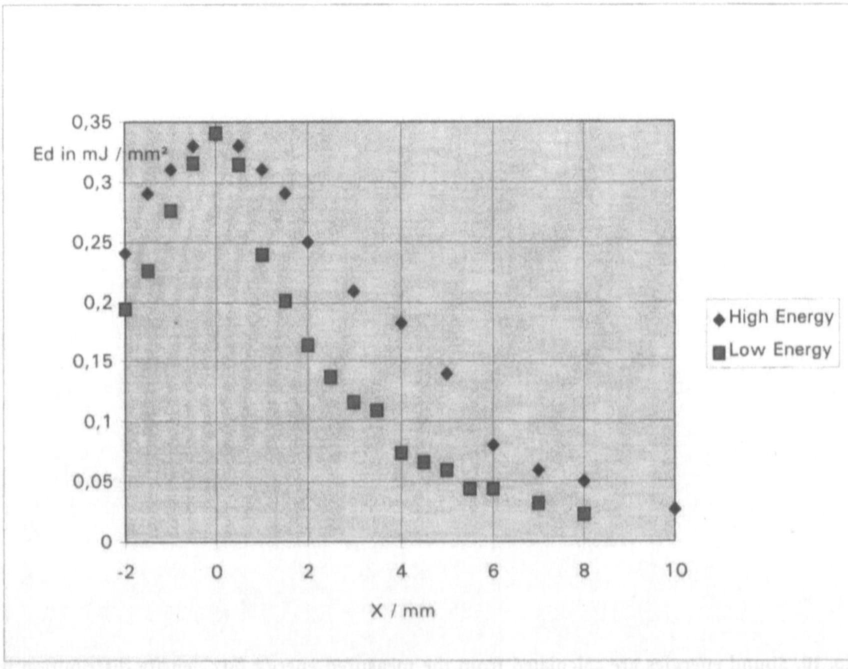

Fig. 11. Comparison of two sound sources adjusted to the same focal energy flux density level. The high energy system has a smaller aperture angle, thus the focal distribution is wider. This leads to significantly higher energy values

ESWL). A comparison of different shock sources is only possible by comparing the effective energies, using the energy values of identical areas.

Sometimes the total energy in the focus is given. This focal total energy is, in the case of areal sound sources, no larger than the primary acoustic energy released by the source if possible losses due to lens parameters are not taken into account. In the case of reflector systems, the focal total energy is lower than the primary acoustic energy; it depends on the percentage of the wave captured by the reflector (in the case of a spark gap source, on the encompassed solid angle).

In the case of other sound sources, losses in the lenses and coupling medium can lessen the focal total energy.

As a general rule: the greater the aperture angle of the system, the higher the focal pressure and the attainable focus energy flux density at a given sound wave excitation. In contrast, the lateral focus dimensions decrease with increasing aperture angle. A sound source with little energy but wide aperture angle can consequently still have a high energy flux density in the focus. The biologically effective areas (see Fig. 11) are, in the case of such a source, considerably smaller than in a system with higher energy but smaller aperture angle.

Effects on biological materials and concrements only occur when certain energy threshold values are exceeded (see section 2.15) [16].

2.9 Primary Acoustic Energy and Electric Energy

As described above, the primary acoustic energy, depending on the sound source, is transferred proportionally to the total energy in the focus.

The electric energy necessary to drive the sound source can be calculated from the charging voltage and the capacity of the storage capacitor. Only a fraction thereof is converted to acoustic energy[8] and it is unsuitable for comparison of different types of sources due to the different electroacoustic efficiency. For the clinical results of a ESWL or ESWA machine the electro-acoustic efficiency has no significance.

2.10 Low- and High-Energy Systems for ESWA

In the literature, there is a differentiation between low- and high-energy strategies in ESWA. The difference is, on the one hand, that in low-energy ESWA local anaesthesia is not administered, so that the maximum stress is defined by the pain the patient experiences. On the other hand, in low-energy treatment, more sessions (typically 3 to 5, but sometimes ten and more) are required.

An objective distinction is possible on the basis of the acoustic effective energy. From the literature we know that low-energy treatment is administered with effective focus energies (6 mm radius of the measuring surface) of up to about 12 mJ. High-energy treatment employs effective energies which are suitable for crushing kidney stones, i.e. from 12 to >50mJ relative to circular effect areas of 6 mm radius.

A differentiation between the two strategies based on the focal energy flux density is however not possible when comparing more strongly focused systems with wide aperture angles and weaker focused systems (typical of kidney lithotripters), as systems with low effective energy can have a quite high focal energy flux density when highly focused. Figure 11 illustrates this context. Although both systems have the same focal energy flux density, the distribution curve of the high-energy system, and therefore its effect area, is considerably wider. Its total energy is thus much higher than the total energy of the low-energy system, when the focal energy flux density is the same in both systems. If both systems are adjusted to have the same total energy, the focal energy flux density of the stronger focused system is significantly higher.

2.11 Dosage

It is not possible on the basis of current knowledge to exactly define how to calculate a sound dosis resulting in a specific effect. In this section, sugges-

---

[8] Given a capacity C and a charging voltage U, $E_{el} = C/2\ U^2$. The electro-acoustic efficiencies of EMSE, piezoelectric shock wave emitter (PESE) and spark gap sources are different, e.g. approx. 1–3% for spark gap as opposed to <0.3% for other sound sources.

tions will, however, be made as to what should be recorded in treatment. In contrast to current practice, in which only the total number of shocks applied and charge levels etc. are listed, this has the advantage of being device-independent and taking into consideration approaches concerning biologically relevant energy parameters. The total effective energy proposed here, as opposed to the summation of the focal energy flux density, allows taking into account the effect area of the appliance. The effect area is considerably larger for high-energy than for low-energy devices (cf. Fig. 11).

In [11], the two energy flux density values 0.1 mJ/mm^2 and 0.3 mJ/mm^2 are cited as the lower thresholds for certain cell effects (see legend of Fig. 10). Looking at the area of the focal energy flux density distribution up to the specific lower threshold value, e.g. 0.1 mJ/mm^2 (with the radius r4 in Fig. 10), one can determine the effective energy at which an energy flux density of at least 0.1 mJ/mm^2 is prevalent. Under the hypothetical assumption that it is highly probable that all cells within this area will show some reaction (in this case, formation of stress fibres), the following equation gives the applied effective total dose E_{01tot}[9]:

$$E_{01tot} = E_1 \cdot S_{z1} + E_2 \cdot S_{z2} + \ldots,$$

where E_1 = effective acoustic energy for energy flux densities >0.1 mJ/mm^2 at device setting (step) 1,
S_{z1} = applied number of shocks at device setting 1,
E_2 = effective acoustic energy for energy flux densities >0.1 mJ/mm^2 at device setting (step) 2,
S_{z2} = applied number of shocks at device setting 2, and so on.

The effective energies causing the postulated effect at each device setting are summed. These energies are determined by the device manufacturers in standardized measuring procedures. From today's point of view, it is of advantage to state the values E_{01tot} for 0.1 mJ/mm^2 and E_{03tot} for 0.3 mJ/mm2 per session. If these values are not available, the calculation of energy dose using predefined effective energies (e.g. calculated for 6 mm area radius) may give an appropriate dose approximation.

[9] The following table shows example data for a hypothetical treatment:

Device setting (step)	Effective energy for threshold E_1 (0.1 mJ/mm)	Number of shocks S_{z1}	Total energy per step $E_1 \cdot S_{z1}$
1	0.1 mJ	50	5.0 mJ
2	0.3 mJ	250	75 mJ
3	0.5 mJ	150	75 mJ
4	1.5 mJ	500	750 mJ
5	4 mJ	600	2400 mJ
6	8 mJ	300	2400 mJ
	Total:	2000 shocks	5780 mJ = 5.78 J

2.12 Spatial Distribution of the Underpressure

To date the exact determination of the underpressure near the focus has been unsatisfactory. At underpressures of only a few MPa, liquids begin to tear up [3] or detach themselves from the surface of a hydrophone and cavitation occurs. Furthermore, some hydrophones react with less sensitivity to underpressure signals, or the latter are forged due to reflections at the hydrophone. The glass fibre hydrophone, which has only recently become available, allows a new approach, which will certainly lead to dependable data in the future.

The signal originating from a spark gap or EMSE source contains no measurable underpressure fractions directly at the source.[10] The underpressure observed in the focus area and along the shock wave axis stems from the edge diffraction wave of the source. This edge diffraction wave is the mirror image of the overpressure signal that radiates from the edge of the focusing system.

As the underpressure signal does not steepen, its amplitude in the focus is usually less (approx. 1/10 of the overpressure signal) than that of the steepened overpressure signal. Its measurable duration is about 2–5 μs.

Whereas overpressure signals experience a positive displacement of the focus due to nonlinear steepening (as mentioned above), one can observe a displacement towards the source in the case of nonsteepened signals. Therefore, the maximum of the underpressure may be a few millimetres in front of the overpressure focus.

Only the piezoelectric source produces a defined primary underpressure signal in addition to the edge diffraction wave. Both underpressure waves coincide in the focus.

Due to the underpressure signal, bubble nuclei are enlarged to bubbles of several hundred micrometers radius. If the underpressure has a sufficient amplitude, new cavitation bubbles are generated due to separation of the liquid. Exact threshold values are however not defined. Depending on the purity and gas content, the threshold lies between -0.5 and –20 MPa for water. For tissue, it is estimated to be between –12 and –16 MPa [9]. The pulse duration of the underpressure signal also plays an important role: the shorter it is, the higher strain amplitudes the tissue can endure.

Evidenced by high-speed photos, it is known that in water cavitation bubbles can be observed on the sound axis way before the focus [10]. If they occur and the intensity at which they occur in tissue is, however, largely unknown.

[10] Although the medium displaced by the overpressure signal must finally flow back, this proceeds so slowly in the case of both the spark-generated gas bubble and the retraction of the EMSE membrane that the occuring underpressures are normally not measurable.

2.13 Generating Therapeutical Shock Waves

In practice, all ESW generators consist of an electrical energy source, an electroacoustic conversion mechanism and a device for focusing the sound waves. To achieve a specific effect, the sound waves must be focused. When employing point sources (e.g. sparks) or cylinder sources, a focusing mirror is used. When employing areal sources, lenses or a self-focusing appliance of partially spherical shape is used.

At the end of each section, the source-specific differences in the generation of the sound waves and their effects on the sound front will be elucidated. It should, however, be noted that no statements can as yet be made regarding the medical and biological relevance of the respective parameters.

2.13.1 Punctiform and Areal Generators

Depending on how the sound is generated, one differentiates between punctiform and areal sources. Punctiform sound sources generate spherically expanding sound waves. Depending on the design, areal sound sources generate plane, cylindrically expanding or spherically converging sound waves.

Each of these forms of expansion of primary sound waves requires a different focusing mechanism. It is normally not possible to deduce the source used from the sound signal measured in the focus of an ESWA source. Specific differences tend to become more apparent in the sound field outside of the focus, as shall be explained in the following.

2.13.2 Generation of Spherical Sound Waves

Spark gap. The first kidney lithotriptors worked with a spark source (Fig. 12). This classic principle is still being used today. In analogy to a spark plug in a car, a lightning flash is generated by feeding high voltage (usually approx. 14–30 kV) to two electrodes under water. This generates a plasma bubble, which leads to the compression of the surrounding liquid. After evacuation of the electric energy store, a vapor bubble remains, which continues to expand with decreasing velocity and finally collapses after some hundred microseconds.

Only the compression wave is emitted during the plasma phase as a useful sound wave. As the primary bubble initially travels at supersonic speed, the sound front of the compression wave is extremely steep from the onset, and therefore a shock wave in the physical sense. Its duration is from 1 μs to about 3 μs.

On the subsequent collapse of the bubble, a weaker sound wave is generated as described above.

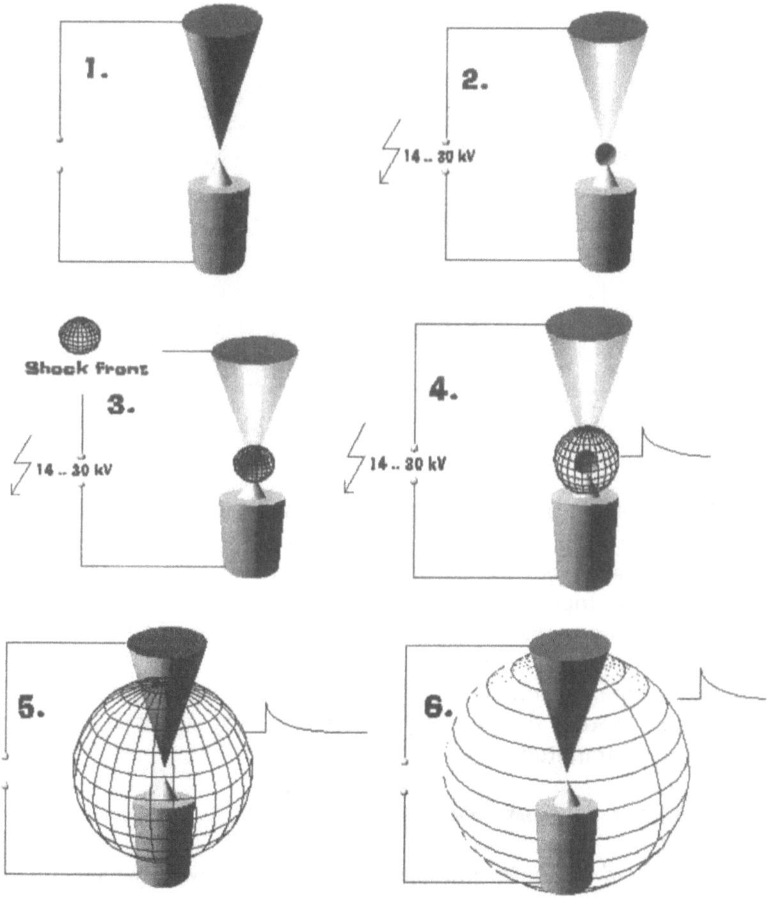

Fig. 12. The first-generation electrohydraulic shock wave generator is a spark gap. After the electrical voltage is applied, a plasma bubble builds up. This bubble shrinks when the electrical energy storage empties. At the same time, the acoustical shock wave begins to propagate outwards in a spherical manner

The high voltage is stored in a capacitor of 40 nF to several hundred nF. Its total energy at the moment of breakthrough is transferred to the developing plasma bubble. The acoustic content is only a few thousandths thereof.[11]

Focusing ellipsoid for spherical waves. An ellipsoid of revolution has the property of mirroring in its second focus all sound events generated in its first focus. If the target, e.g. the calcification, is to be conveyed to the second focus, the ellipsoid has to be adequately cut (Fig. 13). The remaining mirror

[11] The electric primary energy is calculated with a given capacitor C and voltage U according to $E_{el} = C/2U_2$. Popular capacitors in spark gap systems have a capacity of 40–80 nF, so that the primary energy at 14–30 kV charging voltage is between 3.9 and 36 joule per burst. In the case of EMSE systems, the capacitors are usually ten times as large, but the charging voltage is only up to about 20 kV. The charge energies are approx. 20–260 joule.

Fig. 13. A rotationally symmetric ellipsoid focuses the primary spherical shock wave generated at the first focus F1 inside the ellipsoid into the second focus F2, which is positioned inside the tissue

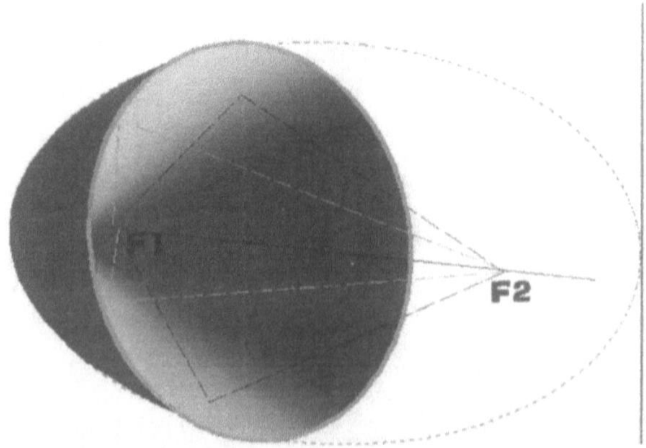

encompasses a certain portion of space of the spherical wave and focuses the former, while the other portion of the spherical wave penetrates the tissue unfocused. The latter portion is observable earlier than the focused shock wave in the second focus, the so-called 'therapeutic focus'[12]. It has an amplitude of <1 MPa to a maximum of 2 MPa. Thus, it is considerably lower than that of the focused shock wave.

Nonlinear steepening processes result in a small displacement of the pressure maximum beyond the geometrical focus F2 (by about 2–5 mm) when increasing sound amplitudes.

Special Properties of the Spark Generator

Primary, unfocused wave. An unfocused overpressure wave which propagates in front of the focused signal by about 40 μs and has a pressure of a few MPa in the area of the focus is typical for a spark source. The focused signal is followed nearly a millisecond later by a quite weak pressure wave which originates from the collapse of the primary gas bubble which developed at breakthrough (Fig. 14). This bubble is a consequence of this principle of generation and bears no relation to cavitation bubbles which may develop elsewhere in the sound field.

"Shock wave from the onset". That they are shock waves in character is typical of spark-generated sound waves. This means that the sound front is extremely steep from the onset, thereby being especially susceptible to attenuation of high frequencies when traveling long distances in tissue, so that one can assume that part of the energy is lost before reaching the focus. Due to the steepening, these high frequencies are continually replenished, which, in turn, leads to further attenuation losses.

[12] In the case of a complete ellipsoid, this portion of the wave would be mirrored on the surface 'behind' the second focus. The time difference between this portion and the focused wave depends on the mirror geometry. It is equivalent to the sound propagation time from focus F1 to the mirror and on to F2 minus the propagation time directly between F1 and F2.

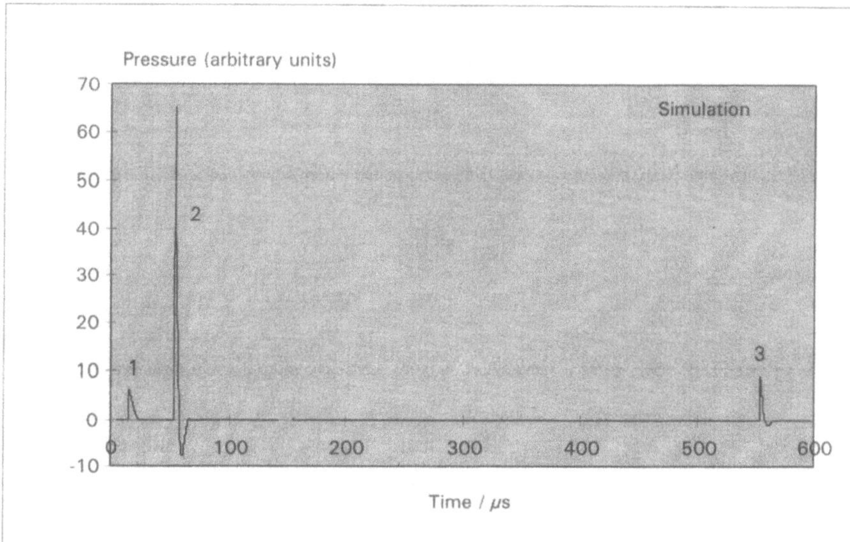

Fig. 14. The focal pressure signal of a focused spark gap source has three components: 1. the direct, unfocused wave, 2. the focused wave, 3. a signal transmitted by the collapsing primary gas bubble

2.13.3 Generation of Plane Sound Waves

Electromagnetic sound source (EMSE). In the EMSE, the principle of which was first described by Eisenmenger in 1962, a slab coil is used. When a pulsiform electric current of several kiloampere passes through the coil it creates a strong magnetic field.

An insulated highly conductive membrane is applied to the coil, in which an eddy current is created by the primary magnetic field, which results in a magnetic field with opposite polarization.

The two magnetic fields cause the membrane to be pushed away (Fig. 15), whereby the water in the area of the membrane is compressed, leading to the emission of a plane overpressure pulse with a time course of a squared half-sine wave (Fig. 16). The pressure on the membrane surface is essentially constant. The duration of the wave is about 2–5 μs.

A capacitor is again used as the electric energy store, which normally has a capacity of several hundred nanofarad and so is considerably greater than in a spark generator. The charging voltage is usually less than in a spark source. Therefore, the electroacoustic efficiency of the two sources is not comparable. A comparison of the charging voltages or of the electric primary energies is therefore not suitable for comparing different ESWA sources.

Lenses. Acoustic lenses are used for focusing in planar sound emitters such as EMSE or piezoelectric converters. Depending on whether the material (e.g.

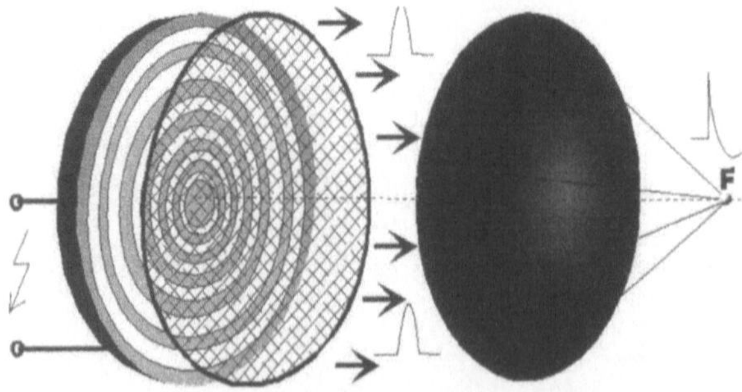

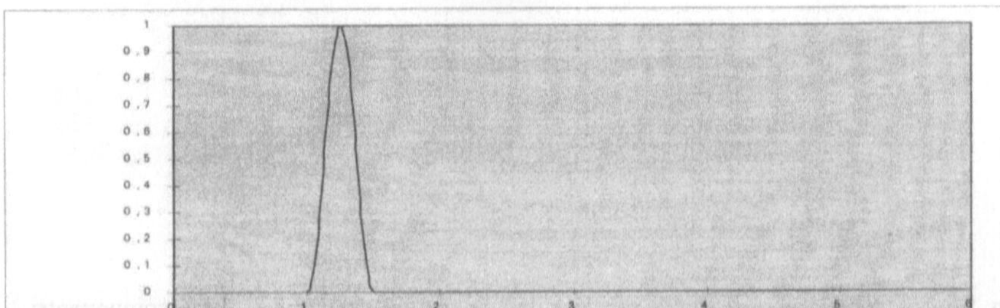

Fig. 15. The electromagnetic shock wave emitter (EMSE) is generating effective ESWA - sound pulses, which are focused to the point F by an acoustic lens. The primary generated wave steepens on its way to the focus

Fig. 16. The acoustic wave generated by a typical EMSE is proportional to the square of the driving electric current [13]. It does not have the same high spectral content as a shock wave and is therefore less attenuated in tissue

perspex or silicone rubber) has a higher or lower sound speed than the transfer medium water, the lense becomes concave or convex.

As the EMSE does not primarily emit a shock wave at all driver settings, the latter develops during travel to the focus, often not before entering the tissue. Because the situation in the focus (layering, attenuation, nonlinearity) is not foreseeable in the individual patient, an exact prognosis of the steepness in the focus is impossible. In-vivo experiments, however, show that the wave may be fully steepened [8]. In the case of sound signals with less than about 25 MPa in the focus, a fully steepened focus signal is not even achieved in water when using common geometries.

Special Properties of the EMSE

Squared sinusoidal time function. The primary EMSE signal initially has the shape of a squared half-sine wave (cf. Fig. 16) with a finite rise time of several hundred nanoseconds. Therefore, it contains only a small portion of higher frequencies and is thus only slightly attenuated in tissue. In the case of low pressures, the typical course is not sufficient to appreciably steepen the signals before reaching the focus, whereas, at higher pressures and with

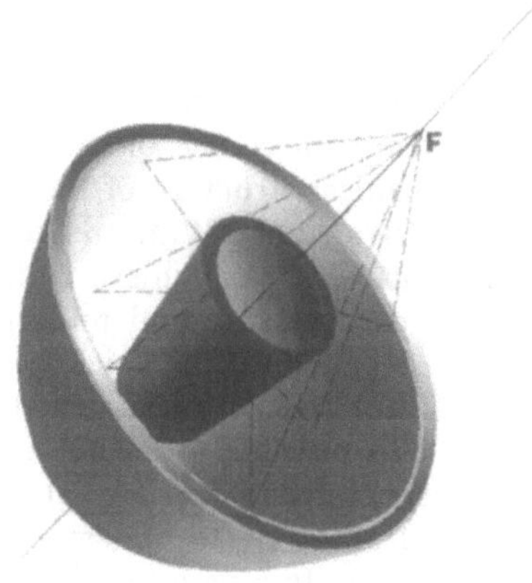

Fig. 17. The cylindrical EMSE source is focused using a paraboloid shaped mirror [14]

ESWA-typical apertures of EMSE systems with lens focusing, shock waves can be measured regularly.

Steepening in the shock tube. To create a steepened signal in front of the lens, one can insert a long shock tube between the EMSE and the lens. During the travel of the wave through the shock tube, the rise time decreases more and more, ideally resulting in a shock wave at the end of the shock tube.

Steepening due to focusing. On its way to the focus the sound wave also steepens, whereby this is supported by the increasing convergence. In a water bath, it is therefore normally possible to register shock waves in the area of the focus in appropriately systems set up (distance lens-focus, initial pressure).

Cylinder EMSE. In this special form of EMSE, the coil is cylindrical and surrounded by a cylindrical membrane. The sound pulse is emitted radially and has the same time course as that of the plane membrane.

Paraboloids for focusing cylindrical waves. The waves of the cylinder EMSE are concentrated in a focus by a paraboloid, whereby only a small section of the paraboloid is used (Fig. 17). As the travel times of the sound from various locations in the cylinder EMSE to the focus can be slightly different, there is a small temporal stretching of the variation of pressure. The rise time of the pressure front is thereby increased, so that, even at high pressure, no shock front may develop in the focus.

2.13.4 Piezoelectric Sound Source

In the case of a piezoelectric sound source, the conversion of electric to mechanical energy takes place in ceramic platelets made of lead zirconate titanate, which, due to the piezoelectric effect when applying a voltage (some hundred volts to several kilovolts), expand or contract.

Mostly, several dozen to several thousand platelets are used, which are arranged close together in a plane or on a sphere-segment-like carrier and emit an altogether wide-area sound front.

The temporal course of the piezo sound wave depends fundamentally on the mechanical structure of the emitter front and backing, as well as on the chosen drive signal. With an acoustically well-adjusted backing, the shortest sound pulse one can achieve without further electric pulse shaping is a wave with an overpressure and underpressure phase. The duration of the signal thereby depends on the thickness of the piezo elements, which is normally chosen as between 1 and 2 μs per half-wave.

It is also possible to create pulse shapes containing several over- and underpressure phases (cf. Fig. 2) by appropriate converter construction. The changes from over- to underpressure create a strong cavitation effect in the focus, leading to severe tissue damage. Possible applications would be in the destruction of tumours [17].

Self-focused structures – Spherical sound sources. It is generally preferred to arrange piezoelectric sound emitters on spherical surfaces. Thus, all sound waves emitted from the individual elements arrive at the centre of the sphere, where the focus forms, simultaneously. The smaller the aperture of the emitting surface, the more the pressure maximum is shifted in the direction of the emitter. This counteracts a positive shift in the direction of the focus caused by steepening. In completely steepened sound waves, the geometrical focus and the pressure maximum usually coincide.

Special properties of the piezo sound source. The piezo sources at first do not generate shock waves but triangularly rising signals. As these only have a small high-frequency content, more or less similar conditions prevail, as for EMSE sources.

In comparison, however, the primary sound pressure of the typical piezo generator is lower. As, due to this, the energy flux density at the piezo converter surface is also considerably lower than in an EMSE, a larger converter surface is required to generate the necessary focus energies.

"Natural" p-. The typical sound signal of the piezo source contains an underpressure portion, whose amplitude is initially similar to that of the overpressure content. However, because the former does not steepen like the overpressure content, a smaller underpressure amplitude is reached in the focus. The underpressure amplitude of the edge diffraction wave also adds to the latter.[13]

[13] If an underpressure portion is initially emitted due to pole-reversed drive of the piezo elements, the total focus signal of the piezo converter comprises the following portions: 1. converter underpressure – 2. (steepened) overpressure – 3. edge diffraction underpressure. It may be presumed that such signals can lead to considerably more severe destruction of tissue due to cavitation. The same applies if the piezo source oscillates with less attenuation and emits several over- and underpressure periods (cf. Fig. 2).

2.14 Practical ESWA

2.14.1 The System

A typical ESWA system comprises the following components:

- Sound generator with electrical driving circuit and coupling cushion (water circuit)
- Sound generator positioning
- Location-finding facilities
- Casing with transformers, controls, impulse generator, etc.

2.14.2 Coupling

Normally, there is a water path between the sound generator and the patient, which terminates at the patient side in a bellows coupling. The water pressure in the bellows is adjustable for coupling. An ultrasound gel is applied between the bellows and the skin of the patient, whereby air bubbles in the gel, which interfere with the sound wave transmission and might cause petechiae due to their caviation effect, are especially to be avoided.

2.14.3 Location Finding

Whereas in renal or gallbladder lithotripsy, in the crushing of a calcification in the shoulder and in the case of a bone fracture the target area can be objectively localized by means of ultrasound or X-ray devices, the physician is dependent on the co-operation of the patient in the palliative therapy of epicondyles and point-of-attachment tendinoses. He normally has the patient point out the location of the greatest pain and then directs the sound waves at that location.

Some systems allow dual imaging. This means that X-rays are used to engage the target precisely and real-time ultrasound is simultaneously used for control, thereby making possible continuous treatment control with minimal exposure to radiation.

X-Ray localization. A location-finding facility must generally be capable of representing the area around the focus in all spatial dimensions. In older lithotriptors this was done with a two-axis X-ray system, whereas newer machines have an isocentric X-ray arm which can be swivelled over the sound focus. This is used to target the focus, whereby the sound source or the patient is moved in the horizontal plane and the latter is AP screened. The X-ray apparatus is then swivelled isocentrically to an oblique position. In this projection, the target can then be adjusted vertically (Fig. 18). It is recommended that during treatment location control is occasionally carried out, especially if the patient is believed to have moved.

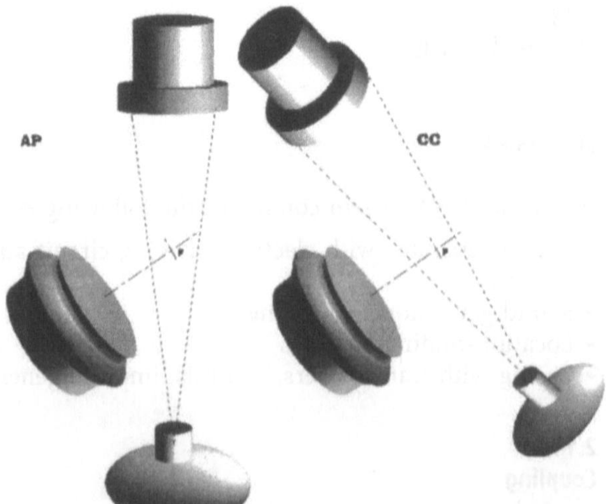

Fig. 18. X-ray targeting is done by first adjusting the target to the X-Y positions of the sound focus in the AP-plane, then swivelling the isocentric X-ray system to a CC-position and adjusting Z component of the target position

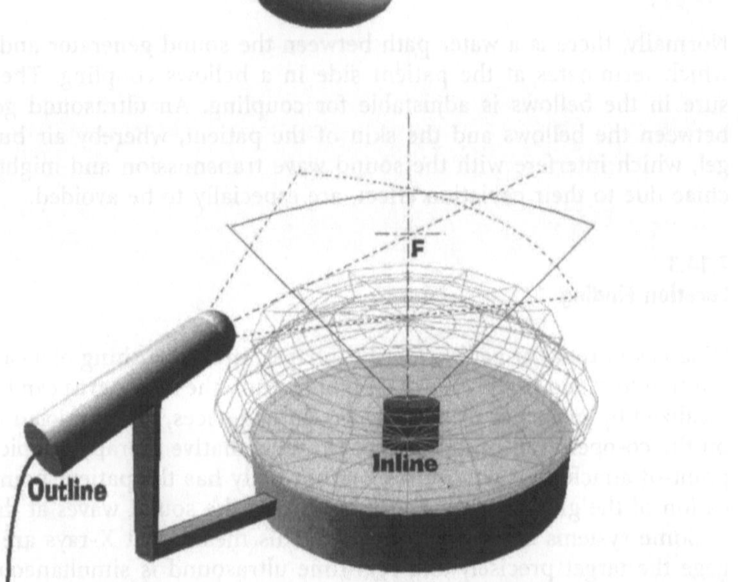

Fig. 19. Ultrasound targeting is done using Inline or Outline imaging systems. Inline systems are positioned on the shock wave source axis inside the coupling cushion. The outline system is fixed to an arm rotating isocentrically around the shock wave focus

Ultrasound localization. Depending on the structure of the imaging ultrasound transducer, one differentiates between inline and outline systems (Fig. 19).

In the inline system, the transducer is situated in the centre of the generator. The transducer can often be swivelled around its axis or axially moved. It is of advantage that the ultrasound image and the treatment source use the same sound window. A disadvantage is that the inline scanner cuts a portion of the therapeutic waves and diffraction waves develop. The resulting energy loss has to be compensated for by increased acoustic primary energy. Furthermore, the image is impaired by the water lead and the coupling pillow, and artefacts can occur, which make localization difficult.

In the outline system the ultrasound scanner is fixed on a movable arm isocentric to the focus. A suitable sound window is attainable by means of an accordingly constructed coupling pillow. As the localization axis and the therapy axis are not identical, a lot more depends on the anatomical orientation. The advantages are that the scanners are easily exchanged, so as to optimally adjust to any therapeutic situation, and that the images are not impaired and free of artefacts.

"Digital" supported ultrasound localization. The problem of the target area not being directly visible in palliative therapies can be overcome by "digital supported ultrasound localization" (DUL) [19]. The locality of the pain is palpated and the device coupled to the locality whilst the finger (Digitus) is still on the spot. One first tunes the ultrasound image to the finger echo. In doing so, the therapy focus comes very close to the centre of the pain. Fine positioning is normally done with the help of information from the patient. This procedure has been proven quite successful in the practice of ESWA therapy.

2.14.4 The Patient

Patient positioning. The patient can be treated sitting or in a lying position. The latter may be of advantage to avoid circulatory problems, especially if local anaesthesia has been administered.

The extremeties can be supported and brought into a suitable and comfortable position by means of an appropriate holder (Fig. 20). This also lessens the possibility of decoupling due to reactions caused by pain or startling.

Safety. The sound energy is nearly entirely reflected from gas-containing tissue. This can lead to severe damage, especially in the lung. Therefore, it

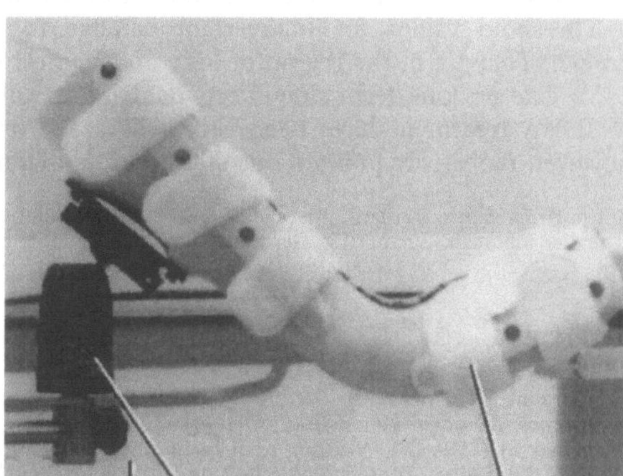

Fig. 20. Holders for arms or legs (see figure) can be used to fixate the extremities and avoid moving of the target (Photo supplied by Dornier Medtech)

should be taken into account in therapy planning that the lung is not in the path of the sound axis, not even farther away from the focus. The safety distance depends on the construction characteristics of the sound source.

The effect of shock waves on nerves is as yet unknown. It has been proved that nerves can be excited by cavitation [5]. Possible damage has to date not been investigated. Therefore, inadvertant exposure of nerves situated near the focus or on the shock wave axis should be avoided. Signs of numbness and other neurological reactions should be taken into careful consideration.

The occurrence of haematomas has been increasingly observed in patients taking haemodilutive drugs. Such medication should be discontinued in good time. In the case of pregnancy, not only the exposure to the X-ray localization procedure necessitates caution. The effect of shock waves (also indirect effects in the case of pain during treatment) on the development of the foetus has still not been sufficiently researched.

For patients with pacemakers, it should be ensured that there is no interference with its operation due to the strong electromagnetic pulses of the therapeutic source. Otherwise, treatment should avoided.

In patients with proneness to dysrhythmia, the ECG should be carefully observed. If necessary, the shock waves can be ECG-triggered.

2.15 Threshold Values in Biological Experiments

The healing effects of ESWAs have as yet not been biophysically understood. First basic research has been carried out with regard to potential damage. Possibly, it may be necessary to intentionally afflict microdamages leading to metaplasia of the diseased tissue so as to bring about later healing.

Threshold values for energy flux density have been ascertained in experiments on human umbilical cords leading to the development of stress fibres and stronger effects on cells [11]. The induction of stress fibres in cells was proven in an umbilical cord model at an energy flux density of 0.1 mJ/mm^2. Detachment of the endothelium occurs at 0.3 mJ/mm^2. One can estimate the specific biological effect area from the focus distribution (cf. Fig. 10).

Threshold values for inadvertant damage to bones are only indirectly known. They lie in the region of high and highest stone crushing doses [21].

To date no long-term side effects or diagnostically identifiable damage due to ESWA treatment have been reported in the orthopaedic literature. It is, however, repeatedly pointed out that accurate diagnosis is imperative [12].

Acknowledgements. I thank my colleagues H. Eizenhöfer, Dr. Forssmann and Dr. Hepp (Dornier Medtech, Germering, Germany) for their valuable comments.

References

1. Stranne SK, Cocks FH, Gettliffe R (1990) Mechanical property studies of human gallstones. J Biomed Mater Res 24:1049–1057
2. Loew M (1994 Die Wirkung extrakorporal erzeugter hochenergetischer Stoßwellen auf den klinischen, röntgenologischen und histologischen Verlauf der Tendinosis calcarea der Schulter. Habilitation thesis, Univ. Heidelberg, Germany

3. Philipp, Delius M, et al. (1993) Interaction of lithotripter-generated shock waves with air bubbles. JASA 5:2496–2509
4. Wiksell, Kinn (1995) Implications of cavitation phenomena for short intervals in extracorporeal shock wave lithotripsy. Br J Urol 75
5. Schelling, Delius M, et al. (1994) Extracorporeal shock waves stimulate frog sciatic nerves indirectly via a cavitation-mediated mechanism. Biophys J 6:133–140
6. Suhr, Brümmer, Hülser (1991) Cavitation-generated free radicals during shock wave exposure: Investigations with cell-free solutions and suspended cells. Ultrasound Med Biol 17:761–768
6a. Gambihler S, Delius M (1992) Influence of dissolved and free gases on iodine release and cell killing by shock waves in vitro. Ultrasound Med Biol 18:617–621
7. Ueberle F (1988) Ein Konzept zur Ultraschall-Ortung und Erkennung von Zielen für Schallpulse hoher Amplitude. Doctoral thesis, Univ. Karlsruhe, Germany
8. Vergunst et al. (1989) Assessment of shock wave pressure profiles in vitro: clinical implications. J Lithotripsy Stone Disease 4:289–298
8a. Vergunst et al. (1990) In vivo assessment of shock wave pressure. Gastroenterology: 1467–1474
9. Herbertz J (1993) Physikalische Grenzwerte für die sichere medizinische Anwendung des Ultraschalls am Menschen. In: DAGA Fortschritte der Akustik. DPG-Verlag
10. Keller, Riedlinger (1990) Vergleich der Kavitation bei verschiedenen Stoßwellengeneratoren. Biomed Tech (Suppl) 35:233–234
11. Steinbach et al. (1993) Effekte hochenergetischer Ultraschallstoßwellen auf Tumorzellen in vitro und humane Endothelzellen in situ: In Chaussy et al. (eds) Die Stoßwelle. Attempto-Verlag, Tübingen, pp 104–109
12. Deutsche Gesellschaft für Stoßwellenlithotripsie (1995) Die Stoßwelle. In: Konsensus-Workshop 4. Attempto-Verlag, Tübingen
13. Eisenmenger (1962) Elektromagnetische Erzeugung von Druckstößen in Flüssigkeiten. Acustica: 1185–1202
14. Weß et al. (1989) Lars, eine großaperturige Leistungsschallquelle für medizinische Anwendungen. DAGA 295–298
15. Delius M, Ueberle F, Gambihler S (1994) Destruction of gallstones and model by extracorporeal shock waves Ultrasound Med Biol 20:251–258
16. Lobentanzer (1991) The concept of acoustic energy in lithotripsy. Dornier User Letter 7:22–26
17. Feigl T, Waldfahrer F, et al. (1995) Destruction of normal and malignant human cells by high-energy pulsed ultrasound. Proc World Congress on Ultrasonics, pp 1087–1090
18. Druckpuls-Lithotripter (1995) German standards draft IEC 87/89A/CDV
19. Bachmann, Rothenberger, Ueberle (1996) in preparation
20. Delius M, Draenert K, et al. (1995) Biological effects of shock waves: in vivo effect of high-energy pulses on rabbit bone. Ultrasound Med Biol 21:1219–1225
21. Kauleskar Sukul et al. (1993) The effect of high-energy shock waves focused on cortical bone. J Surg Res 54:46–51
22. Haupt G, et al. (1992) Influence of shock waves on fracture healing. Urology 39:529–532

PART II

Animal Experiments and Clinical Experiences in Shock Wave Treatment of the Bone

CHAPTER 3

Effect of Extracorporeal Shock Waves on Bone: A Review of Shock Wave Experiments and the Mechanism of Shock Wave Action

M. Delius · K. Draenert · Y. Draenert and M. Börner

3.1 Introduction

Since being introduced to treat of kidney stones in 1980, extracorporeal shock waves have gained worldwide acceptance as the therapy of choice for urinary tract stones. Treating stones at other locations in the human body by shock waves has followed in subsequent years. The first reports of treating pseudarthrosis by shock waves were those of Valchanou and Michailov (1991) and Schleberger and Senge (1992), who thus extended the range of indications for shock wave therapy into a completely new field. Extracorporeal shock waves are now being increasingly accepted as a treatment modality for this disease. More recent indications for shock wave therapy in orthopedics include diseases of the shoulder, foot, and elbow. Their treatment is covered in other chapters of this volume. Present results must still be considered preliminary and require confirmation in future prospective and controlled studies.

The introduction of shock wave therapy into this area poses many new issues to researchers in the field. The changes which shock waves cause in bones, joints, and neighboring soft tissue are not well understood. Even more importantly, the mechanism of action by shock waves on these tissues has not been clarified. To the present there have been only a few initial hints as to what in fact occurs during biological shock wave application. More research must be carried out in the future to shed further light on these basic issues.

This short review considers the findings from experiments in which shock waves have been applied to bone. We discuss the major experiments that have been carried out for this topic. Readers with a special interest in the field and especially those applying shock waves in their clinical practice should urgently study the literature on their own. Some of the questions, especially the effects on bone, should become immediately obvious. These require further experimental clarification.

The review is divided into five sections. After an introduction to the morphological and functional alterations of shock waves on bone (Sect. 2), the three subsequent sections cover topics of special interest: whether shock waves accelerate fracture healing (Sect. 3), whether shock waves facilitate loosening of the bone-cement interface during revision arthroplasty (Sect. 4), and whether shock waves affect epiphyseal bone growth before closure of the epiphyseal growth plate (Sect. 5). The possible mechanisms of action of shock waves and what happens when shock waves are applied to bone are the topics briefly considered in the last section (Sect. 6). In our view, a specific shock wave action, shock wave–gas bubble interaction, is of special importance for this new area.

3.2 Effect of Shock Waves on Bone

A fundamental distinction must be made between the application of shock waves in in vivo an animal experiments (Sects. 2.1, 2.2) and their ex vivo application to explanted bones (Sect. 2.3). In the latter case only the physical effect of shock waves on a material must be considered and not a biological or medical effect.

3.2.1 Rabbit Femur In-vivo

We examined the effect of shock waves on the femur in an in vivo experiment using 19 rabbits (Delius and Draenert 1995). A total of 1500 shock waves were generated from an electrohydraulic lithotripter at high voltage (Table 1) and high pulse energy and on the distal femur epicondylus to a site 1 cm above the ground plate of the patella. The shock wave path traversed directly through the knee joint; this allowed us also to examine the hitherto unknown effect of shock waves on joints. The rabbits were positioned on a Styrofoam support with a hole in its middle through which one of the legs was pulled in a bent position and lowered in a waterbath into the focus of the lithotripter. Under radiographic control the femur was aligned exactly in a vertical position on the vertical axis of the shock wave field. This set-up prevented shock waves from entering the abdominal cavity, which can cause

Table 1. Type of lithotripter, number of discharges (range when there were several experimental groups) and lithotripter voltage or (in two cases) energy density of the experiment

Experiment	Lithotripter type	Shock wave no. (range)	Voltage or energy density (range)
Delius and Draenert (1995)	Dornier XL1	1500	27.5 kV
Augat and Claes (1992)	Dornier Compact	500	14 kV
Kaulesar Sukul et al. (1993)	Siemens Lithostar	5000-10000	0.23–0.60 mJ/mm^{-2}
Haupt et al. (1992)	Dornier XL1	500	14 kV
Johannes et al. (1994)	Siemens Lithostar	4000	0.54 mJ/mm^{-2}
Seemann et al. (1992)	Dornier XL1	250–1200	18 kV
Augat and Claes (1995)	Dornier Compact	300–3000	16 kV
Forriol et al. (1994)	Siemens Lithostar	500	0.47–1.2 mJ/mm^{-2}
Weinstein et al. (1988)	Dornier HM3	3200	20 kV
May et al. (1990)	Dornier HM3	3000	25 kV
Braun et al. (1992)	Dornier Compact	150–300	18–23 kV
Schreurs et al. (1991)	Siemens Lithostar	100–2000	18 kV
Lewis (1992)	Dornier HM3	1000	20 kV
Stranne et al. (1993)	Dornier HM3	3200	20 kV
Stranne et al. (1992)	Dornier HM3	2000	20–26 kV
Yeaman et al. (1989)	Dornier XL1	1500	20 kV
Van Arsdalen et al. (1991)	Dornier HM3	1000	18 kV

Table 2. Fluorescent dyes, color of the dye under epi-illumination, administration interval (days after shock wave application), and interval from shock wave application to the endpoint of the experiment

Dye	Color	Administration (days)	Endpoint (days)
–	–	–	6
Oxytetracycline	Yellow	5–11	11
Calcein blue	Blue	12–18	41
Alizarin komplexon	Red	19–25	59
Calcein green	Green	26–32	85

No dye was administered to the first group dissected after 6 days and only a single dye (oxytetracycline) to the second group dissected after 11 days. The other groups were given all dyes

gut, liver, and even lung hemorrhages, which is a known side effect after shock wave application to these tissues.

The rabbits were divided into five groups, and the interval between shock wave application and dissection varied between 6 and 85 days (Table 2). This wide range was chosen to demonstrate both the acute shock wave effects and their long-term effects on bone remodeling. The latter were investigated by four-color polychrome sequence labeling with four fluorescent dyes over the next month. Following a waiting period of 3 days after shock wave application each of the dyes was administered over the course of 1 week. No dye was administered to the group dissected 6 days after shock wave application and only a single dye at dissection 11 days after shock wave application. At the endpoint of the experiment the legs were perfused and examined radiologically. The medial epicondylus was cut into 500-μm serial sections which included the area of the focus and the ground plate of the patella. They were then examined under a fluorescence microscope by epifluorescent light.

Skin ulceration was observed in all rabbits at the shock wave entry site at the knee. Femoral fractures were found in the upper third of the femur in 16% of the rabbits; no cause was found for their generation. Cases were also encountered of muscle hematomas, petechial hemorrhages, and scarring in the upper thigh. However, all knee joints were completely normal and showed no change. Radiologically there were single or multiple lucencies in the focal area in 30% of the examined femoral bones. There were no signs of fractures or alterations of the compact bone.

Evaluation of the changes 6 days after shock wave application revealed three prominent findings at the compact and trabecular bone:

- Periosteal detachment with subperiosteal hemorrhage. This sometimes encompassed a major part of the epiphysis. More importantly, bone marrow content and marrow fat was pressed out of the marrow canal under the periosteum (Fig. 1).
- Both diffuse hemorrhages and hematomas were found in the marrow canal. The former were more extensive; the latter were principally in the focal area and were not larger than a few millimeters.

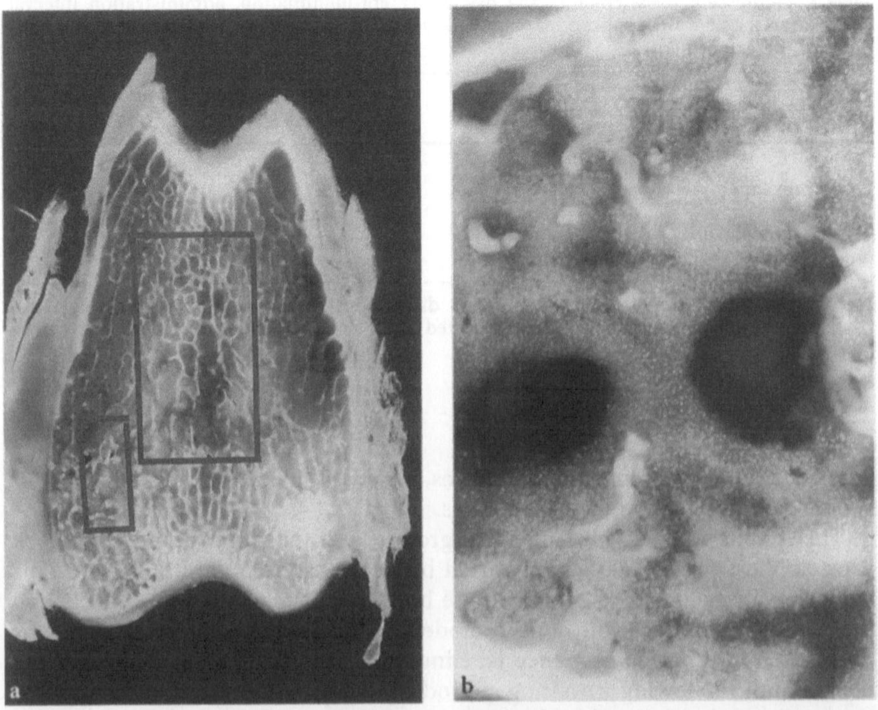

1

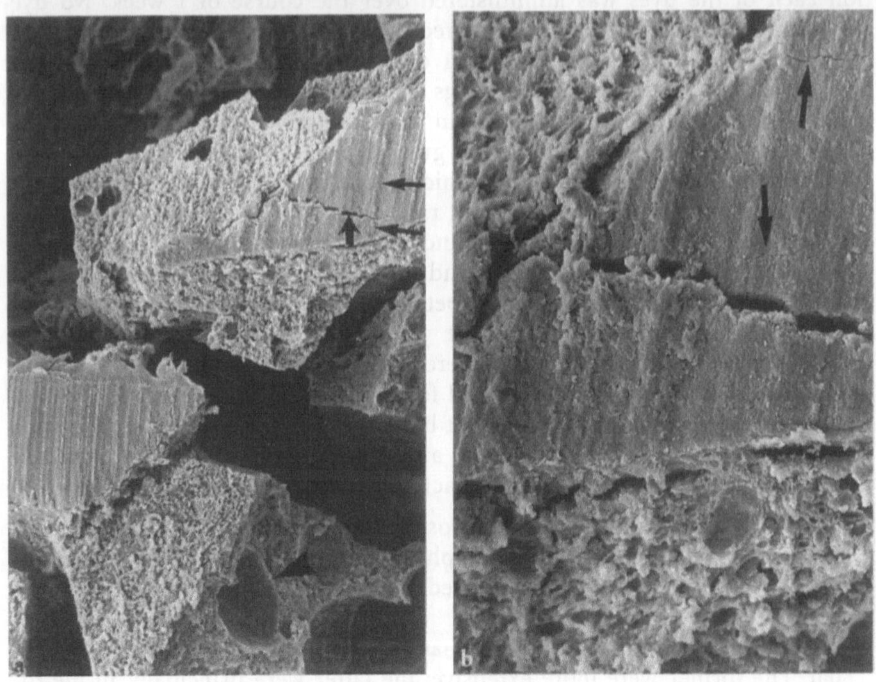

2

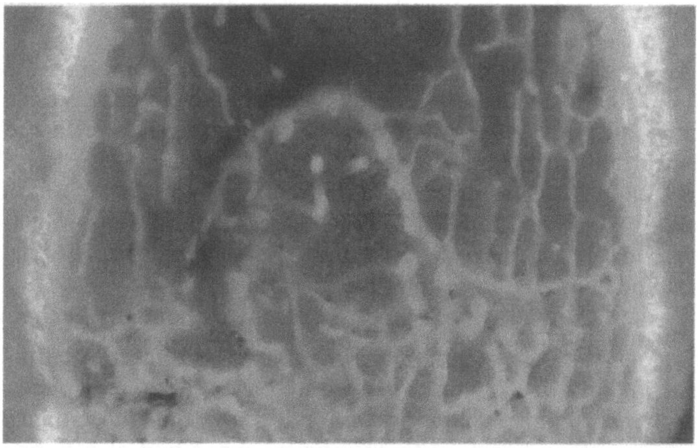

Fig. 3. Strong periosteal reaction 11 days after shock wave application. The bright areas indicate the tetracycline label in the newly formed bone. Spongiosal trabecular fractures are visible in the center

- Bone trabecles in the marrow canal were multiply fractured and were sometimes split into small fragments (Fig. 2). Fragments were dislocated, some of them out of the focus in the direction of the periphery of the epicondylus. Electron microscopy clearly revealed fractures of trabecles even at sites which had not been observed under the light microscope (Fig. 3). These changes were not observed either in cortical bone or at the patellar ground plate.

Examination of the other treatment groups illustrated the further development of these bone lesions over the following periods after shock wave application:

- After 11 days: the tetracycline label revealed the periosteal apposition of new bone. This was a prominent reaction which sometimes completely encompassed the circumference of the cortex. The trabecular bone in the

Fig. 1 a, b. Rabbit femur 6 days after shock wave application. The marrow is hemorrhagic in the center and at both lateral sides. Marrow contents have been pressed out of the marrow under the periosteal space. Multiple fractures of trabecles with dislocation of the fragments in the middle are seen in the center within the two rectangles. **b** Detail of **a** under higher magnification. Two hemorrhages are visible in the center, as well as diffuse hemorrhages

Fig. 2 a, b. Two bone trabecles in the femoral epiphyseal bone (in the upper right and lower left quadrant) surrounded by marrow tissue. Upon scanning electron microscopic view, the trabecles have diameters of 90 μm. A fracture is visible at the tip of the trabecle on the right (*large arrow*). Examination of the slides under light microscopy had not shown this type of fracture. The wavy pattern of the saw blade at the trabecle (*small arrow*) which is nearly perpendicular to the direction of the fracture gap indicates that the fracture cannot have been caused by the blade during cutting of the bone. The holes (*triangle*) indicate fat cells. **b** Higher magnification of the fracture gap from **a.** Ground substance is visible at the upper and lower sides of the picture and also in the gap. Smaller fracture lines are visible in the right upper part of the figure (*small arrows*)

marrow appeared rarefied and resorbed, with empty areas lacking the usual spongiosal architecture.

- After 41 days: the periosteal reaction was even more prominent, and there was also an endosteal reaction. Osteophytes had been generated at the distal femur epicondylus, some of them with bizarre shapes. In the marrow the resorption had further proceeded.
- After 59 days: a strong prominent thickening of the cortex was found; its thickness had almost doubled in some cases. Finally, there was apposition of new bone at the marrow trabecles. The center of the epiphysis, however, remained empty and showed no reaction.
- After 85 days (3 months): the picture remained essentially unchanged.

The obvious findings of this experiment were the fragmentation of bony trabecles in the marrow cavity, with an only partial and incomplete regeneration even 3 months after shock wave application, and the strong periosteal reaction with profound cortical thickening by apposition of new bone, which was probably a consequence of the subperiosteal bleedings. One may speculate that such a periosteal reaction also occurs in the treatment of a pseudarthrosis and accelerates healing; however, this hypothesis has not been tested. Shortcomings of the experiment include: (a) it could not answer the question of whether shock waves can generate cortical fractures in vivo because the fractures had not occurred in or near the focus but further away at the proximal femur, and (b) its design did not rule out the control of possible systematic errors such as those caused by the animal's movements during shock wave application after fixation of the leg. There was also the danger resulting from the transport of marrow contents under the periosteum: however, again, it was not examined how much marrow spilled over into the circulation, or what consequences this had. The same result, the washout of marrow fat of a cortical bone, was also noted after shock wave application to the bone-cement interface (see Sect. 4.3).

3.2.2
Sheep Calcaneus In-vivo

The effect of shock wave application on bone changes and new bone formation was also investigated in another in vivo experiment using sheep by Augat and Claes (1992). Here 500 shock waves were applied to the calcaneus of three of these animals at a considerably lower energy than in the previous experiment (Table 1). Three fluorescent dyes were used for polychrome sequence labeling, and the histological examination 6 weeks after shock wave application was combined with bone densitometry. Only a small focal destruction of the trabecular architecture was found in a single case. There was no new bone formation, even at the periosteum.

The reasons for the absence in this report of many of the previously described bone changes are not clear. It may be concluded that the threshold for generation of bone damage was just only barely reached at the low pulse energy used in this experiment. This may also explain why no periosteal hemorrhage was found in this case.

3.2.3
Rabbit Femur Fixated

The experiment carried out by Kaulesar Sukul et al. (1993) differed from the above in vivo experiments and was performed with a different purpose. The study examined what happens when shock waves are applied to bare bones positioned in the focus of a shock wave field where the overlying tissue has been removed. Table 1 lists the energy flow of the lithotripter employed in this experiment, which was varied over a wider range. The number of shock waves was also varied and was extremely high in some cases. Shock waves were applied to explanted tibiae and femora of rabbits which had been conserved for an unreported time in formaldehyde solution. Either 5000 or 10000 shock waves were focused exactly in a waterbath to the interface of the bone diaphysis with the surrounding water. Visible bone changes were documented photographically with increasing numbers of shock waves. It was found that shock waves of high pulse energy induced complete fractures at high large shock wave numbers, splitting off of the bone ends or cutting round holes into the cortex. Lower pulse energies merely loosened small bone chips from the bone surface or caused no visible change at all.

The dependence of the shock wave effect on the pulse energy is now a well-established fact and has been demonstrated both for stone fragmentation and for the lytic effect of shock waves on cells (Delius et al. 1994, 1995). In principle this should be also the case for bone. In contrast to these results, the fracturing of a bone cortex can be achieved only with a considerably higher energy. Mechanical properties of bone, such as compressive and tensile stress and strain, may have been responsible. The experiment differed from the in vivo experiments of this section because cavitation (see Sect. 6) occurred in the water along the long axis of the shock wave field, and the bone surface was always in direct contact with it. Surface effects such as the generation of petechial skin hemorrhages, for example, from shock waves, are known to be generated at the interface of water and skin. These are greatly enhanced when the water in the lithotripter tub has not been degassed. This type of event occurs less often in the in vivo situation. The effects of this experiment may also have been greatly facilitated by the experimental design. Dry bones should have had an effect that was greater by an order of magnitude. Dried kidney and gallstones are well known to behave in this way.

3.2.4
Summary

Application of shock waves to bone in vivo can generate hematomas and diffuse hemorrhages, fragmentation of bony trabecles in the marrow, and the transport of marrow content under the periosteum when high voltage and high pulse energy are applied. The experimental data has not to date been supported by further data, and the number of investigations on the topic is still limited. Several other experiments on the topic have so far been published only in abstract form. The experiment with the lower pulse energy suggests that most of the changes found by the high shock wave energy do not occur at low energy.

3.1 Effect of Shock Waves on Fracture Healing

The previous section reports results of experiments on the effect of shock waves on normal viable bone. The effects on bone have also been examined to determine whether shock waves can facilitate the natural repair of a fracture. These experiments required adequate animal models and different approaches, such as creating an experimental fracture or a burr hole.

3.3.1 Rat Humerus Fracture

The first experiment on this topic was that carried out by Haupt et al. (1992) which examined a fracture of the humerus caused in 40 rats by manual compression of the limb. A total of 100 shock waves from an electrohydraulic lithotripter were applied at five different intervals (2, 5, 9, 14, and 19 days) after generating the fracture. Controls were treated identically but without shock wave application. The fractures were examined radiologically at weekly intervals in a blinded manner to monitor the progress of healing.

The endpoint of the experiment was reached after 35 days, at which time there was no difference in the breaking strength of the bones. Histologically there was also no difference between the groups, and neither hemorrhages nor necrosis within the bones was observed. Only the evaluation of radiographs revealed a significant difference in the progress of healing.

3.3.2 Dog Radius Osteotomy

In another experiment of this kind Johannes et al. (1994) used dogs to establish a model of delayed fracture healing that was considered especially suited to investigating the treatment of pseudarthrosis by shock waves. The fracture gap remains wide after osteotomy of the distal radius, and callus formation does not take place over the following 12 weeks. One-half of the ten dogs with this pretreatment were then treated with 4000 shock waves from an electromagnetic lithotripter (Table 1); the other half served as controls.

After 12 weeks radiological examination showed bony bridging of the fracture gap in all treated dogs but in only one of the control dogs. The bridging was confirmed histologically. The authors emphasized the good clinical results obtained from pseudarthrosis treatment but did not examine either the acute changes which the shock waves had caused nor their time course. No functional investigations were performed.

These were positive results for the use clinical use of shock waves to accelerate fracture healing especially in view of the treatment of pseudarthrosis. They findings have, however, been questioned by the negative results of other investigations.

3.3.3
Rabbit Tibial Osteotomy

The experiment reported in Sect. 3.1. was repeated in a similar way and with the same type of lithotripter by Seemann et al. (1992) but with a different experimental design: a burr hole was drilled at the proximal tibia and both fibulae were cut by osteotomies. Shock wave treatments varying in number from one to ten were performed over the following 17 days; the number of discharges varied between 250 and 1200 (Table 1). Fracture healing was examined in the following days with various methods.

Densitometric analysis revealed no significant difference between the various treatment groups and the controls. The breaking strength of the bones increased in the groups after shock wave application, as expected; however, again, there was no difference to the controls. Analysis of calcium and collagen content also yielded no significant results. The authors concluded that fracture healing is not accelerated by shock waves, at least not with the pulse energy used in this experiment.

3.3.4
Sheep Tibial External Fixation

Another contribution to the topic of whether shock waves facilitate fracture healing came relatively recently from a thorough investigation by Augat and Claes (1995). These authors used an established experimental model and generated a controlled lesion. In 18 sheep an osteotomy was performed of the diaphysis of the tibia, and the fracture gap was fixed by an external fixation device. Various groups of sheep were then treated at different pulse energies by shock waves from an electromagnetic lithotripter focused into the fracture gap. A group treated identically but without shock wave application served as controls (Table 1).

After 9 weeks the fracture gap was examined biomechanically, radiologically, and histologically. The authors found no difference in the areas of callus between the shock wave treated group and the control group. The tensile strength also did not differ significantly between the groups. However, at one of the four examined sites the tensile strength was significantly lower, i.e., bones tended to break earlier, in the shock wave treated group than in the control group. This was in contrast to the expected result. The authors concluded that shock wave application tends to deteriorate fracture healing, an opinion which is also supported by the report below.

3.3.5
Sheep Tibial Osteotomy

The largest study of this kind was performed in lambs by Forriol et al. (1994). Two different protocols were used to treat 37 lambs by osteotomy. In the first the cortex of the proximal tibia was fenestrated with a rectangular window, and in the second three holes were drilled in a line along this bone. After 14 days 500 shock waves were applied to the defect by an electromagnetic lithotripter (Table 1). A part of the animals not receiving shock waves served as a control group. Three weeks after treatment the bones were prepared for histological and radiological examination.

No quantitative evaluation of the results was reported. The authors report in the shock wave treated groups no effect on the periosteal surface but the formation of new trabecular bone at the endosteal surface. This formation contrasted clearly to the case among control animals, in which the healing of the defects was further advanced. In agreement with the previous experiment it was concluded that shock wave application delays bone healing. Endosteal new bone formation was tentatively explained by the fact that the shock wave energy had been lower at sites where endosteal new bone formation was recorded than at the lesion sites where the energy directly applied to the defect had been higher, and where no appropriate reaction was observed. The very short duration of the experiment – only 4 weeks after shock wave application compared to 12 and 9 weeks in the experiments in Sects. 3.4 and 3.5 – may require further clarification.

3.3.6
Summary

The experiments presented above found no acceleration of fracture healing by shock waves. There was only one positive finding, and this was in part based only on a radiological aspect and not on functional tests. A major difference is also the choice of animal models. It is known that fracture healing of rabbits and rats differs from that in sheep and dogs and probably also in humans. Delayed fracture healing by shock waves has been found repeatedly and cannot be denied.

3.4
Shock Waves for Revision Arthroplasty to Loosen the Bone-Cement Interface

Possible applications of extracorporeal shock wave treatment were proposed even before renal and biliary lithotripsy had been clinically introduced, including its use in organs such as the eye and at bones. It was conjectured that shock waves could allow faster removal of old, impacted bone cement from the bony canal in revision arthroplasty by loosening the bone-cement interface. The technique was hoped to improve a procedure that is normally time consuming and tedious for the surgeon. It was not considered a drawback to this application that polymethylacrylate has an acoustic impedance of 1.9×10^6 rayl and is acoustically similar to muscle tissue while bone has an impedance of $1.45–6\times10^6$ rayl with a wide variability of trabecular bone (Jacobsen and Webster 1974).

3.4.1
Cement Removal

In one of the first experiments on this topic Weinstein et al. (1988) examined the physical effect of shock waves on the involved materials and their connection, i.e., the cement-bone interface. Twelve canine femora were freed of all adherent tissue and cut proximally; a canal was then drilled and filled with bone cement. These compound specimens were exposed after 24 h to 3200 shock waves from an electrohydraulic lithotripter. The discharges were applied to eight points around the interface. The specimens were then cut into slices with a diamond saw and examined by electron microscopy. The shear strength was assessed by measuring the force necessary to force the central cement specimen out of a transverse bone slice.

The shear strength was found to be significantly decreased by 40% after shock wave application. Histological examination revealed loosened bone and cement fragments in a widened gap between the two interface layers and microfractures in the spaces, which were widened to 1–5 μm diameter. The authors concluded that shock waves should be a valuable adjunct for revision arthroplasty.

3.4.2 Implant Removal

A very similar experimental design was employed shortly thereafter by May et al. (1990). Canine femora were again used. A channel was drilled, filled with bone cement, and treated 24 h later with 3000 shock waves. In contrast to the previous experiment, however, the strength of the compound material at the bone-cement interface was not determined by cutting the test specimens into slices. Instead, the tension was measured by pulling out a steel rod which had been implanted into the femur. Its impedance of course differed considerably from that of the cement, and these results are therefore not directly comparable.

As in the previous section on fracture healing, there are also negative reports of experiments on shock wave application for revision arthroplasty. The results of these argue against the above positive findings and call the concept into question again. We reached a similar conclusion after preliminary experiments on the topic more than 12 years ago (unpublished).

3.4.3 Cement Removal

Braun et al. (1992) used the same design as that in the above experiment to examine femoral segments. Human specimens were used and were exposed in an electrohydraulic lithotripter. A steel rod had been implanted as in the above experiment. Shock wave application did not generate any radiological change and did not change the amount of force necessary to press the implanted cylinders out of segments. Microscopic examination of the specimens revealed neither microfractures nor dislocated bone trabecles at the interface. Most remarkable was a cloudy material which appeared in the water of the lithotripter waterbath during shock wave application. Under the microscope it was seen to consist of fat droplets and fat cells which had been washed out of the marrow or the bone-cement interface. The danger of a spillover of marrow content into the circulation and its possible deleterious consequences was clearly recognized and addressed. This is in agreement with the bone changes found after shock wave application to bone in vivo.

Similar to the study of the effects of shock waves on bone itself by putting bare bones into the waterbath (Sect. 2), researchers have also examined what shock waves do to bone cement itself when specimens are exposed to it in the lithotripter waterbath without any bone.

3.4.4 Bone Cement Disks

In one of the first approaches Schreurs et al. (1991) exposed disks of bone cement to 2000 shock waves from an electromagnetic lithotripter. Morphological examination afterwards revealed an area of increased porosity at the upper surface of the disk in the focus. A closer view under the scanning microscope revealed small craters, some of which had a ringlike shape. These were undoubtedly generated by cavitation in the waterbath in the focus. The lesions were smaller than the pore sizes usually found in bone cement. An effect of shock waves on the mechanical properties of the cement could not be excluded; however, the specimens were not tested mechanically.

3.4.5 Bone Cement Cylinders

Lewis (1992) also tested bone cement mechanically. Bone cement cylinders were polymerized as rods and then cut with a saw and sanded down to pieces of a defined geometry. Shock wave exposure was performed with 1000 discharges from an electrohydraulic lithotripter. In the subsequent mechanical test the fracture toughness was significantly lowered, by the small extent of 14%. This result was taken as confirming the applicability of shock waves for revision arthroplasty.

The experiment not only demonstrated a negligible difference between treated and untreated test specimens but also used an excessively low number of test objects. Moreover, the position of the test object in the shock wave field was not reported. The inner surface of the test cylinder with a chevron notch may have been changed by cavitation as in the experiment above. It is also possible that the special geometry of the conelike shape facilitated the occurrence of microfractures in the specimens from a direct shock wave effect (see Sect. 6). No further examination was performed with respect to these questions.

3.4.6 Mechanical Properties of Bone

Loosening the bone-cement interface by shock waves was examined again in a comprehensive experiment by Stranne et al. (1993). This study asked whether the mechanical properties of bone itself differ after shock wave application. Here 28 canine femora were employed, and the design was the same as that above, with implantation of steel rods. Some of the specimens were exposed to 3200 shock waves from an electrohydraulic lithotripter, and the rest served as controls. In contrast to the other investigations, here the major issue was not the compressive or tensile forces required to remove the implant. The cement was removed mechanically thereafter from both the shock wave treated bones and the controls, which had been cemented but not exposed to shock waves. This took a very long time (4.5 h per specimen!), and the time required did not differ between the femora exposed and those not exposed to shock waves. The torsional strength of the bones was then tested mechanically and compared to control femora which had not been treated with cement or shock waves. No statistically significant differences were found between the groups. The loosening of the bone-cement interface had not taken place as originally hypothesized.

3.4.7
Implant Removal

In a further experiment Stranne et al. (1992) examined the removal of femoral implants in the absence of bone cement. Titanium cylinders were implanted into the femur of rabbits. The femur was removed 15 weeks later and exposed to 2000 shock waves in an electrohydraulic lithotripter with the implant in place. The push-out force of the bone cylinder was assessed as described above. There was no difference between the implants and controls. Microfractures were observed neither by radiology nor by electron microscopy. The authors concluded that the interface between bone and prosthesis had not been markedly loosened.

3.4.8
Summary

From the numerous reports discussed above it does not appear that shock waves can be used as an adjunct in orthopedic surgery to loosen the bone-cement interface. Studies show no positive results, regardless of whether implants had been inserted or not. Any new efforts in this area would require new approaches and new ideas.

3.5
Shock Wave Application to the Growing Bone

Among the questions concerning the effects of shock waves on bone, one was examined as early as the late 1980s: whether shock waves have an affect on the growing bone.

3.5.1
Rat Femur

A key report on this topic was that of Yeaman et al. which appeared in 1989. The proximal tibiae of 18-week-old rats were exposed to 1500 shock waves from an experimental electrohydraulic lithotripter (Table 1). The bones were examined histologically 2, 4, or 10 weeks after shock wave application. The result was striking since focal alterations were found in 44% of the 18 examined bones, consisting of focal dysplasias of the epiphyseal plate. In two cases the dysplasias were extensive, and the legs of these rats were clearly shortened! No change in the epiphyseal plate was found in the control rats, and there was no difference in the diameters of their epiphyseal plates.

This experiment established that shock waves can affect bone growth when administered before the closure of the epiphyseal plate. It led to shock wave therapy before closure of the epiphyseal plate being added to the list of contraindications of orthopedic shock wave applications. Despite the impact of this experiment it has not been repeated, and other shock wave parameters such as the dependence of epiphyseal dysplasias on the discharge number or pulse energy have not been examined. Moreover, the result cannot be extrapolated directly to the human situation because the bones of different species differ not only in terms of mechanical properties such as cortical thickness and spongiosal architecture but also in their acoustic parameters. It is well known from ultrasound experiments that the choice of the animal species determines the occurrence of certain types of lesion such as lung hemorrhage.

3.5.2 Rabbit Femur

These problems were also known to Van Arsdalen et al. (1991), the authors of the second experiment in this area which also dealt with bone growth after shock wave application. Here 1000 shock waves were applied from an electrohydraulic lithotripter to the femoral head of six young rabbits (Table 1). At dissection 6 months later their weight had doubled. No difference was found in the length of the femur, and the diameter of the femoral head was comparable to that in the control group. There were no histological abnormalities. When one compares the physical shock wave parameters of this experiment with those in the above experiment and considers the differences noted between various animal species (weight difference in rabbits and rats greater that one order of magnitude), the result does not appear completely unexpected.

3.5.3 Summary

Shock waves can inhibit bone growth before closure of the epiphyseal plate.

3.6 Mechanisms of Shock Wave Action

Since the clinical introduction of lithotripsy substantial research has been carried out to evaluate the mechanisms of stone fragmentation by shock waves and the generation of tissue damage. Two possible causes of these effects have been proposed: a direct shock wave effect and cavitation (reviewed in Delius 1994).

3.6.1 Direct Shock Wave Effect

Stone fragmentation was the first clinical shock wave application, and its mechanism of action was considered clear even in the beginning: due to its high pressure and its short rise time the shock wave generates such compressive and tensile forces within the stone and at its interfaces between the stone and the surrounding medium that it leads to fracture. This suggests that microfractures which are naturally present in a stone are subsequently enlargened by successive shocks until the material fails by fatigue.

There are many examples of a direct shock wave effect in material research. Detonation of a charge, for example, at the base of a plexiglas cone, leads to fracture of the cone tip: during its upward propagation the pressure wave in the material is reflected at the conical walls as a tensile wave. The tension increases progressively during the propagation of the wave to the tip until it exceeds the strength of the material: the tip is blown off. A direct shock wave effect has also been observed when shock waves are applied to glass and plaster spheres: horizontal material layers are spalled off in slices at defined distances from their rounded tops (Delius and Gambihler 1991). Another example of a direct shock wave effect is the splitting off of the tips of cholesterol gallstones with a tetrahedral shape after several shock waves.

3.6.2 Cavitation and Shock Wave–Gas Bubble Interaction

Cavitation is defined as the generation and movement of gas or air bubbles in a fluid or in tissue. The bubbles expand from invisibly small micron- or submicron-sized gas particles called cavitation nuclei, grow to a certain size, and collapse again. During this process high pressures and temperatures are generated for a short period. The collapse of a cavitation bubble in the fluid at a near-by surface can cause a small crater in the material. Cavitation is of great physical and economical importance, for example, in turbine blades and ship propellers because it can erode and eventually destroy even hard metals. Cavitation is found along the long axis of the shock wave field in the waterbath of a lithotripter and can be easily photographed. It is the primary process which destroys cells when shock waves are applied to cells in a suspension and is also primarily involved in the fragmentation of gallstones by shock waves (Delius and Brendel 1988).

Shock wave–gas bubble interaction is a special form of cavitation and occurs when a lithotripter shock wave hits a gas bubble (Philipp 1994). The bubble is compressed, and the bubble wall then moves as a bullet, with a speed of up to several hundred meters per second. Foils can be penetrated.

The primary lesion of tissue damage by shock waves is vessel wall destruction principally that of veins, with concomitant hemorrhage and the generation of thrombi. Today it is thought to be caused largely by cavitation. We now have evidence that primarily shock wave–gas bubble generation is involved in this process. The shock wave effect is completely suppressible by minimal static excess pressure in the exposed vessel. This is interpreted such that the gas bubbles become smaller due to the pressure, and that shock wave–gas bubble interaction can therefore no longer occur (Delius 1997).

3.6.3
Possible Mechanism of the Shock Wave Action on Bone

The question arises as to which is the actual mediator of the biological shock wave effects - cavitation or a direct shock wave effect? This question, however, is not in fact posed at the present since only few of the above experiments have revealed positive or expected results. No experiments to date have directly addressed the question. Further research is urgently needed to clarify the matter if shock wave application is to become a standard procedure.

Although the present models of shock wave action do not allow defininte conclusions to be drawn, we can make the following final observations on this topic:

- The nature of bone changes in vivo after shock wave application (see Sect. 2.1) argues strongly in favor of a cavitation-mediated mechanism. Skin ulceration is certainly mediated this way; this occurs particularly in the water of the lithotripter tub. The pressing out of marrow from the marrow cavity may indicate the volume expansion of cavitation bubbles in the marrow, and the generation of hemorrhages in the periosteum and the marrow and the generation of trabecular fractures with their dislocation can be explained by cavitation and shock-wave gas-bubble interaction in the lithotripter focus.
- There is a possible involvement of direct shock wave effect in generating the fractures described after application of the shock waves to bare bone (Sect. 2.3); however, this has not yet been confirmed.
- Shock wave–gas bubble interaction may also be responsible for another effect which is important in the orthopedic application of shock waves and which has never been mentioned: the pain experienced during shock wave application. Experiments in which frog nerves were exposed to shock waves have shown that shock waves can generate sum action potentials leading to depolarization of the nerve. This has also been shown to be due to shock wave–gas bubble interaction (Schelling et al. 1994).

Should shock wave application to bones become accepted one day as a standard therapy, further research must attempt to clarify what it is that shock waves in fact do, and why they do it.

References

1. Augat P, Claes L (1992) Einfluß von Stoßwellen auf spongiösen Knochen. Annual Report of the Gesellschaft für Biomedizinische Technologien, Ulm, 4:25–27
2. Augat P, Claes L, Suger G (1995) In vivo effect of shock-waves on the healing of fractured bone. Clin Biomech 10:374–378
3. Braun W, Claes L, Rüter A, Paschke D (1992) Effects of extracorporeal shockwaves on the stability of the interface between bone and polymethylmethacrylate: an in vitro study on human femoral segments. Clin Biomech 7:47–54

4. Delius M (1994) Medical applications and bioeffects of extracorporeal shock waves. Shock Waves 4:55–72
5. Delius M (1997) Minimal static excess pressure minimises the effect of extracorporeal shock waves on cells and gallstones. Ultrasound Med Biol 23:611–617
6. Delius M, Draenert K, Al Diek Y, Draenert Y (1995) Biological effects of shock waves: in vivo effect of of high energy pulses on rabbit bone. Ultrasound Med Biol 21:1219–1225
7. Delius M, Gambihler S (1991) Effect of shock waves on gallstones and materials. In: Paumgartner G, Ferrucci J, Burhenne J (eds) Lithotripsy and related techniques for gallstone treatment. Proceedings of the 3rd International Symposium on Biliary Lithotripsy, Mosby Year Book, St. Louis, pp 27–33
8. Delius M, Ueberle F, Gambihler S (1995) Acoustic energy determines haemoglobin release from erythrocytes by extracorporeal shock waves in vitro. Ultrasound Med Biol 21:707–710
9. Delius M, Ueberle F, Gambihler S (1994) Destruction of gallstones and model stones by extracorporeal shock waves. Ultrasound Med Biol 20:251–258
10. Forriol F, Solchaga L, Moreno JL, Canadell J (1994) The effect of shockwaves on mature and healing cortical bone. Int Orthop18:325–329
11. Haupt G, Haupt A, Ekkernkamp A, Gerety B, Chvapil M (1992) Influence of shock waves on fracture healing. Urology 39:529–532
12. Jacobson B, Webster JG (1977) Medicine and clinical engineering. Prentice-Hall, Englewood Cliffs
13. Johannes EJ, Kaulesar Sukul DM, Matura E (1994) High energy shock waves for the treatment of non-unions: an experiment on dogs. J Surg Res 57:246–252
14. Kaulesar Sukul DM, Johannes EJ, Pierik EG, van Eijck GJ, Kristelijn MJ (1993) The effect of high energy shock waves focused on cortical bone: an in vitro study. J Surg Res 54:46–51
15. Lewis G (1992) Effect of lithotripter treatment on the fracture toughness of acrylic bone cement. Biomaterials 13:225–229
16. May TC, Krause WR, Preslar AJ, Vernon Smith MJ, Beaudoin AJ, Cardea JA (1990) Use of high-energy shock waves for bone cement removal. J Arthroplasty 5:19–27
17. Philipp A, Delius M, Scheffcyk C, Vogel A, Lauterborn W (1993) Interaction of lithotripter-generated shock waves with air bubbles. J Acoust Soc Am 93:2496–2509
18. Schelling G, Delius M, Gschwender M, Grafe P, Gambihler S (1994) Extracorporeal shock waves stimulate frog sciatic nerves indirectly via a cavitation-mediated mechanism. Biophys J 66:133–140
19. Schleeberger R, Senge T (1992) Non-invasive treatment of long-bone pseudarthrosis by shock waves (ESWL). Arch Orthop Trauma Surg 111:224–227
20. Schreurs BW, Bierkens AF, Huiskes R, Hendrikx AJ, Slooff TJ (1991) The effect of the extracorporeal shock wave lithotriptor on bone cement. J Biomed Mat Res 25:157–164
21. Seemann O, Rassweiler J, Chvapil M, Alken P, Drach GW (1992) Effect of low-dose shock wave energy on fracture healing: an experimental study. J Endourol 6:219–223
22. Stranne SK, Callaghan JJ, Cocks FH, Weinerth JL, Seaber AV, Myers BS (1993) Would revision arthroplasty be facilitated by extracorporeal shock wave lithotripsy? Clin Orthop 287:252–258
23. Stranne SK, Callaghan JJ, Fyda TM, Fulghum CS, Glisson RR, Weinerth JL, Seaber AV (1992) The effect of extracorporeal shock wave lithotripsy on the prosthesis interface in cementless arthroplasty. J Arthroplasty 7:173–179
24. Valchanou VD, Michailov P (1991) High energy shock waves in the treatment of delayed and nonunion of fractures. Internat Orthopaedics (SICOT) 15:181–184
25. Van Arsdalen KN, Kurzweil S, Smith J, Levin RM (1991) Effect of lithotripsy on immature rabbit bone and kidney development. J Urol 146:213–217
26. Weinstein JN, Oster DM, Park JB, Park SH, Loening S (1988) The effect of the extracorporeal shock wave lithotriptor on the bone-cement interface in dogs. Clinical Orthop Rel Res 235:261–267
27. Yeaman LD, Jerome CP, McCullough DL (1989) Effects of shock waves on the structure and growth of the immature rat epiphysis. J Urol 141:670

CHAPTER 4

The Influence of Shock Waves on Epiphysial Growth Plates: First Results of an In-Vivo Study with Rabbits

S. Lüssenhop · D. Seemann · M. Hahn and L. Meiss

4.1 Introduction

Differences in leg length are a routine problem in daily orthopaedic practice. Length differences up to about 3 cm are usually compensated conservatively by using arch supports or orthopaedic shoes. Larger differences in length are treated surgically. A discontinuation of growth can, for example, be achieved by epiphysiodesis according to Phemister, and a temporary retardation of growth by clasping after Blount. Both methods are burdened by uncertainty in prognosis and the usual risks of surgical treatment. A non- or minimally invasive method would avoid or minimize the latter.

In the past, a multitude of conservative and minimally invasive methods to influence growth have been tested, e.g. arteriovenous shunts [14], venous stasis [14], interruption of epi-or metaphysial blood supply [31], sympathectomy [2, 10], obstruction of the medullary artery [6, 16], resection of the periosteum [16, 23, 29], percutaneous curettage [5] or forage [8, 22], CO_2 laser [21], electrocauterization [26], X-rays [18, 24], heat [25], cold [4], ultrasound [9], implantation of various materials [23, 34], electricity and electromagnetic fields [3, 33]. In individual cases, satisfactory results were achieved. They were, however, never prognosticable or even constantly reproducible, so that there is still no alternative to standard surgical treatment [11, 27].

Various studies have pointed out the positive effect of shock waves on the healing of bones [12, 30, 32]. As far as known, the effect of shock waves on epiphysial growth plates was first studied in 1989. Yeaman et al. directed shock waves at the proximal tibia epiphysis of 5-week-old Sprague-Dawley rats. In the rats treated, 44% showed focal shock-wave-induced dysplasia of the epiphysial growth plates, which lead to a closure of the epiphysis and a shortening of the tibia in 17% (defect >1 mm). However, a systematic study of the specific influence of shock waves on bone growth in the epiphysis has to date not been carried out. The aim of this study was to make a statement concerning possible, perhaps dose-dependent growth retardation in epiphyses due to the influence of shock waves by applying these in various doses. An early ossification of the epiphysis as a reaction to the epiphysial damage was expected [18–20, 26].

4.2 Materials and Methods

4.2.1 Selection of the Experimental Animals

Experiment 1 was carried out with 18 100-day-old and experiment 2 with 18 120-day-old White New Zealand rabbits.

The skeletal development of rabbits is very similar to that of humans, which means that the results obtained in rabbits can be well applied to humans [13].

In this study, the proximal tibia epiphysis was chosen as the target for shock wave application, because it has been studied in many other works on similar problems. The results of this study are therefore comparable with those of other studies.

The growth profile of the rabbit tibia displays a continuous strong growth up to about day 90. The growth rate then slowly decreases. The proximal and distal tibia epiphysis finally ossify between day 150 and day 225 [1, 13].

The rabbits were 100 and 120 days old at the onset of the study. The criteria for choosing this age was that the animals were still to be growing and that the epiphyses had to be wide enough to still be able to securely centre the focus of the shock waves in the epiphysis. Shock wave treatment of younger rabbits with longer remaining growth time was therefore ruled out.

Sex-specific differences in growth were avoided by choosing only females.

4.2.2 Setup of the Experimental Apparatus

The Shock Wave Generator Osteostar. The experimental system Osteostar (Siemens, Erlangen) was used for the application of the shock waves.

The Osteostar comprises a modified SIREMOBIL X-ray image conversion system coupled with a shock wave generator. Shock waves can so be applied under X-ray control.

The shock waves are generated electromagnetically. Individual shock waves are emitted and focused. They are transmitted by means of water-filled coupling bellows which can be positioned near the target. The bellows are coupled with the movable c-arc of the SIREMOBIL, which enables exact centering of the target in the focus (cf. Sect. 4.2.4). One can choose from 19 energy levels (0.08–1.20 mJ/mm^2).

Construction of a fixing Apparatus for positioning the Rabbits. It was necessary to construct a special fixing apparatus which enabled bringing the right proximal tibial epiphysial growth plate into the centre of the focus and retaining it there during application of the shock waves. The epiphysial growth plate was to be treated from the lateral direction, so as to allow capturing possible axis deformities due to shock wave application both qualitatively and quantitatively well.

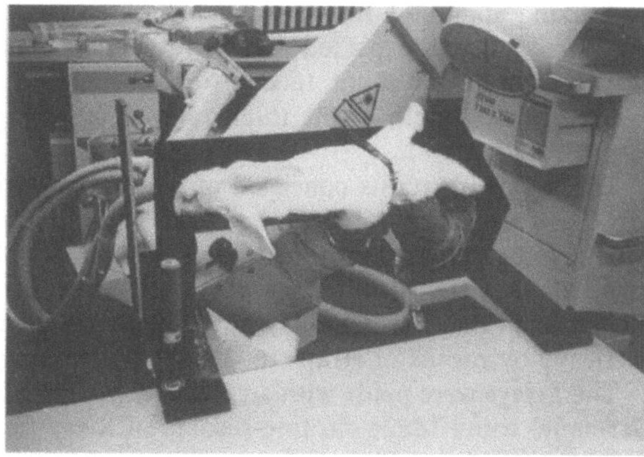

Fig. 1. Principle experimental setup (for the left hind leg). The rabbit is lying in aprone position on the fixing device; the hind leg to be treated is hanging into a water-filled tube. The hind leg is screened in the anteroposterior ray path by means of the c-arc. The shock wave head is coupled to the water-filled tube

The apparatus had to meet the following requirements:

1. Reproducible fixation of the rabbits
2. Fixation of the rabbits allowing lateral treatment of the right proximal tibial epiphysial growth plate
3. Exact positioning of the right proximal tibial epiphysial growth plate in the focus
4. Lossless transmission of the shock waves

The fixing apparatus consisted of a wooden table, under which in a corner a plexiglass tube with one open end was attached. The closed end of the plexiglass tube pointed downwards at an angle of 45° (Fig. 1).

The transmission of the shock waves from the Osteostar to the tube was to be as complete as possible. On the other hand, the tube had to be stable enough to resist the mechanical stress due to the shock waves. Therefore, a plexiglass tube with small wall thickness (3 mm) was chosen.

The rabbit was lying on the table in a prone position, so that its right hind leg protruded into the tube via an opening in the table. The left hind leg lay pointing backward to the left of the opening. The front legs were stretched forward, with the rabbit's head resting on them. Breast, behind and the left hind leg were fixed to the table by means of adjustable straps.

Distilled water was filled into the tube, whereby attention was paid that the water level was above (2–3 cm) the proximal tibial epiphysial growth plate

4.2.3
Acquisition of X-ray Images

To capture possible shock wave effects, X-ray images in the standard planes were taken. So as to be able to compare the anteroposterior X-rays of the right and left tibia, as well as the tibiae of the different age groups, with one another, the hind legs of the rabbits had to be positioned in the same way and such that the position could be reproduced. The position of the tibiae was always to be parallel to the X-ray plate, so that no projection-based errors in measurement would occur.

A fixing apparatus was constructed which could be adjusted to the growing rabbits. It was expected that there would be approximately a doubling in body weight (from about 1600 g to about 3200 g) and an increase of about 3–4 cm in the length of the thighs and tibia during the measurement period (age: 100–240 days).

The X-ray apparatus consisted of a base plate with two positioning blocks for the tibiae. The rabbits were laid with their backs on the base plate, whereby the thighs were positioned upright at the positioning blocks. The knee joints were bent at a right angle over the edge of the positioning blocks, such that the tibiae lay horizontally on them. The paws were attached vertically by means of straps to slender positioning plates.

The X-rays were made with an HOX 125 A (Fritz Hofmann GmbH, Erlangen, Germany) using 18×24 cm fine-resolution X-ray film. The distance focus–film was 74 cm and the distance focus–object (top edge of tibia) was 62 cm.

4.2.4
Definition of the Location of the Effect of the Shock Wave

The right proximal tibial epiphysial growth plate was treated from a lateral direction. The focus was centred on the middle of the growth plate.

The c-arc of the Osteostar was swivelled around its orbital axis such that the coupling bellows were exactly lateral to the growth plate (the fixing device was tilted laterally by 45°; correspondingly, the orbital adjustment of the c-arc was 45°).

The epiphysial growth plate is best represented radiologically with a ray path perpendicular to the tibia. As the tibia was directed by the fixing device at an angle of 45°, the c-arc was swivelled by the same angle around its sagittal axis. The growth plate was visible as a thin radiolucent line in this projection.

4.2.5
Test Procedure

The experiments were carried out on 18 female 100-day-old (Group 1) and 18 120-day-old (Group 2) White New Zealand rabbits. In Group 1, the right proximal tibial epiphysial growth plate was treated laterally once with 2000 level-19 (1.20 mJ/mm^2) shock waves. In Group 2, the same was treated twice with a total of 4000 level-19 (1.20 mJ/mm^2) shock waves.

One day before shock wave application the right lateral knee joint and the adjacent regions of the femur and tibia were shaved, so as to prevent an energy loss in the transmission of the shock waves due to possible inclusion of air in the fur.

After administration of anaesthesia, the rabbit was positioned in a special fixing device and the right proximal tibial epiphysial growth plate subsequently centred in the focus.

Six animals of each group were killed after 3, 6 and 12 weeks for micro- and macroscopical examination and for the making of X-ray images of all (right and left) tibiae.

The rabbits were kept individually in wire cages at a room temperature of 25°C (±5°) and an average humidity of 55 (±10)%. The day and night rhythm corresponded to the seasonal conditions, or, when necessary, was regulated by means of artificial lighting from 07:00 to 19:00.

4.2.6
Representation of the Shock Wave Effect

A disorder in the area of the proximal tibial epiphysial growth plate induced by shock wave treatment must, under the given experimental setup, lead to differences in length and/or axis deformities. To detect and quantify them, X-rays were made of the hind legs of each rabbit before and 3, 6 and 12 weeks after shock wave application. To do so, short-term anaesthesia (ketamin base, xylacin) was administered to the rabbits and then X-ray images made in the anteroposterior and mediolateral ray paths, whereby a special fixing device was used. This made it possible to position the tibiae in a redproducible fashion and thereby rendering them comparable. The anteroposterior images were made with separate cassettes, so as to avoid projection error. The lateral images were made by laying the lateral side of the hind legs on the X-ray plate. Rotation errors were avoided by extension of the paws.

To be able to detect growth deformities at all levels, the following parameters were determined radiologically:

1. Length of the tibia
2. Angle of the tibia head/shaft angle in the frontal plane
3. Angle of the tibia head/shaft angle in the sagittal plane
4. Mediolateral diameter of the tibia head
5. Anteroposterior diameter of the tibia head

The means of the right and left tibiae, respectively, were calculated for each treatment group and compared with each other using the t-test (two-sided, paired samples).

A more detailed analysis of the growth behaviour was done by determining the growth rates of the individual right and left tibiae from the X-ray images. The growth rates were calculated for the periods: shock wave application to third week after, third to sixth week and sixth to twelfth week. To do so, for example, for the parameter "length of the tibia", the linear growth of the tibia was measured after 3, 6 and 12 weeks, and from this, the difference between growth of the right tibia minus growth of the left tibia was calculated. The result was how much more or less the right tibia had grown to the left tibia within the respective period.

Finally, the morphological changes caused by the shock wave application were represented. The surface integrity of the growth plate and the adjacent portions of the epi- and metaphysis were assessed macoscopically. Morphological changes of the epiphysial growth plate were examined macroscopically, radiologically and histologically.

4.3
Results

After treatment all the rabbits had a local, sometimes extensive haematoma at the entry point of the shock waves (Fig. 2). About 30% of the animals displayed skin lesions of pinhead size in the area of the haematoma. All of these lesions healed without consequences within 14 days under local wound treatment.

The macroscopical assessment of the freshly prepared tibia heads of the animals killed after 3, 6 and 12 weeks did not bring to light any visible damage or obvious deformation on the treated side of the tibia head or tibial shaft in either in Group 1 (2000 shock waves) or in Group 2 (4000 shock waves). There was especially no development of osseous bridges visible from the exterior in any of the cases.

The analysis of the standardized X-rays did not result in any statistically significant difference in either Group 1 or Group 2 between the treated right tibiae and the left tibiae serving as comparisons for the parameters "length of the tibia, mediolateral diameter of the tibia head", "anteroposterior diameter of the tibia head" and "tibia head/shaft angle in the sagittal plane".

As concerns the parameter "tibia head/shaft angle in the frontal plane", a significant valgus deformity of the right tibia in comparison to the left before and 3 weeks after treatment was encountered in Group 1. Although valgus growth of the right and left tibia was observed during the entire period

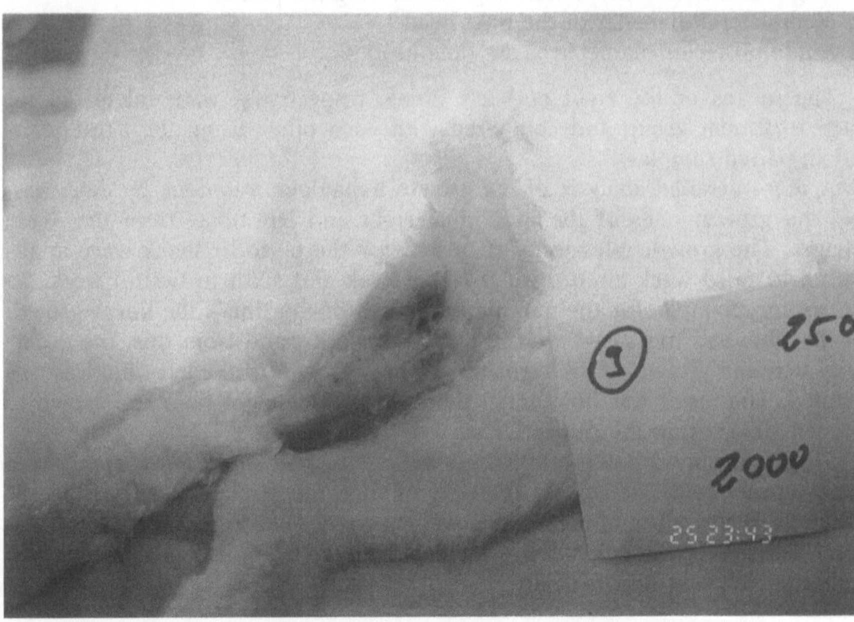

Fig. 2. Haematoma in the treated right hind leg (2000 shock waves with an intensity of 1.2 mJ/mm^2

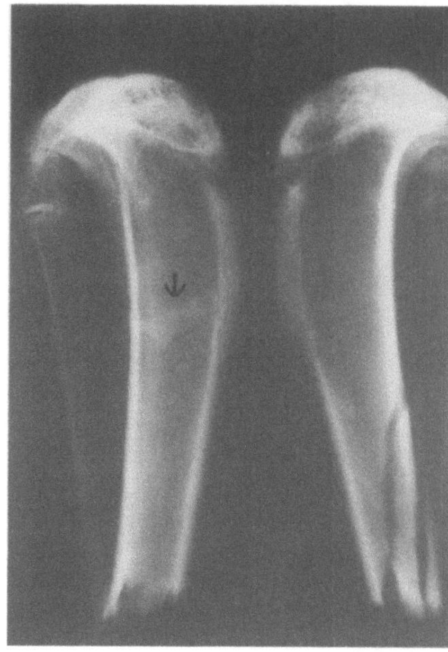

Fig. 3. Example of an ossification (arrow) spreading across the medullary cavity on the treated side 12 weeks after treatment

of observation in Group 1, a deviant varus growth of the treated right tibia was observed in 80% of the rabbits at the treated right side between the third and sixth week of observation.

Further analysis of the X-rays did not reveal any peculiarities worth mentioning in Group 1.

With regard to the absolute values, all parameters were the same on both sides in Group 2. An increase in valgus deformity as in Group 1 was not found.

On viewing the growth rates, a side-different, nonsignificant trend towards valgus growth on the right was found between time of treatment and 3 weeks after treatment. In contrast to Group 1, during the course of the experiment, an osseous structure leading across the medullary cavity of the treated right tibia was found in 8 of the 18 cases, which moved away relatively from the epiphysial growth plate during further growth (Fig. 3). Damage or obvious variations in calibre of the actual epiphysial growth plate were not found.

Histologically, it was a lamellar ossification (Figs. 4 and 5).

4.4 Discussion

The aim of this study was to investigate the possibility of nonsurgical influence on growth in epiphysial growth plates by means of shock wave therapy.

An experimental study with two groups of 18 White New Zealand rabbits each was carried out. The right proximal tibial epiphysial growth plate of the animals in Group 1 was treated laterally once with 2000 shock waves of 1.20

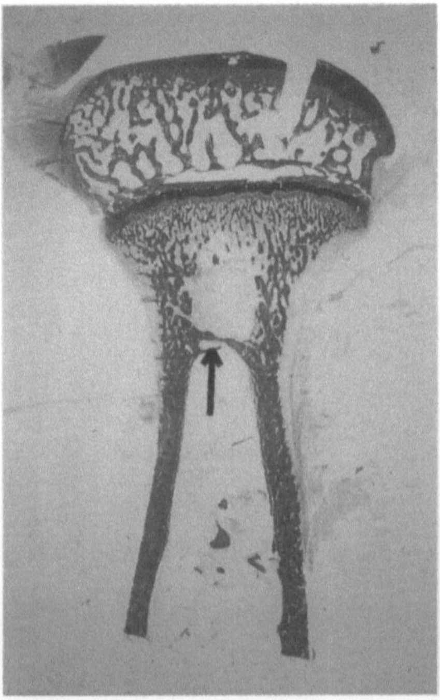

4

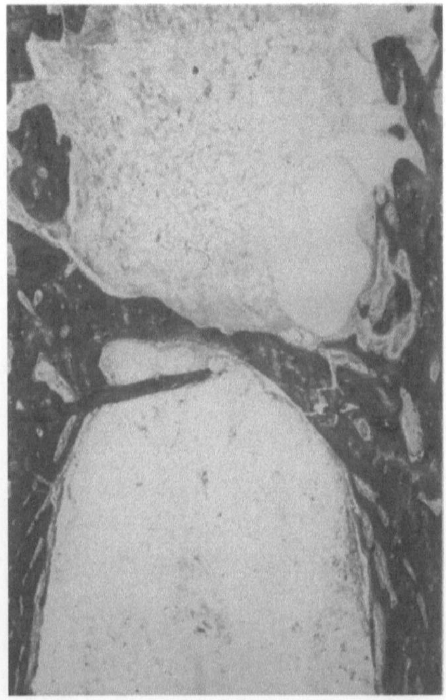

5

Fig. 4. Histological preparation of the right proximal tibial epiphysial growth plate 6 weeks after treatment, not decalcified, toluidine blue stain, lens magnification. In the shock wave path, an ossification (arrow) across the medullary cavity is visible, which has moved relative to the intact epiphysial growth plate in the distal direction

Fig. 5. The same preparation as in Fig. 4 in threefold magnification. This is a lamellar ossification

mJ/mm^2. In Group 2, the animals received 2000 shock waves of 1.20 mJ/mm^2 in each of two sessions 14 days apart.

The effect of the shock waves was represented by means of X-ray images in two planes 3, 6 and 12 weeks after treatment. The image objects were measured (length of the tibia, tibia head/shaft angle in the frontal and sagittal plane, anteroposterior and mediolateral diameter of the tibia head) and the treated epiphysial growth plate examined radiologically and macroscopically with regard to shock-wave-induced morphological changes. Each left tibia was used for reference.

In Group 1, although valgus growth of the right and left tibia prevailed throughout the entire period of observation, a deviant varus growth of the treated right tibia was observed in 80% of the animals between week 3 and week 6. The growth deviation was below statistical significance, allowing only to speak of a trend. A corresponding trend to increased valgus growth was observed in Group 2 within the first 3 weeks after treatment.

The observed effect in Group 1 appears to be caused by a partial stimulation of growth of the lateral portion of the epiphysial growth plate by shock wave treatment. Interface effects of the shock waves at the interface cartilage-bone in the lateral portion of the epiphysial growth plate, as well as a pronounced perifocal haematoma at the entry point of the shock waves into the lower leg (lateral), may have caused an increase in blood supply and a subsequent stimulation of growth of the lateral epiphysial growth plate.

Shock-wave-induced influence on the growth with regard to the other parameters was not observed. Furthermore, no radiologically or macroscopically evident changes in the treated epiphysial growth plate were found at any time.

This was different in Group 2. In addition to a trend towards increased valgus growth within the first 3 weeks after treatment, an ossification in the medullary cavity, which ran across in the direction of shock wave application, was found in 8 rabbits. These changes moved away relative to the epiphysial growth plate with growth and were classified as cicratrization within the medullary cavity.

The intended effect of a bridge developing over the epiphysial growth plate was not achieved with the shock wave doses applied here. Even a partial injury near the growth plate, as is assumed with respect to the changes observed in Group 2, does not lead to greater growth disturbances. A dose-dependent influence of epiphysial growth plates due to shock waves is assumed. Whether this effect can lead to growth manipulation with higher doses remains to be seen.

References

1. Alberius P (1986) The correlation between craniofacial and long-bone growth: an experimental investigation in normal bones. Am J Anat 177:519–525
2. Barr JS, Stinchfield AJ, Reidy JA (1950) Sympathic ganglioectomy and limb length in polymyelitis. J Bone Joint Surg 32A:793–802
3. Becker OR, Sparado JA, Marino AA (1977) Clinical experiences with low-intensity direct-current stimulation of bone growth. Clin Orthop 124:75–83
4. Bierens de Haan B, et al. (1986) The effects of cold upon bone growth: a preliminary study. Ann Plast Surg 16(6):509–515
5. Bowen J, Johnson WJ (1984) Percutaneous epiphsiodesis. Clin Orthop 190:170–173
6. Brookes M (1957) Femoral growth after occlusion of the principle nutrient canal in day-old rabbits. J Bone Joint Surg 39B:563–571
7. Broughten NS, Dickens DRV, Cole WG, Menelaus MB (1989) Epiphysiolysis for partial growth arrest. J Bone Joint Surg 71:13–16
8. Canale ST, Russel TA, Holcomb RL (1986) Percutaneous epiphysiodesis: experimental study and preliminary clinical results. J Pediatr Orthop 6:150
9. Duarte LR (1983) The stimulation of bone growth by ultrasound. Arch Orthop Trauma Surg 101:153
10. Goetz RH, Toit JG du, Swart BH (1955) Vascular changes in poliomyelitis and the effect of sympathectomy on bone growth. Acta Med Scand Suppl 306:56–83
11. Grill F, Chochole M, Schultz A (1990) Beckenschiefstand und Beinlängendifferenzen. Orthopäde 19:244–262
12. Haupt G, Haupt A, Ekkernkamp A, Gerety B, Chvapil M (1992) Influence of shock waves on fracture healing. J Urol 6:529–532
13. Heikel HVA (1960) On ossification and growth of certain bnes of the rabbit, with a comparison of the skeletal age in the rabbit and in man. Acta Orthop Scand 29:171–184
14. Keck SW, Kelly PJ (1965) The effect of venous stasis on intraosseous pressure and longitudinal bone growth in the dog. J Bone Joint Surg 47A:539–544
15. Kember NF (1960) Cell division in endochondral ossification: a study of cell proliferation in rat bones by the method of tritiated thymidine autoradiography. J Bone Joint Surg 42B:824

16. Kuijpers-Jagtman AM, Bex JHM, Maltha JC, Daggers JG (1988) Longitudinal growth of the rabbit femur after vascular and periosteal interference. Anat Anz Jena 167:349–358
17. Langenskiöld A, Edgren W (1950) Imitation of chondrodysplasia by localized roentgten ray injury – an experimental study of bone growth. Acta Chir Scand 99:353–373
18. Langenskiöld A, et al. (1989) Regeneration of the growth plate. Acta Anat 134:113–123
19. Lee EH, Gao GX (1993) Management of partial growth arrest. Physis, fat or silastic. J Pediatr Orthop 13:368–372
20. Mäkelä EA, Vainnionpää S, Vihtonen K, Mero M, Rokkanen P (1988) The effect of trauma to the lower femoral epiphysial plate. J Bone Joint Surg (Br) 70B:187–191
21. Morein G, Gassner S, Kaplan I (1978) Bone growth alterations resulting from application of CO_2-laser beam to the epiphysial growth plates. Acta Orthop Scand 49:244–248
22. Ogilvie JW (1986) Epiphysiodesis: evaluation of a new technique. J Pediatr Orthop 6:147
23. Pease CN (1952) Local stimulation of growth of long bones. J Bone Joint Surg 34A:1–24
24. Phillips RD, Kimeldorf DJ (1966) Age and dose of bone growth retardation induced by X-irridation. Radiol Res 27:384–396
25. Ring PA, Lee J (1958) The effect of heat upon the growth of bone. J Pathol Bact 75:405
26. Rosen MA, Beer Kj, Wiater JP, Davidson DD (1990) Epiphysiodesis by electrocautery in the rabbit and dog. Clin Orthop 256:244–253
27. Saxer U, Simunovic V (1975) Möglichkeiten des operativen Beinlängenausgleichs. Ther Umsch 32(5):306–311
28. Silverskiöld N (1934) Über Längenwachstum der Knochen und Transplantation von Epiphysenscheiben. Acta Chir Scand 75:77
29. Solá CK, Silberman FS, Cabrini RI (1963) Stimulation of the longitudinal growth of long bones by periosteal stripping. J Bone Joint Surg 45A:1679–1684
30. Sukul K, Johannes EJ, Pierik EGJM, Eijck GJWM van, Kristelijn MB (1993) The effect of high-energy shock waves focused on cortical bone: an invitro study. J Surg Res 54:46–51
31. Trueta J, Amato VP (1960) The vascular contribution to osteogenesis. J Bone Joint Surg 42B:571–587
32. Valchanou VD, Michailov P (1991) High-energy shock waves in the treatment of delayed nonunion of fractures. Int Orthop (SICOT) 15:181–184
33. Roermund PM van, et al. (1991) Bone growth and remodeling after distraction epiphysiolysis of the proximal tibia of the rabbit. Clin Orthop 266:304–312
34. Wilson CL, Percy EC (1956) Experimental studies of the epiphysial stimulation. J Bone Joint Surg 38A:1097–1104
35. Yeaman LD, Jerome CP, McCullough DL (1988) Effects of shock waves on the structure and growth of the immature rat epiphysis. J Urol 10:670–672

CHAPTER 5

Osteorestoration via Shock Wave Application. A new Possibility of Treating Disturbed Bone Union

J. Haist

Abstract. The so-called osteorestoration via shock wave application is a relatively new method in the treatment of disturbed fracture healing. To date 62 areas in 60 patients with a diagnosis of pseudo-arthrosis have been treated. The results have been surprisingly good, whereby a dependence on the kind of pseudo-arthrosis has been observed. Indications and contra-indications can be specified from the experience in application.

5.1 Introduction

Despite increasing optimization of the conservative, and especially surgical treatment of fractures, delayed bone union up to therapy-refractory pseudo-arthrosis still represents a typical, albeit rare complication in some fractures.

Treatment of disturbed osseus healing is still based to a great extent on operative methods, such as freshening of the fracture ends, autogenous or homologous spongiosaplasty and osteosynthetic stabilization.

For the patient, this means another operation with all its possible complications.

Often the local soft-tissue situation limits the manner of operative intervention.

In conservative treatment, one is faced with the dilemma of long-term, sometimes month-long immobilization of the extremity with the well-known negative effects on cartilage, mineralization of the bone and movability of the joint. So-called functional treatments with special orthotic devices mean long-term therapy for the patient and often fail due to the lack of compliance of the patient.

In the past two decades, it has often been tried to influence fracture healing in various ways.

First of all, there were physical methods, especially the application of electromagnetic forces, which were used in the osteogenesis (Bassett 1984; Kraus 1984; Paterson et al. 1977; Werhan 1991). It is under discussion that the process considered osteogenetic mostly takes place on the cellular level (Kraus 1984; Werhan 1991).

Since the beginning of the 1980s extracorporeal shock wave treatment, or for short, lithotripsy, of gallstones and especially kidney stones has become an established therapy (Chaussy et al. 1984; Forssmann et al. 1977).

It is estimated that more than 2,000,000 patients worldwide have undergone this therapy. The minimal invasiveness and lack of complications in this treatment has pushed surgical stone therapy more and more into the background, the latter now being restricted to special indications.

Due to the small stress for the patient, lithotripsy is nowadays favoured as an outpatient treatment.

In the past 10 years, three physically different principles have been used to generate extracorporeal shock waves.

The machines of the last generation generate the shock waves via electromagnetic systems which transmit an electromagnetic impulse by sudden activation of a metal membrane. The shock wave is transmitted via an internal water-filled lead, focused by means of an acoustic lense and coupled to the patient by a flexible membrane.

The electromagnetic shock wave systems have in the meantime established themselves in the field of lithotripsy. The various machines of the big manufacturers (Siemens, Storz, Dornier, HTM and Philips) differ only in marginal physical characteristics.

The positive influence of extracorporeal shock waves on osteogenesis in the sense of an increased callus formation has already been described in earlier, partly experimental and partly clinical works (Ekkernkamp et al. 1992; Graff 1989; Haupt 1990; Schleberger and Senge 1992).

5.2 Patients and Methods

Since January 1991, 62 pseudo-arthroses with various locations in 60 patients were treated with shock waves.

All of the patients had either undergone unsuccessful surgery several times or had been treated conservatively over a long period, whereby the last operation had been carried out at least 6 months before. In correspondence with the clinical frequency, tibial pseudo-arthroses were by far the most often treated cases (38). The other locations were distributed nearly ubiquitously:

Radius in 4 cases
Mid- and proximal femur in 7 cases
Subcapitular humerus in 2 cases
Metatarsal bone in 3 cases
Navicular bone in 8 cases

A prerequisite for osteorestoration is analgesia, which is carried out corresponding to the location either as IV regional, 3-in-1 block, peridural anaesthesia or insufflation anaesthesia.

The machines used were: an experimental machine by Siemens called Osteostar (Fig. 1), a series model typically used in urology called Lithostar (Siemens) and, for four tibial pseudo-arthroses, a mobile machine typically used in athopaedics called Minilith (Storz).

Depending on the size of the area to be treated, between 2000 and 10200 pulses of various energies were applied, whereby it was undertaken to make use of the submaximal available energy between 0.25 and 1.2 mJ/mm^2.

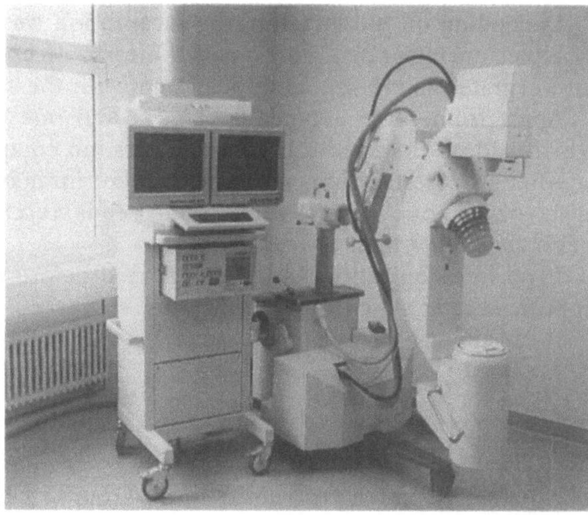

Fig. 1. Osteostar by Siemens

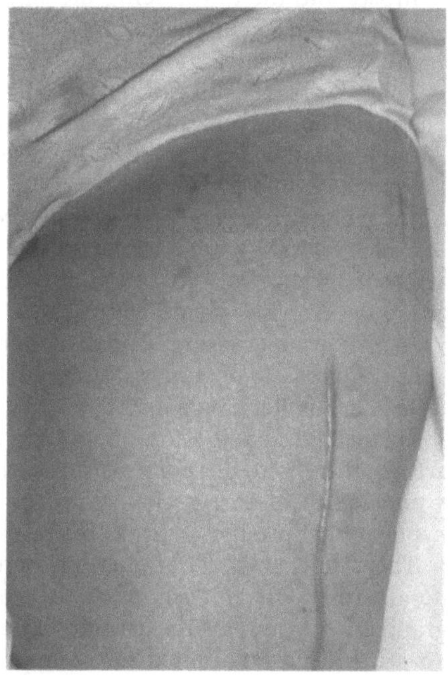

Fig. 2. Small haematoma after high energy shock wave therapy

The fracture ends were treated with 300 pulses each at a distance of 1 cm. The fissure itself was subsequently treated, also at a distance of 1 cm, whereby the shock waves were applied with an angle of incidence of approximately 30°. Additionally, 200 pulses of the energy level used were applied at a distance of 1 X-ray-cm to supposedly intact periosteum about 1.5 cm distal and proximal of the fissure.

Depending on the location, the localization was carried out with the help of either an integrated c-arc or, if the form of pseudo-arthrosis allowed, via an integrated inline sonographic system with the sector scan technique.

Apart from some cutaneous (Fig. 2) and one extensive deep haematoma which had no therapeutical consequences, no complications were observed.

After osteorestoration, all patients were immobilized with various plaster casts or orthotic devices until an osseous reaction was proven; however, never for longer than 8 weeks.

If no immobilization had been effected before treatment, this regime was continued after shock wave application.

X-ray controls were carried out at periods of 2–4 weeks.

5.3 Results

The patients were classified in three groups. The first group consisted of posttraumatic pseudo-arthroses, the second of postoperative pseudo-arthroses and the third, being the smallest group to date, of special cases.

In addition, a differentiation between hypertrophic and atrophic pseudo-arthroses was made.

There were 48 successful therapies as opposed to 14 unsuccessful ones. The duration of bone union was on average 34 days.

Bone union was observed in 24 cases with 26 areas in the group with post-traumatic pseudo-arthroses ($N = 33$). Osteorestoration had no effect in 9 cases. All of the failures were from the subgroup of atrophic pseudo-arthroses.

Osteorestoration was successful in 18 cases of the postoperative pseudo-arthroses group ($N = 23$). Here also, the failures ($N = 5$) belonged to the sub-group of atrophic pseudo-arthroses.

In the group of special cases, there was one success (fibrous dysplasia) and 3 failures. Two patients suffered from osteogenesis imperfecta and one from morbus Recklinghausen.

Further differentiation between atrophic and hypertrophic pseudo-arthroses leads to 12 failures in the group of atrophic pseudo-arthroses with a population of 15 patients. With the exception of 2 cases, all patients with hypertrophic pseudo-arthroses were treated successfully.

The criterion of differentiation between atrophic and hypertrophic pseudo-arthrosis was not so much the conventional X-ray image as the scintigraphic behaviour of the pseudo-arthrosis. Considerably accumulating pseudo-arthroses were allotted to the hypertrophic group, whereas little or no accumulation lead to allotment to the atrophic group.

A residual vitality of the pseudo-arthrosis thus appears to be an important prerequisite for the success of the method.

5.4 Cases

1. A 38-year-old patient who had undergone pendulum osteotomy of the left tibia in July 1991 (Fig. 3a). Due to the absence of bone union, shock wave

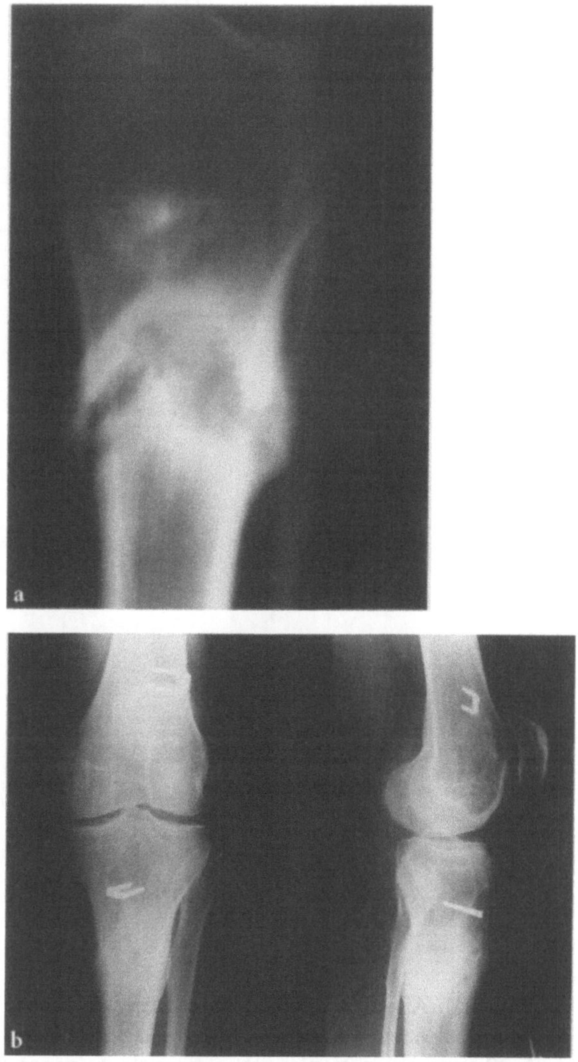

Fig. 3a, b. a Tibial pseudo-arthrosis, 7 months after surgical treatment, **b** 6 weeks after shock wave therapy complete bone consolidation

therapy was carried out 7 months later. Complete bone union was achieved within 6 weeks (Fig. 3b).
Technical data: Osteostar, 4100 pulses at 0.96 mJ/mm^2.

2. A 41-year-old patient who had undergone a valgus correction osteotomy of the right tibia in March 1990. No adequate ossification was observable by September 1991, so that osteorestoration was carried out (Fig. 4a). Within 10 weeks, complete ossification was achieved (Fig. 4b).
Technical data: Osteostar, 3600 pulses at 0.90 mJ/mm^2.
3. A 47-year-old patient with radius pseudo-arthrosis persisting for more than 7 months. Shock wave therapy was carried out in December 1991 (Fig. 5a). After only 5 weeks, a significant osseous reaction was observed

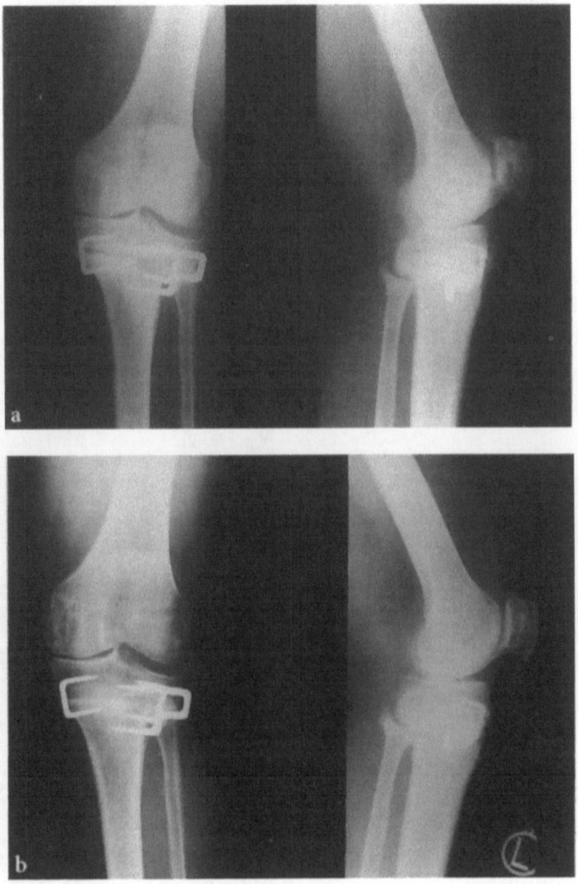

Fig. 4a,b. a Pseudo arthrosis 9 months after tibia osteotomy, **b** 10 weeks after shock wave complete bone consolidation

(Fig. 5b). After 10 weeks, the fracture was completely ossified (Fig. 5c). Technical data: Osteostar, 2900 pulses at 0.90 mJ/mm^2.

4. A 29-year-old patient with a persistent (more than 12 months) navicular pseudo-arthrosis, although extensive conservative treatment had been carried out. Shock wave therapy was undertaken in January 1996 (Fig. 6a). Bone union was observed 8 weeks later (Fig. 6b).
Technical data: Minilith, 4100 pulses at 0.25 mJ/mm^2.

5.5 Discussion

On the background of rapid developments in medicine and technology attempts are being made to replace surgical treatment by nonivasive methods.

Osteorestoration via shock wave application is a nonivasive method for treatment of disturbed bone union.

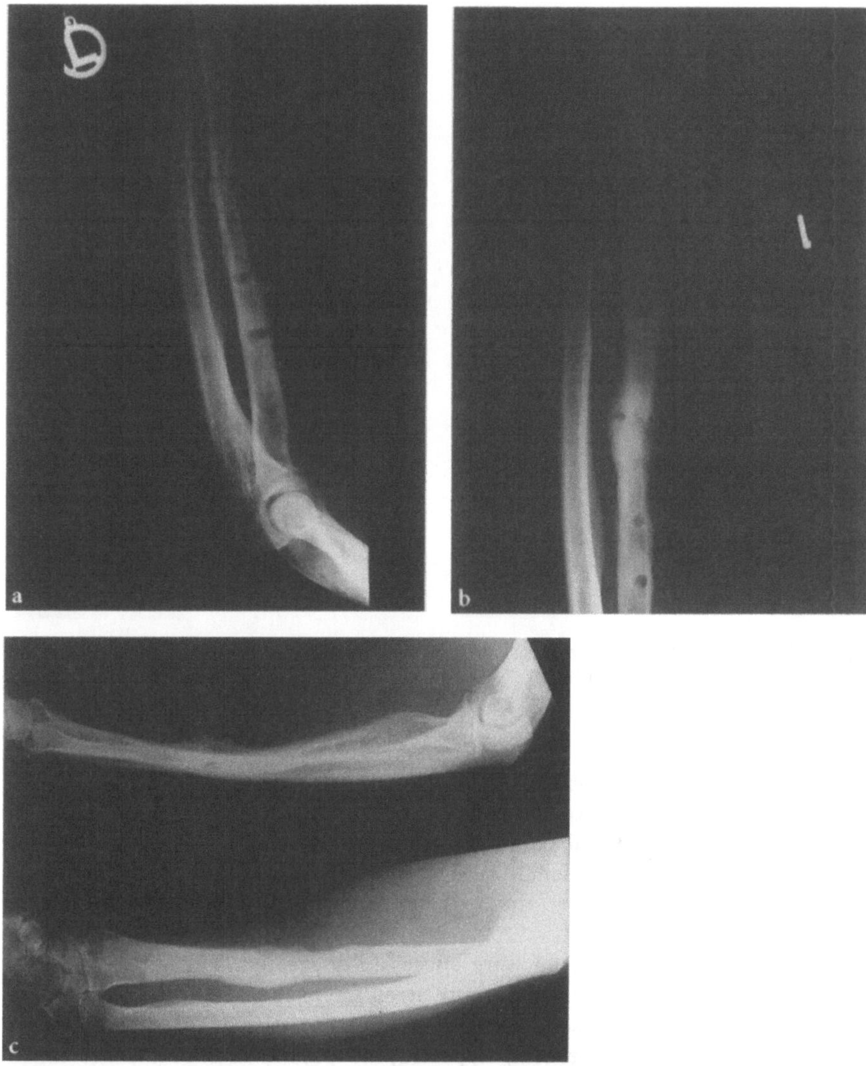

Fig. 5 a–c. **a** 7 months old radius pseudo-arthrosis of the naviculare bone, **b** 8 weeks after shock wave therapy complete bone consolidation

Other authors have already proven the positive effect of shock waves on osteogenesis (Ekkernkamp et al. 1992; Graff 1989; Haupt et al. 1990; Valtschanov et al. 1989).

As concerns the biological effect of shock waves on the bone, there are various hypotheses (Graff 1989; Lingemann et al. 1989; Schleberger and Senge 1992).

Schleberger and Senge (1992) discuss the possibility of a transformation of local connective-tissue cells and as an alternative angiogenesis with callus formation similar to the normal behaviour in fractures.

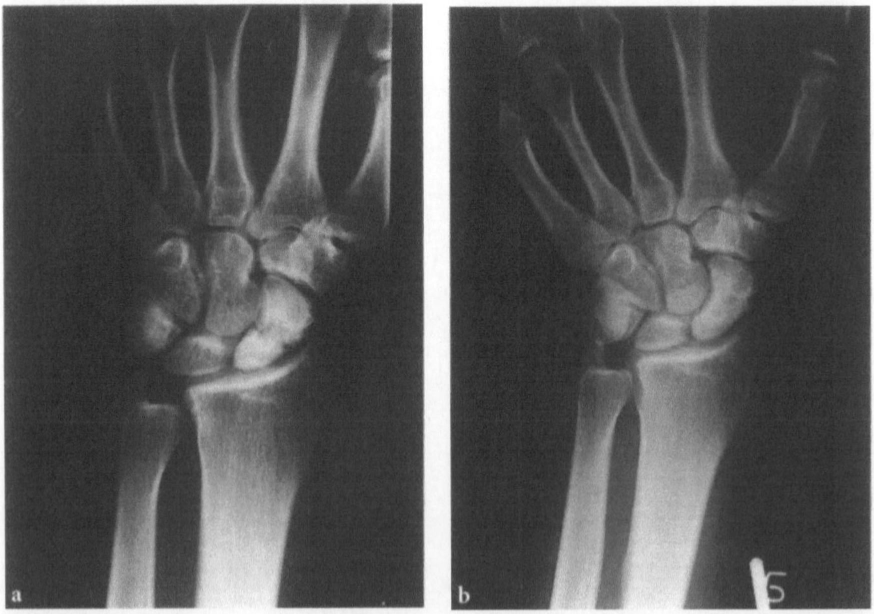

Fig. 6. a 12 months old pseudo-arthrosis of the naviculare bone, **b** 8 weeks after shock wave therapy complete bone consolidation

The simultaneous occurrence of osteosynthesis does not constitute a contra-indication after the experiments we have carried out, as a loosening of the osteosynthetic material could be ruled out, even when high-frequencies were applied (Haist and Reichel (1991)).

Our results clearly show the extraordninarily positive effect of shock waves on bone union.

Of 62 pseudo-arthroses, 48 were successfully treated. The total of 14 failures were mostly from the subgroup atrophic pseudo-arthroses. Only two scintigraphically active pseudo-arthroses did not display ossification after shock wave therapy. In general, hypertrophic pseudo-arthroses react much better and faster to osteorestoration than atrophic pseudo-arthroses.

A disproportionately high number of failures (three of four) occurred in the group of special cases. Therefore, it appears that an intact osseous potential is a prerequisite for the success of osteorestoration. The effects of shock waves in connective tissue were impressively demonstrated in an animal model with induced delayed wound healing (Haupt and Chvapil 1990). Here, the epithelization of the induced wound was considerably greater after shock wave application than in the group subjected to conventional wound healing. The stimulation of the epithelization was observed as dose-dependent when applying low energies. The effects manifest themselves in an increase in granulation and vascularization.

The advantages of osteorestoration as compared to the established methods are obvious. On the one hand, the patient is not subjected to the stress of an operation, and on the other hand, long terms of immobilization can be considerably shortened.

Of course, the patients treated to date constitute an inhomogeneous group as such, so that final conclusions do not appear permissible.

Haist et al. (1992), Sukul et al. (1992) and Valchanov et al. (1989) describe dose-dependent defects in the cortical layer and spongiosa with microfractures and the development of small perifocal haematomas. These are factors which promote osteoneogenesis in the sense of new or increased callus formation.

In our histological preparations, we found dose-dependent corticospongy defects and microfractures in the treated fracture ends.

The changes in fat marrow described by Braun et al. (1992) were not observed by us.

One indication for osteorestoration in our view are patients with posttraumatic pseudo-arthroses, who have been operated unsuccessfully several times or have undergone unsuccessful conservative therapy. A special case is navicular pseudo-arthrosis, which is treated after failure of conservative therapy. Osteorestoration is also indicated for patients who develop pseudo-arthrosis postoperatively, e.g. after corrective osteotomies or arthrodeses.

Pseudo-arthroses in fibrous dysplasia, osteogenesis imperfecta and morbus Recklinghausen constitute special cases of application (Table 1).

In addition to universally valid contra-indications such as pregnancy, blood coagulation diseases and intake of immunosuppressive agents, specific contra-indications are infected and unstable pseudo-arthroses. In such cases, the therapy of choice is surgery. Following Schleberger and Senge (1992) and Yeaman et al. (1989), shock wave application to pseudo-arthroses in the vicinity of the epiphysis in the growing years appears to us to be contra-indi-

Table 1. Contra-indications for osteorestoration

1. Infected pseudo-arthroses
2. Unstable pseudo-arthroses
   - insufficient immobilization
   - lack of / insufficient osteosteosynthesis
3. Pseudo-arthrosis near epiphysis in children
4. Pseudo-arthrosis near joints

Table 2. Indications for osteorestoration

1. Posttraumatic pseudo-arthroses
   - several unsuccessful operations / conservative treatments
   - special case: navicular pseudo-arthrosis
2. Postoperative pseudo-arthroses
   - corrective osteotomies:
1. tibia
2. femur
   - delayed bone union
   - arthrodeses
3. Special cases
   - pseudo-arthrosis in fibrous dysplasia
   - pseudo-arthrosis in osteogenesis imperfecta
   - pseudo-arthrosis in morbus Recklinghausen

cated, because of possible damage to the latter. Pseudo-arthroses in the vicinity of joints are not treated due to the possible damage to the subchondral lamella. In the case of pathological fractures, osteorestoration should not be undertaken. Here, there is the possibility of opening vessels near tumours which could give rise to intravascular spread of tumour cells (Table 2). Notwithstanding the ongoing discussion and experimental and clinical research concerning the mode of action and the range of indications for osteorestoration, the principle of this undoubtedly careful and possible effective method should be noted.

One aspect concerning the application of a new method of treatment of disturbed bone union is certainly the proof of cause and effect. However, no mode of action has yet been defined in osteorestoration. Due to the increasing number of patients treated, new insights can be expected in the near future.

References

1. Bassett CAL (1984) The development and application of pulsed electromagnetic (PEMFs) for ununited fractures and arthrodeses. Orthop Clin North Am 15:61
2. Braun W, Claes L, Rüter A, Paschke D (1992) Einfluß von Stoßwellen auf die Festigkeit des Verbundes von Knochen und Polymethyl-Methacrylat. Z Orthop 130:236
3. Chaussy W, Schmiedt E, Jocham D (1984) Extracorporeal shock wave lithotripsy (ESWL) for treatment of urolithiasis. Urology: 59
4. Dahmen PD, Meiss L, Nam VC, Franke R, Gonchars V (1993) Neue Wege in der Schmerztherapie – Einsatz der extrakorporalen Stoßwellentherapie (ESWT) zur Behandlung von knochennahen Schmerzen und Weichteilschmerzen. Special publication of the presentation by Dr. Dahmen at the DGOT Congress, Munich, Germany
5. Dahmen PD, Meiss L, Nam VC, Skruodies B (1992) Extrakorporale Stoßwellentherapie (ESWT) im knochennahen Weichteilbereich an der Schulter. Extr Orthop 11:25–27
6. Ekkernkamp A, Bosse A, Haupt G, Pommer A (1992) Der Einfluß der extrakorporalen Stoßwellen auf die standardisierte Tibiafraktur am Schaf. In: Ittel TH, Siebert HG, Mathias HH (Eds) Aktuelle Aspekte der Osteologie. Springer, Berlin Heidelberg New York, pp 307
7. Forssmann B, Hepp W, Chaussy W (1977) Eine Methode zur berührungsfreien Zertrümmerung von Nierensteinen durch Stoßwellen. Biomed Tech 22:164
8. Graff J (1989) Die Wirkung hochenergetischer Stoßwellen auf Knochen und Weichteilgewebe. Habilitation thesis, Ruhr Universität Bochum, Germany
9. Haist J, Reichel W (1991) Einsatz der ESWL bei der osteosynthetisch versorgten Pseudarthrose. Eine experimentelle Studie. Lecture given at 40th Annual Meeting of the Northwest German Orthopaedists, Cologne, Germany
10. Haist J, Reichel W (1991) Die Stoßwellenbehandlung der pathologisch verzögerten Frakturheilung. Erste klinische Erfahrungen. Lecture given at the 3rd Symposium of the Orthopaedic University Hospitals Erfurt and Mainz, Mainz, Germany
11. Haist J, Ziegler P (1991) Shock wave therapy of pathologically disturbed fracture healing. An alternative to surgical treatment. Bilateral Czechoslovak-German Symposium on Clinical and Experimental Orthopaedics, Prague, Czechoslovakia
12. Haist J, Rumler F, Witzsch U, Burger RA, Heine J (1992) Die extrakorporale Stoßwellenbehandlung als Therapie der gestörten Bruchheilung und Pseudarthrosenbildung nach kniegelenksnahen Umstellungsoperationen. Symposium Gonarthrose, Nürnberg, Germany
13. Haist J, Reichel W, Witzsch U, Bürger RA (1992) Die extracorporale Stoßwellentherapie. Eine Möglichkeit der Behandlung der gestörten Frakturheilung. Lecture given at 41st Annual Meeting of the Northwest German Orthopaedists, Cologne, Germany
14. Haist J, Steeger D, Witzsch U, Bürger RA, Haist U (1992) The extracorporeal shock wave therapy in the treatment of disturbed bone union. 7th International Conference on Biomechanical Engineering, Singapore, Malaysia

15. Haist J, Steeger-Keitz D von (1994) Die Stoßwellentherapie der Epicondylopathia radialis et ulnaris. Ein neues Behandlungskonzept knochennaher Weichteilschmerzen. Special publication for German Congress of Orthopaedists, Wiesbaden, Germany
16. Haupt G, Haupt A, Gerety B, Chvapil M (1990) Enhancement of fracture healing with extracorporeal shock waves. Lecture given at AUA Annual Meeting, New Orleans, La.
17. Haupt G, Chvapil M (1990) Effects of shock waves on the healing of partial-thickness wounds in piglets. J Surg Res 49:45
18. Kraus W (1984) Magnetfeldtherapie und magnetisch induzierte Elektrostimulation in der Orthopädie. Orthopäde 13:78
19. Lingemann JE, McAteer JA, Kempson FA, Evon AP (1989) Bioeffects of extracorporeal shock wave lithotripsy. Endurology 1:89
20. Paterson DC, Carter RF, Maxwell GM, Hillier TM, Ludbrook J, Savage JP (1977) Electrical bone growth stimulation in an experimental model of delayed union. Lancet 181:1278
21. Schleberger R, Senge T (1992) Nichtinvasive Behandlung diaphysärer Pseudarthrosen mit der Stoßwelle (ESWL). In: Ittel TH, Siebert HG, Mathias HH (Eds) Aktuelle Aspekte der Osteologie. Springer, Berlin Heidelberg New York, pp 311
22. Sukul Kaulesar DMKS, Johannes EJ, Pierik EGJM, Eick GJM van, Kristelijn MJE (1992) The effect of shock wave application on bones: an in vitro study. J Surg Res 53
23. Valchanov V, Michailov P, Patrashkov T (1989) New possibilities of high-energy shock waves for treatment of disturbed bone union. Poster World Congress on ESWL and Endurology, Kyoto, Japan
24. Valchanov V, Michailov P (1991) High-energy shock waves in the treatment of delayed and nonunion of fractures. Int Orthop (SICOT 15:181
25. Werhan C (1991) Biophysikalische Grundlagen der Anwendung zur Beeinflussung der Osteogenese. Z Orthop 129:118
26. Yeaman LD, Jerome CP, McCullough DL (1989) Effects of shock waves on the structure and growth of the immature rat epiphysis. J Urol 141:670

CHAPTER 6

Extracorporeal Shock Waves in the Treatment of Pseudarthrosis, Tendinosis Calcarea of the Shoulder, and Calcaneal Spur

R. Diesch · G. Haupt

6.1 Introduction

The introduction of extracorporeal shock waves for the treatment of urolithiasis revolutionized urinary stone therapy [1, 2]. Further applications have included stones elsewhere in the body, such as gall bladder, pancreas, and salivary glands [3–5]. We have evaluated the effect on shock waves on wound and fracture healing in experimental models since 1986 and confirmed for the first time the osteogenetic potential of shock waves [6–8].

The lack of a fracture to heal within 6 months defines pseudarthrosis [9]. Some 0.5%–10% of bone fractures become pseudarthrosis [10]. Often a combination of soft tissue and bone lesions hinder the healing processes. The standard therapy of pseudarthrosis is (re-)osteosynthesis with spongiosa plastic; many patients must undergo repeated surgeries, with a consequently increased risk of infection and operative failure.

Due to the osteogenetic potential of shock waves we tested their effect in the treatment of pseudarthrosis. In addition, since 1993 we have treated tendinosis calcarea of the shoulder and plantar calcaneal spur based on shock wave effects on soft tissue described by others [11–13]. These soft tissue diseases are often associated with continuous pain both with and without activity.

6.2 Material and Methods

A total of 172 consecutive patients with pseudarthrosis were treated by extracorporeal shock waves. Each patient had had at least one unsuccessful surgical attempt to treat pseudarthrosis and was scheduled for repeat surgery. There were 57 women and 115 men; the mean age was 41±15.4 years (range 7–79 years).

Only patients with hyper- or oligotrophic pseudarthrosis were included; the indication for spongiosa plastic was mandatory. Patients were excluded if they suffered from atrophic or infected pseudarthosis, if there was a large defect (>6 mm), or if it they had a pseudarthrosis of the os naviculare. General contraindications were blood coagulation disorders, pregnancy, and tumor-related pseudarthrosis or lung tissue in the shock wave focal area.

Of the 172 cases of pseudarthrosis 142 were posttraumatic, and 30 had developed after osteotomy. There were 33 cases at upper extremities (humerus 14, forearm 18, hand 1) and 139 at lower extremities (femur 36, lower leg 65, foot 38).

We treated 199 patients with therapy-resistant tendinosis calcarea and 48 with plantar calcaneal spur by means of extracorporeal shock waves. The mean duration of pain before treatment was 39 months; all patients suffered from pain with and without activity. All patients with tendinosis calcarea had radiologically visible calcfications in the rotatory cuff. Follow-up was conducted with a patient questionnaire including a visual analog scale for pain and activity of daily life.

Shock wave treatments were performed with 2000–3000 shock waves at an energy density in the focal area of 0.30–0.35 mJ/mm^2 for pseudarthrosis and 800–1000 shock waves at up to 0.20 mJ/mm^2 for soft tissue treatments. For shock wave generation an Ossatron (HMT, Switzerland), MFL 5000 (Philips, Germany), or Compact S (Dornier, Germany) was used. An integrated expandable water cushion with synthetic membrane was used for coupling in each device. Positioning of the area of interest in the focus was X-ray guided with a C-arm. In 122 patients we administered a single treatment, in 40 two treatments, and in 10 three treatments. The majority were treated under general anesthesia.

After shock wave therapy all pseudarthroses were stabilized with a cast or brace if no internal or external osteosynthetic stabilization had been performed earlier. The patients were followed clinically and radiologically.

6.3 Results

Patients with tendinosis calcarea had a mean of 2.2 shock wave treatments, and those with calacaneal spur had 1.8. We were able to follow-up 78% of patients.

Subjective treatment results are summarized in Table 1. Complete radiological consolidation was shown by 66% of the pseudarthrosis patients after shock wave treatment: 72% in those with posttraumatic pseudarthrosis and 43% in those with pseudarthrosis after osteotomy. The rate of healing depended on the location of the pseudarthrosis; pseudarthroses at the lower extremity had a higher success rate.

The only complications observed were intracutaneous hematomas, which are know from urology to accompany extracorporeal shock wave treatment.

Table 1. Results of subjective evaluation

	Tendinosis calcarea		Calcaneal spur	
	n	%	*n*	%
Completely satisfied	128	64	32	66
Satisfied	41	20	7	14
Not satisfied	26	13	9	18

6.4 Discussion

The effects of shock wave on bony tissue were investigated by Graff and coworkers as early as 1986 in a study on the side effects of shock waves on tissues during shock wave treatment of ureteral and renal stones. They performed transmission measurements both in vitro and in vivo in pigs, rabbits, and beagle dogs. Bleeding and necrosis as in a blunt trauma were seen at 48 h, followed by aseptic bone marrow necrosis, and osteocyte damage, and osteoneogenesis. This represented the physiology of fracture healing without preexisting fracture [11, 14–16]. Our own study of the effect that shock waves have on fracture healing also revealed osteoneogenesis, thus stimulating fracture healing by shock waves [6, 8]. This effect was verified in a standardized fracture model [17–20]. Johannes et al. have reported similar results [21]. A pseudarthrosis model showed healing to be enhanced by shock waves [22]. Other experiments using lower energies, however, have not demonstrated shock wave induced osteoneogenesis [23, 24].

The first clinical data on the treatment of pseudarthrosis with shock waves were reported by Valchanov et al. [25]. Of 82 treatments 70 were reported as successful; however, their specification of patients, treatment, and follow-up were incomplete [26]. Bürger et al. found only 35% healing and 21% callus formation in 37 patients [27–31]. In the same group Haist reported the importance of the pseudarthrosis type: while all patients with hypertrophic pseudarthrosis reached complete healing after shock wave therapy only 3 of 13 patients with atrophic pseudarthrosis had sufficient results [32].

Schleberger [33] and Schleberger and Senge [34] postulated stabilization of the pseudarthrosis after shock wave treatment providing only axial pressure on the pseudarthrosis and achieved a treatment success in 41 of 45 patients. They recommended orthesis; however, osteosynthetic material can also be used without compromising safety or success [35, 36]. To our knowledge, the data presented here are on the largest series of pseudarthrosis cases yet treated by extracorporeal shock waves. Although three different instruments were used, these data can be pooled since the manufacturers of the devices report them to have similar energy density (0.34–0.35 mJ/mm^2).

The soft tissue treatments were performed with higher energy densities than those described by other authors [37–40]; treatments were therefore performed under local anesthesia. The need for repeated treatments was significantly lower in our patients. Thus one might speculate that treatment success is correlated with the amount of energy used, which can be administered in small number of treatments at higher energy density or in a greater number of treatments at lower energy density. In our hands, the higher energy density approach revealed stable success rates for up to 4 years.

6.5 Conclusions

Shock wave therapy for hypertrophic pseudarthrosis is effective. It is noninvasive and, in case of failure, does not compromise any invasive therapy. It has a low complication rate and can be performed on an outpatient basis. Compared to the alternative surgical treatment it is very cost effective and has very high patient acceptancy. Shock wave therapy is valuable as a first-line treatment of hypertrophic pseudarthrosis.

For soft tissue treatments (calcific tendinitis and clacaneal spur) extracorporeal shock waves are used at various energy densities with similar short-term success. Both regimens are interesting new modalities; the higher energy density approach sustains success rates of up to 4 years.

References

1. Chaussy C, Eisenberger F, Wanner K, Forssmann F, Hepp W, Schmiedt E, Brendel W (1976) The use of shock waves for the destruction of renal calculi without direct contact. Urol Res 4:175
2. Chaussy C (1982) Extracorporeal shock wave lithotripsy. Karger, Basel
3. Iro H, Schneider H, Födra C, Waitz G, Nitsche N, Heinritz HH, Benninger J, Ell C (1992) Shockwave lithotripsy of salivary gland stones. Lancet 339:1333–1336
4. Sauerbruch T, Delius M, Paumgartner G, Holl J, Wess O, Weber W, Hepp W, Brendel W (1986) Fragmentation of gallstones by extracorporeal shock waves. New Engl J Med 314:818–822
5. Sauerbruch T, Holl J, Sackmann M, Werner R, Wotzka R, Paumgartner G (1987) Disintegration of a pancreatic duct stone with extracorporeal shock waves in a patient with chronic pancreatitis. Endoscopy 19:207–208
6. Haupt G, Haupt A, Gerety B, Chvapil M (1990) Enhancement of fracture healing with extracorporeal shock waves. J Urol 143:23
7. Haupt G, Ekkernkamp A, Chvapil M, Haupt A, Gerety B (1991) Der Einfluß extrakorporaler Stoßwellen auf die Knochenbruchheilung. Hefte zur Unfallheilkunde, 220:524
8. Haupt G, Haupt A, Ekkernkamp A, Gerety B, Chvapil M (1992) Influence of shock waves on fracture healing. Urology 39:529–532
9. Rüter A (1986) Frakturen. In: Jäger M, Wirth CJ (eds) Praxis der Orthopädie. Thieme, Stuttgart, pp 338–344
10. Jäger M, Wirth CJ (1986) Pseudarthrosen. In: Jäger M, Wirth, CJ (eds) Praxis der Orthopädie. Thieme, Stuttgart, pp 338–345
11. Graff J (1989) Die Wirkung hochenergetischer Stoßwellen auf Knochen und Weichteilgewebe. Thesis, Ruhr-Universität Bochum
12. Dahmen GP, Meiss L, Nam VC, Franke R, Gonchars V (1992) Extrakorporale Stoßwellentherapie (ESWT) im knochennahen Weichteilbereich an der Schulter. Erste Therapieergebnisse. Extracta Orthopaedica 15:25
13. Loew M, Jurgowski W (1993) Erste Erfahrungen mit der Extrakorporalen Stoßwellen-Lithotripsie (ESWL) in der Behandlung der Tendinosis calcarea der Schulter. Z Orthop 131:470–473
14. Graff J, Richter K-D, Pastor J (1987) Wirkung von hochenergetischen Stoßwellen auf Knochengewebe. Verh Ber Dtsch Ges Urol 39:76
15. Graff J, Richter K-D, Pastor J (1988) Effect of high energy shock waves on bony tissue. Urol Res 16:252
16. Graff J, Berding C, Beck M (1989) Transmission of shock waves through bone: Is it possible to treat iliac ureteral stones with patient in supine position? In: Lingeman JE, Newman D (eds) Shock wave lithotripsy. Plenum, New York, pp 115–120
17. Ekkernkamp A, Haupt G, Knopf H-J, Püllenberg P, Muhr G, Senge T (1991) Effects of extracorporeal shock waves on standardized fractures in sheeps. J Urol 145:257A
18. Ekkernkamp A (1992) Die Wirkung extrakorporaler Stoßwellen auf die Frakturheilung. Thesis, Habilitationsschrift, Ruhr-Universität Bochum
19. Ekkernkamp A, Bosse A, Haupt G, Pommer A (1992) Der Einfluß der extrakorporalen Stoßwellen auf die standardisierte Tibiafraktur am Schaf. In: Ittel T, Sieberth G, Matthiass H (eds) Aktuelle Aspekte der Osteologie. Springer, Berlin Heidelberg New York, pp 307–310
20. Haupt G, Ekkernkamp A, Püllenberg P, Senge T (1992) Einfluß extrakorporal erzeugter Stoßwellen auf standardisierte Tibiafrakturen im Schafmodell. Urologe 31:A43

21. Johannes, EJ Kaulesar Sukul DM, Pierik EG, Kristelijn MJ, van Eijck GJ, Bras J (1992) Non-operative treatment of non-unions in bone with extracorporeal shock waves. Eur Surg Res 24:24
22. Johannes EJ Kaulesar Sukul DM, Matura E (1994) High-energy shock waves for the treatment of nonunions: an experiment on dogs. J Surg Res 57:246–252
23. van Arsdalen KN, Kurzweil S, Smith J, Levin RM (1991) Effects of lithotripsy on immature bone and kidney development. J Urol 146:213–216
24. Seemann O, Rassweiler J, Chvapil M, Alken P, Drach GW (1992) Effect of low-dose shock wave energy on fracture healing: an experimental study. J Endourol 6:219–223
25. Valchanow V, Michailow P, Patrashkov T (1989) New possibilities of HM-3 lithotriptor for treatment of disturbed bone union. 7th World Congress on ESWL and Endourology, Kyoto
26. Valchanou VD, Michailov P (1991) High energy shock waves in the treatment of delayed and nonunion fractures. Internat. Orthopaedics (SICOT) 15:181–184
27. Bürger RA, Witzsch U, Haist J, Karnosky V, Ahlers J, Hohenfellner R (1992) Extracorporeal shock wave therapy of pseudarthrosis. J Urol, 147:260A
28. Bürger RA, Witzsch U, Haist J, Grebe P, Hohenfellner R (1993) Die extrakorporale Stoßwellentherapie – eine neue Möglichkeit zur Behandlung von Pseudarthrosen. In: Chaussy C EF, Jocham D, Wilbert D (eds) Stoßwellenlithotripse, Aspekte und Prognosen. Attempto, Tübingen, pp 127–130
29. Witzsch U, Bürger RA, Karnoski V, Haist J (1992) Hochenergie-Stoßwellenbehandlung – eine Methode zur Therapie von Pseudarthrosen. Urologe 31:A43
30. Bürger RA, Witzsch U, Haist J, Karnosky V (1991) Extrakorporale Stoßwellenbehandlung bei Pseudarthrose und aseptischer Knochennekrose. Urologe 30:A48
31. Bürger RA, Witzsch U, Haist J, Karnosky V, Hohenfellner R (1991) Extracorporeal shock wave therapy of pseudo-arthrosis and aseptic osteonecrosis. J Endourol Volume 5:548
32. Haist J (1995) Die Osteorestauration via Stoßwellenanwendung. Eine neue Möglichkeit zur Therapie der gestörten knöchernen Konsolidierung. In: Chaussy C, Eisenberger F, Jocham D, Wilbert D (eds) Die Stoßwelle – Forschung und Klinik. Attempto, Tübingen, pp 157–161
33. Schleberger R, Senge T (1991) Nicht-invasive Behandlung nach Versagen der Frakturheilung durch Stoßwellen. In: Ittel T, Sieberth G, Matthiass H (eds) Aktuelle Aspekte der Osteologie. Springer, Berlin Heidelberg New York, pp 311–317
34. Schleberger R, Senge T (1992) Non-invasive treatment of long bone pseudarthrosis by shock waves (ESWL). Arch Orthop Trauma Surg 111:224–227
35. Schleberger R (1995) Anwendung der extrakorporalen Stoßwelle am Stütz- und Bewegungsapparat im mittelenergetischen Bereich. In: Chaussy C, Eisenberger F, Jocham D, Wilbert D (eds) Die Stoßwelle – Forschung und Klinik. Attempto, Tübingen, pp 166–174
36. Haupt G, Katzmeier P (1995) Anwendung der hochenergetischen extrakorporalen Stoßwellentherapie bei Pseudarthrosen, Tendinosis calcarea der Schulter und Ansatztendinosen (Fersensporn, Epicondylitis). In: Chaussy C, Eisenberger F, Jocham D, Wilbert D (eds) Die Stoßwelle – Forschung und Klinik. Attempto, Tübingen, pp 143–146
37. Rompe JD, Küllmer K, Eysel P, Riehle HM, Bürger R, Nafe B (1996) Niedrigenergetische extrakorporale Stoßwellentherapie ESWT beim plantaren Fersensporn. Orthop Praxis 32:271–275
38. Rompe JD, Rumler F, Hopf C, Nafe B, Heine J (1995) Extracorporeal shock wave therapy for the calcifying tendinitis of the shoulder. Clin Orthop 321:196–201
39. Haist J, von Keitz-Steeger D (1996) Shock wave therapy in the treatment of near to bone soft tissue pain in sportsmen. Int J Sports Med 17:S79
40. Dahmen GP, Franke R, Gonchars V, Poppe K, Lentrodt S, Lichtenberger S, Jost S, Montigel J, Nam VC, Dahmen G (1995) Die Behandlung knochennaher Weichteilschmerzen mit Extrakorporaler Stoßwellentherapie (ESWT) Indikation, Technik und bisherige Ergebnisse. In: Chaussy C, Eisenberger F, Jocham D, Wilbert D (eds) Die Stoßwelle – Forschung und Klinik. Attempto, Tübingen, pp 175–184

Clinical Experience with Shock Wave Therapy of Pseudarthrosis, Delayed Fracture Healing, and Cement-Free Endoprosthesis Loosening

W. Schaden

Abstract. Since January 1995 a total of 53 patients with nonunions or delayed fracture healing has been treated with high-energy shock waves in the Meidling Trauma Center. Correct immobilization of the fracture was carried out after shock wave treatment. Follow-up examinations were conducted at least 3 months after treatment (3 months–2 years). In 31 cases (59%) a single treatment with shock waves resulted in bony consolidation with a simultaneous decrease in pain symptoms. Apart from negligible local reactions (swelling, hematomas, petechial hemorrhages), no complications were observed. The treatment is not invasive; personnel and technical requirements are not problematic. We therefore conclude that the extracorporal shock wave therapy should be the first choice of treatment for nonunions and delayed fracture healing before extensive surgery is considered.

7.1 Introduction

Since January 1995 a total of 53 patients with nonunions or delayed fracture healing has been treated with extracorporal shock wave therapy. The fractures had persisted for an average of 98.8 weeks (range 3–352). The patient series was composed of 20 women (mean age 56.8 years, range 17–85) and 33 men (mean age 45.3 years, range 10–82). The mean age for the overall series was 51.05 years. At the time of shock wave therapy 44 patients (83%) had received prior surgical treatment at least once, on average twice. Osteosynthesis material such as screws, plates, marrow pins, wires, and cerclages was present in 32 fractures (60%) at the time of treatment.

The Ossatron system from the company HMT was used to produce the shock waves. Treatment was carried out under general anesthesia in 26 patients (49%) and under regional anesthesia in 27 (51%; plexus 14 patients, 26.4%; spinal 13 patients, 24.5%). Depending upon the location of the fractures 1000–12000 impulses of 16–28 kV were applied. The level of shock wave energy was determined by bone volume and fracture size (Table 1).

It is imperative that the fracture is correctly immobilized after shock wave treatment. The fractures of 26 patients (49%) were immobilized with a cast or orthopedic brace. Patients with osteosynthesis material with signs of loosening were also immobilized with a plaster bandage. The type of immobilization was chosen individually depending on location and type of fracture. Clinical and radiological follow-up examinations were conducted after 4, 8

Table 1. Shock wave energy in relation to bone volume and fracture size

Location	Shock waves	kV	Shock wave direction
Upper arm	2500–4000	20-28	2–4
Ulna	1000–2000	24	2–4
Radius	1500	24	3
Hand/Foot	1000–1500	20	1–3
Femur	4000–8000	28	4–16
Lower leg	2500–12000	24-28	2–24
Hip endoprosthesis	4000–8000	28	8–16
Pelvic osteotomy	8000	28	16

Table 2. Results according to fracture localization and case numbers

Location	Total	Consolidated	Not consolidated
Lower leg	17	10	7
Ulna	7	5	2
Upper arm	5	1	4
Scaphoid	5	3	2
Femur	3	2	1
Radius	2	1	1
Talus	2	2	
Knee	2	0	2
Ankle	1	1	
Elbow	2	1	1
Thumb	1	0	1
Metatarsus	1	0	1
Femoral neck	1	1	0
Pelvic osteotomy	1	1	0
Hip endoprosthesis	3	3	0
Total	53	31	22
%	100%	59%	41%

Table 3. Possible causes of the 22 nonconsolidated fractures (41%)

	n	%
Unsuitable	9	17
No or inadequate fixation	2	3.6
Reoperation too soon	2	3.6
New trauma	1	1.8
Not definable	8	15
Total	22	41

and 12 weeks. The total follow-up period for all patients was at least 3 months (3 months–2 years)

A total of 31 (59%) fractures were consolidated. We observed a pronounced correlation between therapeutic success, applied energy, and sufficient fracture immobilization. Table 2 shows the results according to fracture localization and case numbers; the possible reasons for nonconsolidation (22 patients, 41%) are listed in Table 3. Therefore, if exact indications are applied, and continuous therapy is conducted correctly, the failure rate can be reduced to 15%. The last 13 patients were treated accordingly, with a resulting fracture healing in 11 (84.6%).

Radiological examination of two of the three patients with hip endoprostheses showed loosening in the shaft. After an initially unproblematic postoperative period complaints were expressed in these two cases after 9–20 months. Extracorporal shock wave therapy had been conducted here after 13 and after 26 months, respectively. The third patient suffered from complaints 4 months after endoprosthetic surgery; no radiological signs of loosening were found. Extracorporal shock wave therapy had been applied 8 months postoperatively. Laboratory analysis showed no infection in any of the three patients. Progress was similar in these three cases: symptoms were almost completely eliminated directly after treatment but reached the initial level after 4–6 weeks. After 8–10 weeks symptoms disappeared (the total disorder-free period is now 22, 10, and 18 months, respectively).

The only side effects that occurred were local swelling, hematomas, and, very seldom, petechial hemorrhages. No cases of infection or damage to blood and nerve vessels occurred. The treatment is noninvasive, and personnel and technical requirements are very simple. Therefore we conclude that the application of extracorporal shock wave therapy should be the first choice of treatment for nonunions and delayed fracture healing before extensive surgery is conducted. Due to the low risk a wide range of indications should be included. Furthermore, repeated treatment should also be considered if necessary.

7.2 Case Studies

Case No. 1. A 17-year-old woman suffered a lower leg fracture in an automobile accident and was treated primarily in an external clinic (Fig. 1A). After 12 months the plate and distal interlocking screws in the intra-medullary pin were removed, and a fibula osteotomy was conducted. Spongioplasty in the area of the tibia fracture was also carried out (panel B). Because of fistulation and puriform discharge the pin was removed, and fistula revision surgery was conducted 2 months later. The upper leg was then immobilized (panel C) in a cast. This was removed after 8 weeks, and the patient was mobilized with partial weightbearing, which caused the fracture to bend (panel D). Correction of the position was performed and high-energy shock wave therapy was followed by immobilization in an upper leg cast for 8 weeks. Radiological and clinical examination of the fracture showed consolidation; the patient was allowed to mobilize with partial loading (panel E). Panel F shows the treated leg 8 months after shock wave treatment.

Case No. 2. A 45-year-old woman had fallen out of a chair and suffered a scaphoid fracture. Figure 2A shows the wrist joint after 4 months of immobilization in a cast including the proximal phalanx of the thumb. The fracture gap is still visible and may have increased, with formation of a posttraumatic cyst. Shock wave therapy was applied at this time, followed by immobilization for 6 weeks. During this period the scaphoid fracture had healed. Panel B shows the same wrist 12 weeks after shock wave treatment.

Case No. 3. A 46-year-old man suffered a comminuted lower leg fracture in a motorcycle accident. The fracture was treated with a fixateur externe on the day of the accident (Fig. 3A). After 8 weeks the fixateur was removed and the leg was immobilized (panel B). After 9 months pseudarthrosis was diagnosed, and high-energy shock wave treatment was applied (panel C). Figure 3 also shows: computed tomography at the time of shock wave treatment, with a pseudarthrosis gap visible in all cuts (panel D); X-ray 8 weeks after shock wave treatment at the time of cast removal (panel E); X-ray 4 months after treatment (panel F); and computed tomography 4 months after shock wave treatment (panel G). Consolidation is visible in all computed tomography cuts.

Case No. 4. A 53-year-old man had fallen from an 18-m-high crane approx. 28 years previously and suffered a distal comminuted fracture of the lower leg. After primary extension and fixation therapy an arthrodesis was conducted 1 year after the accident. Evidently the fracture never consolidated, but by wearing orthopedic shoes the patient was able to continue working in construction. After a distortion trauma that occurred 1 year ago the patient suffered increasing pain. Figure 4A shows an X-ray of the non union at the time of high-energy shock wave treatment. Panel B shows an X-ray after the fixation cast was removed 16 weeks after shock wave treatment; there are notable signs of consolidation. Panels C and D show computed tomography images of the same leg shortly before and 16 weeks after shock wave treatment, respectively.

Case No. 5. Figure 5A shows the hip of a 64-year-old woman with coxarthrosis 8 months after endoprosthetic surgery. The patient suffered all clinical signs of endoprosthetic loosening without infection. The radiological examination showed no gap. The complaints were localized in the area of the shaft tip, to which high-energy shock waves were applied. Panel B shows the hip 3 months after shock wave therapy, with notable spongiosa accumulation around the shaft tip; panel C shows the hip 20 months after treatment.

Case No. 6. Figure 6A shows the hip of a 66-year-old woman who had suffered a femoral neck fracture and received endoprosthetic surgery. After a complaint-free period of 10–12 months increasing pain symptoms developed. Evident loosening in the area of the endoprosthetic shaft was visible radiologically. Figure 6A shows the X-ray 13 months after surgery at the time of high-energy shock wave treatment. Panel B shows the hip 9 months after treatment; there is no change radiologically, but the patient had been free of complaints since the 8th week after shock wave application.

Case No. 7. Figure 7A shows the right hip of a 67-year-old woman who received endoprosthetic surgery after a femoral neck fracture. After 1 year without disorder the patient complained of increasing pain upon pressure.

Radiological analysis showed discrete signs of loosening at the proximal and distal ends of the shaft. High-energy shock waves were applied 26 months after endoprosthetic surgery (panel A). X-rays taken 2 months (panel B) and 7 months (panel C) after treatment show only a slight radiological difference, but the patient has suffered from hardly any pain since 9 weeks after shock wave treatment.

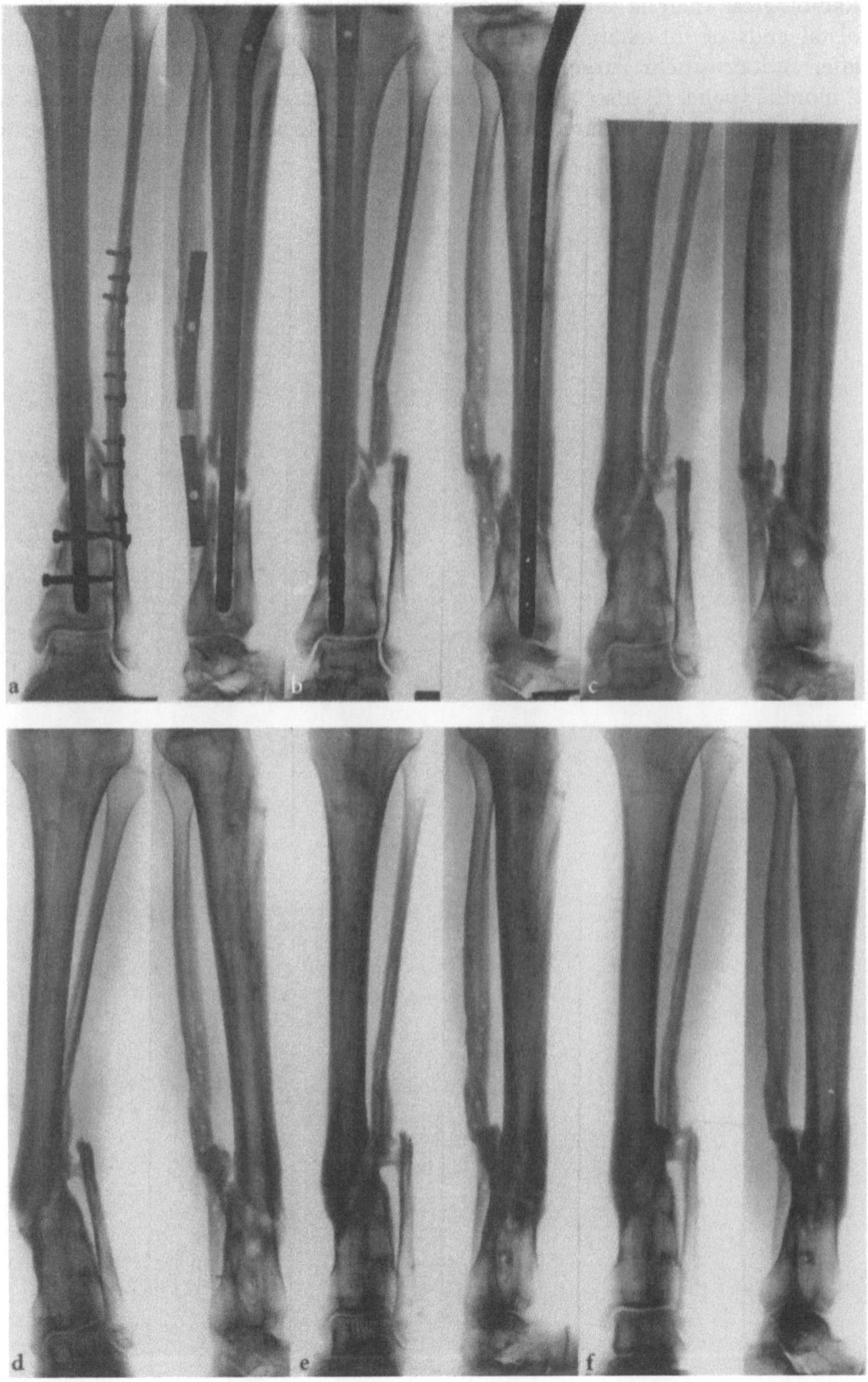

Case 1 Fig. 1 a–f

Case 2 Fig. 2a,b

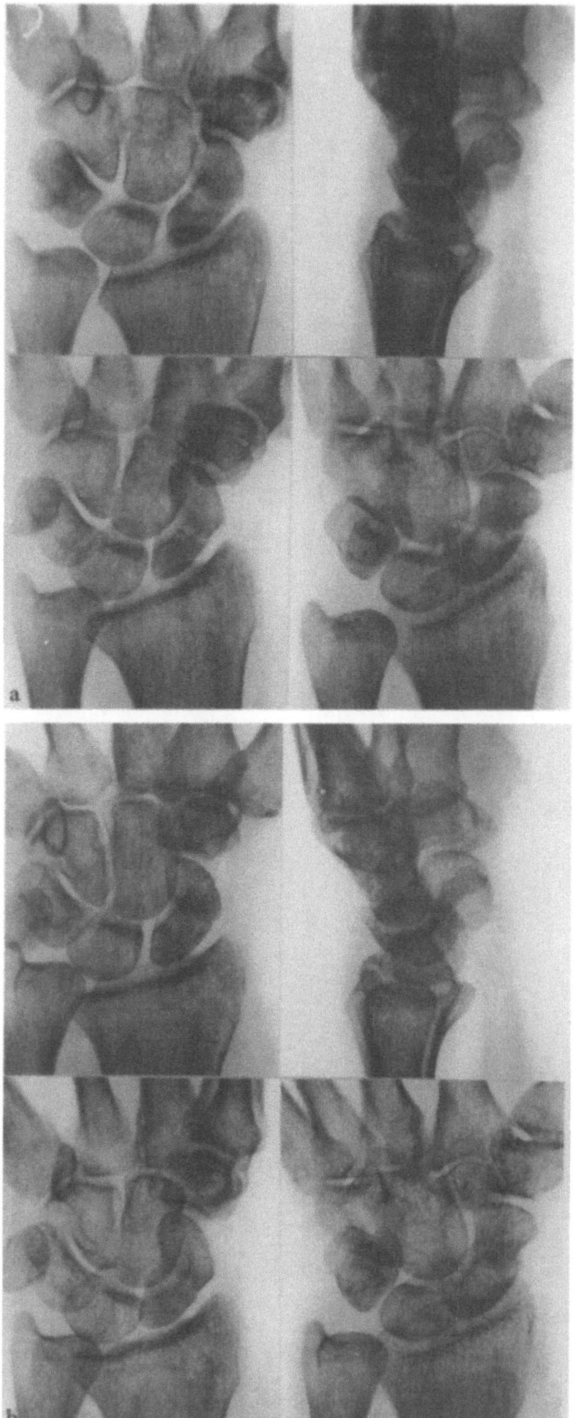

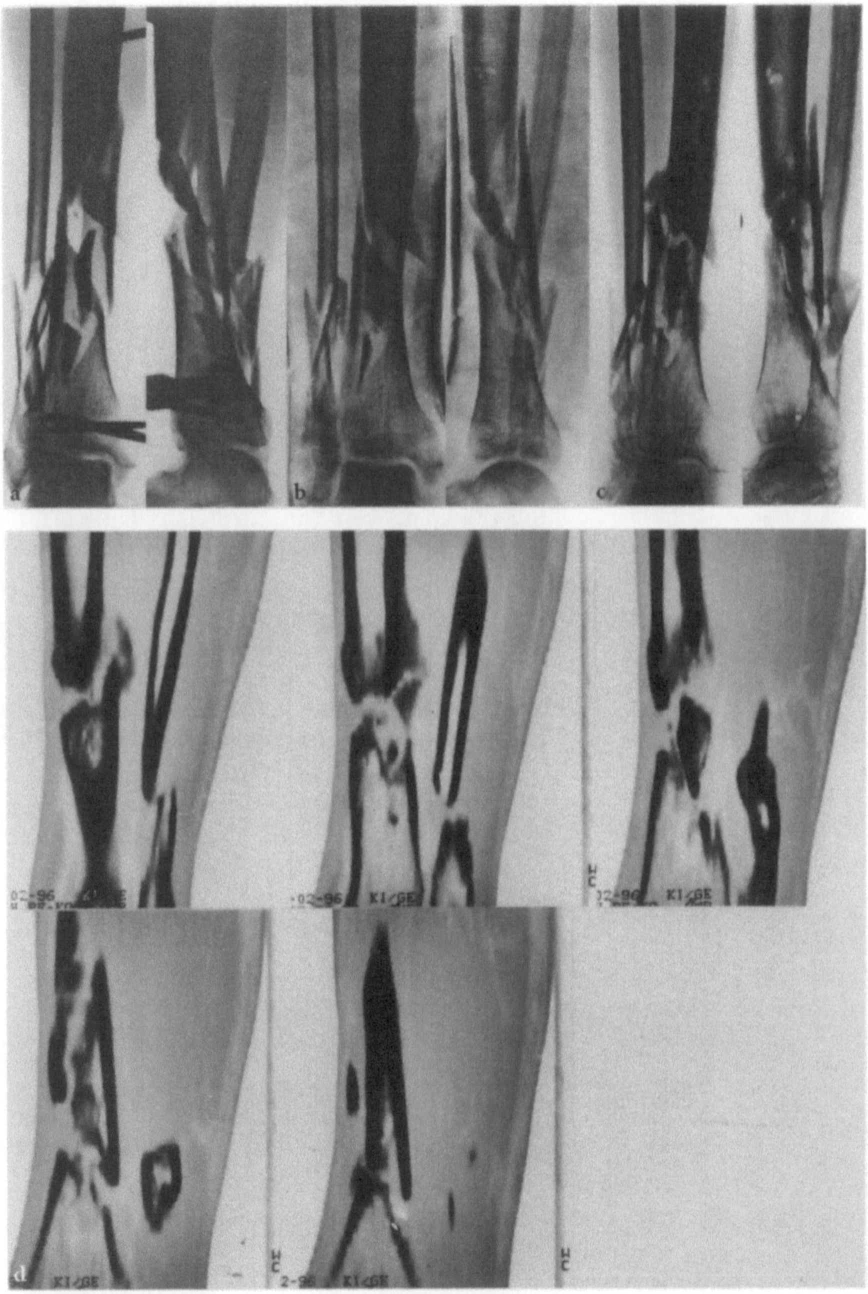

Case 3 Fig. 3a–d

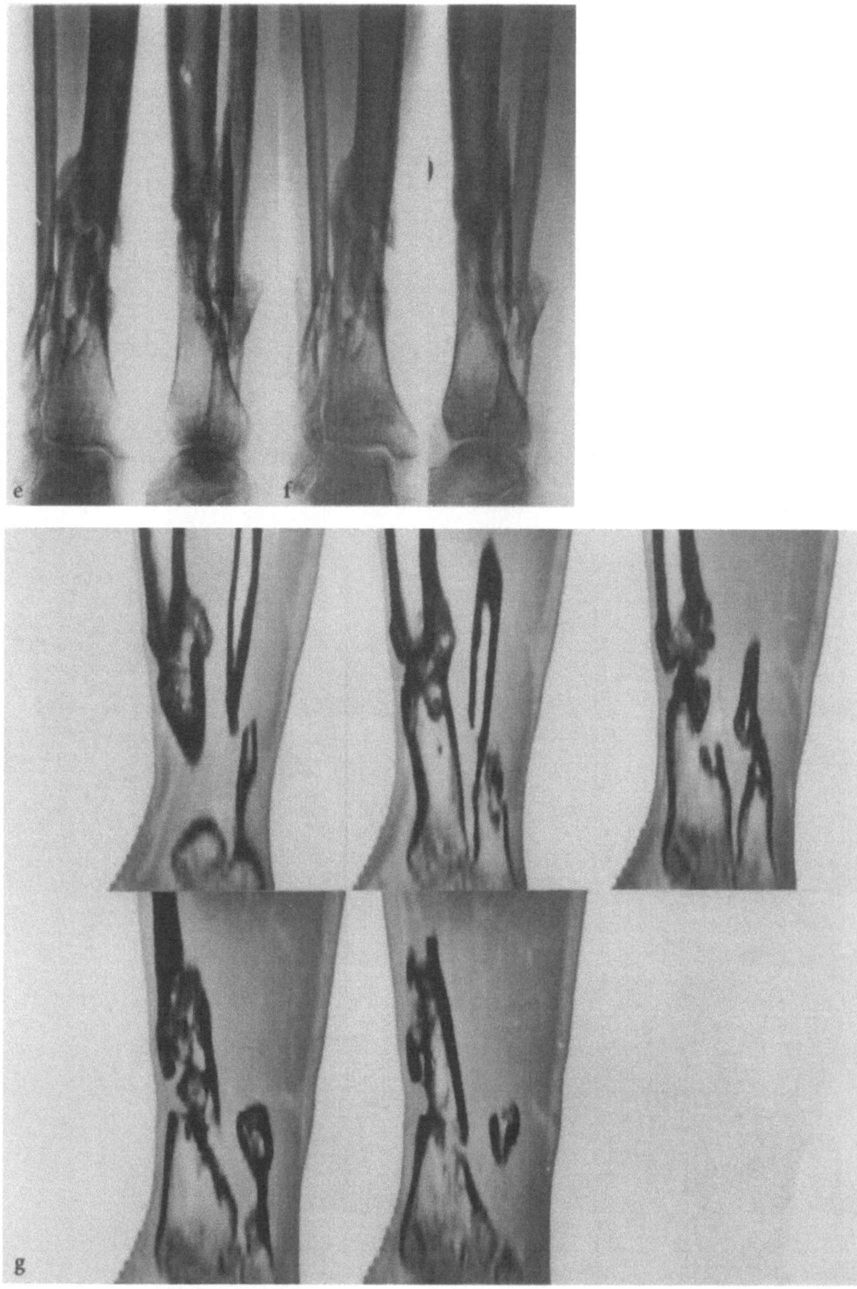

Case 3 Fig. 3e–g

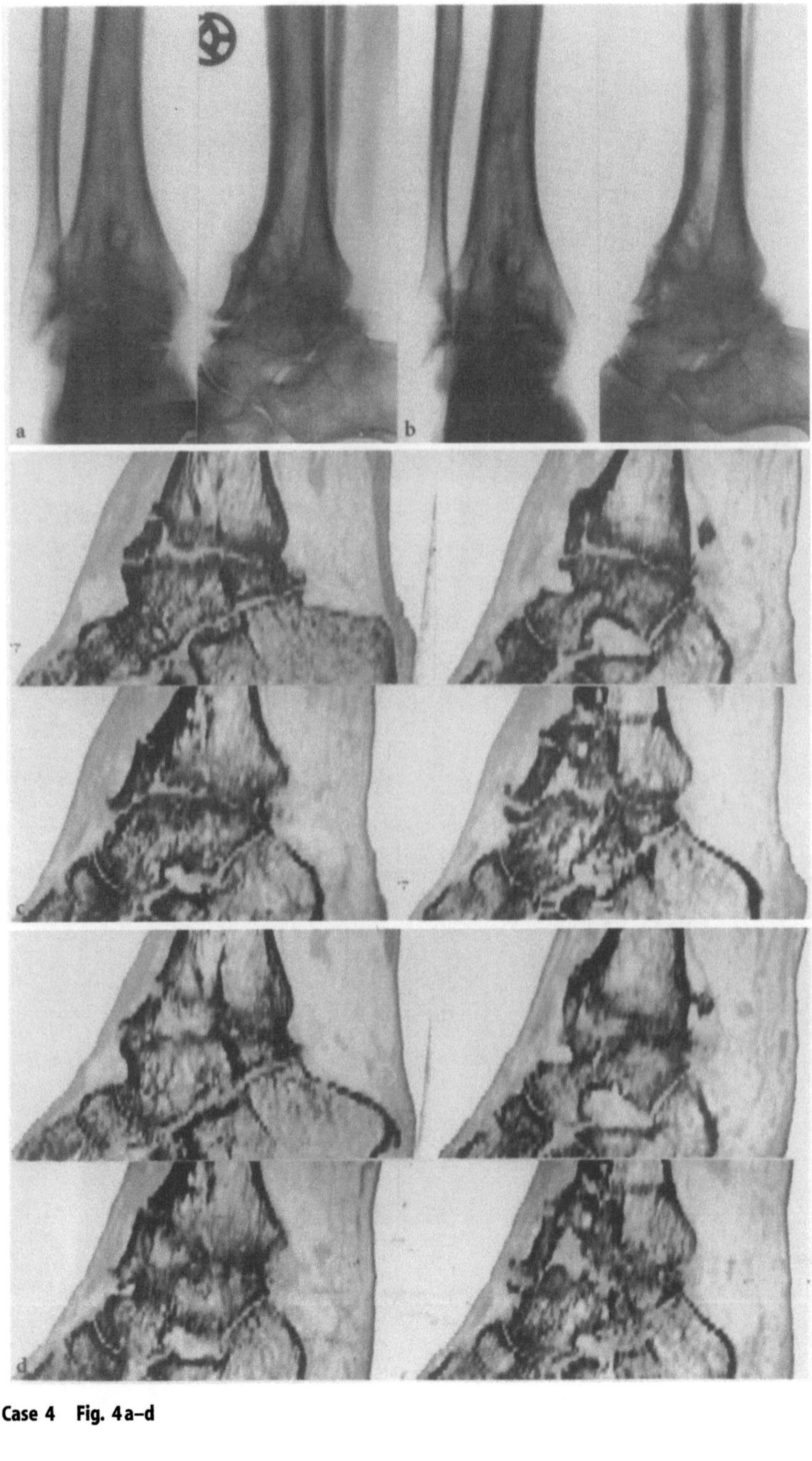

Case 4 Fig. 4 a–d

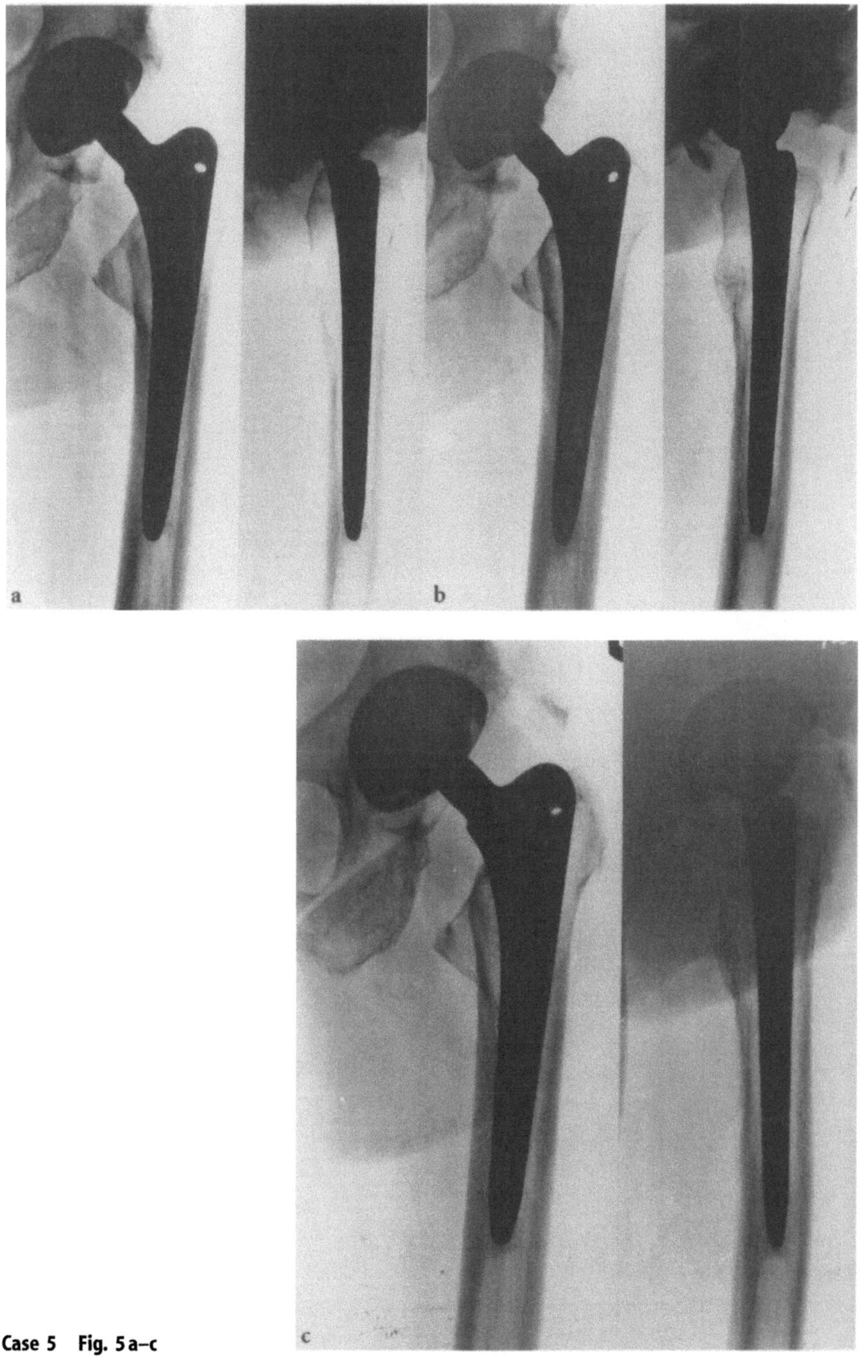

Case 5 Fig. 5 a–c

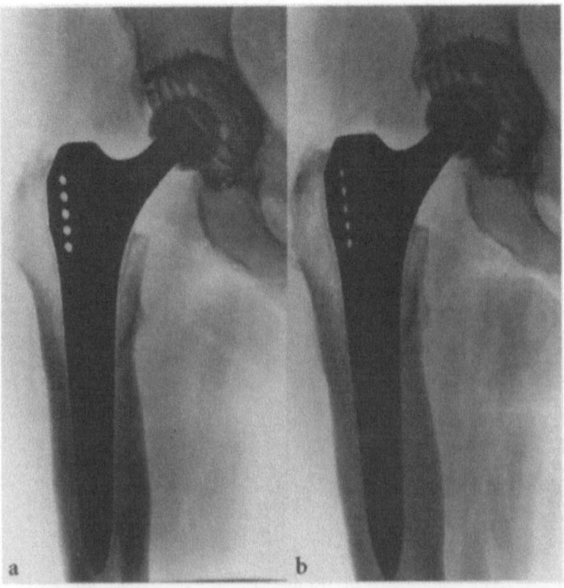

Case 6 Fig. 6a–b

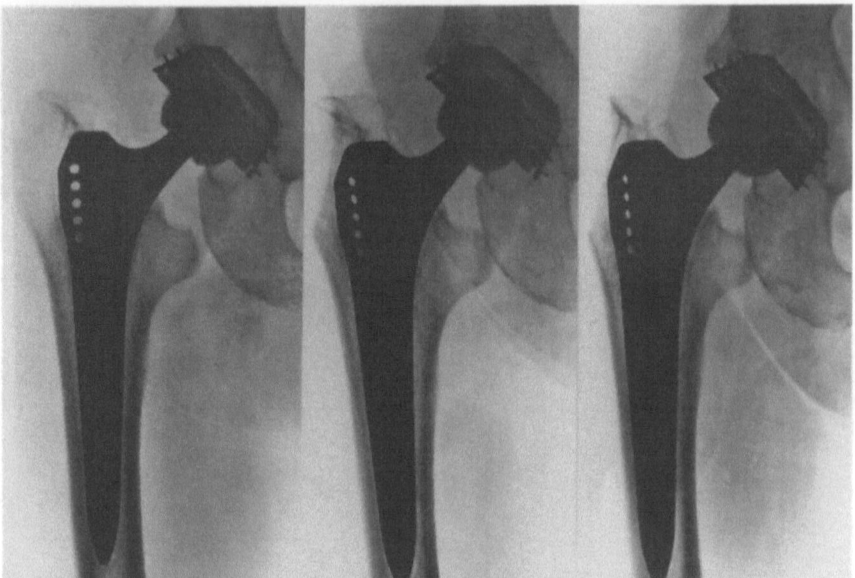

Case 7 Fig. 7a–c

Results with Extracorpeal Shock Wave Therapy in Bone and Soft Tissue Pathologies

S. Russo · S. Gigliotti · C. de Durante · R. Canero · D. Andretta and B. Corrado

8.1 Introduction

The possibility of aging bone tissue biologically by means of extracorporeal shock wave therapy (ESWT) has been well demonstrated by experimental studies both in vitro and in animal models [4, 5, 9, 10]. The positive results obtained with ESWT in treating nonunions [2, 7, 8, 13, 16, 18] and tendinopathies has recently led to increased scientific interest. We present our protocols for these treatments and discuss our results in a homogeneous group of patients

8.2 Materials and Methods

8.2.1 Bone Tissues

A total of 125 patients aged 17–63 years were treated with ESWT. The affected bones were: clavicule, 2; humerus, 3; phalanx, 14; metacarpal, 64; hamate, 1; ulna, 4; radius, 2; femur, 13; tibia, 10 (congenital cases, 3). The nonunion had lasted an average of 29 months (not longer than 5 years). Local anesthesia was administered only to patients with carpal scaphoid noninion. The relative carpal height and the carpal indexes were evaluated when the carpal scaphoid was affected to exclude alterations in these parameters. Standard and comparative X-rays were used, and the areas of lesion were examined by magnetic resonance imaging (MRI), which also allowed evaluation of the vitality and vascularization of the nonuinion bone fragments.

The pressure field of shock waves used in ESWT depends upon the size of bone to be treated and the size of tissue of nonunion. Only one or two treatments may be necessary for small bones with diameters not exceeding those of the pressure field, while larger bones require more applications. Table 1 presents our treatment protocol. The decision to cease treatment or to carry out a further phase of treatment is based to the osteogenetic response observed in the X-ray and MRI. Treatment is followed by immobilization with a cast or external fixation. This is kept in place until MRI and X-ray show consolidation.

Our electromagnetic system was the Modulith SL 20 (Storz, Kreuzling, Switzerland). This system directs a power of 1 mJ/mm^2 to the focal point. Due to the small size of the area (6–28 mm) it is possible to aim very exactly and thus avoid damage to nearby neural and vascular structures. The angle

Table 1. ESWT protocol

- Small bones
  - First treatment phase
    - Applications:
      - Two applications (24–48 h), 4000 impulses, 0.7–1.0 mJ/mm^2
    - Immobilization:
      - Carpal scaphoid: cast for 30+20 days
      - ther small bones: cast or external device for 30 days
    - X-ray control at 30–50 days:
      - Total fusion: stop treatment
      - Partial fusion: second treatment phase
      - No fusion: second treatment phase
  - Second treatment phase
    - Applications:
      - Partial fusion: two applications (24-48 h), 4000 impulses, 1.0 mJ/mm^2
      - No fusion: two applications (24-48 h), 4000 impulses, 1.0 mJ/mm^2
    - Immobilization:
      - Carpal scaphoid: cast for 30+20 days
      - Other small bones: cast or external device for 30 days
    - X-ray control at 30–45 days:
      - Total fusion: stop treatment
      - Partial fusion: stop treatment
      - No fusion: failure – stop treatment
- Other bones
  - First treatment phase
    - Applications:
      - Four applications (24–48 h), 4000/5000 impulses, 1.0 mJ/mm^2
    - Immobilization:
      - Cast or external device for 30 days
    - X-ray and MRI control at 30 days:
      - Total fusion: stop treatment
      - Partial fusion: second treatment phase
      - No fusion: second treatment phase
  - Second treatment phase
    - Applications:
      - Four applications (24–48 h), 4000/5000 impulses, 1.0 mJ/mm^2
    - Immobilization:
      - Cast or external device for 30 days
    - X-ray and MRI control at 30 days:
      - Total fusion: stop treatment
      - Partial fusion: third treatment phase
      - No fusion: third treatment phase
  - Third treatment phase
    - Applications:
      - Four applications (24–48 h), 4000/5000 impulses, 1.0 mJ/mm^2
    - Immobilization:
      - Cast or external device for 30 days
    - X-ray and MRI control at 30 days:
      - Total fusion: stop treatment
      - Partial fusion: single applications aimed at the peripheral areas
      - No fusion: MRI and new treatment only in cases of improved signal

of incidence of the waves can be modified by 90°/120° for each application. The pressure field is aimed toward the nonunion tissue and the opposite bone fragments. Those areas with a marked ischemia, as demonstrated by MRI, are specifically treated as well as sclerosis areas.

8.2.2
Soft Tissues

Our system is a small lithotriptor (Minilith, Storz) built specifically for orthopedic applications and equipped with an echographic scan system inserted in the impulse mechanism. This is situated at the end of an articulated arm that can easily reach any area to be treated. The energy produced varies from 0.03 to 0.25 mJ/mm^2. The focus size of the pressure field is 34×25 mm, with the focus depth ranging between 0.5 and 4 cm. The frequency at which shock waves are triggered can be varied between 60–90 and 120 shocks/min. The arm is equipped with three controls for carrying out fine movements in three directions, thus rendering the system ideally suited to reach the most varied treatment zones with maximum accuracy.

We rely on two parameters to focus on the target area: an objective one consisting of the ultrasound localization of the damaged zone, and a subjective one representing the focus of maximum pain perceived by the patient during the treatment. We have obtained the best results with 1500–2000 impulses and a frequency of 120 shocks/min at 0.03–0.12 mJ/mm^2. Each treatment takes about 12–15 min and is performed on an outpatient basis, and the number of treatment sessions vary between two and five, separated by a period of 2 days in acute cases and 7 days in chronic cases. Only 20% of patients require a light local anesthesia. None these values of course is definitive, and each may be modified according to further experiences.

The following pathologies were those treated over an 8-month period: radial epicondylitis, 129; ulnar epicondylitis, 18; shoulder tendinopathies, 82; achilleus tendinopthies, 27; painful heel, 36; knee tendinopathies, 12. Initially we applied ESWT only in patients who had previously undergone other types of noninvasive treatments but without success. In view of the encouraging results obtained we then extended the indications and used ESWT as a first-line therapy.

Absolute side effects included infective tenosynovitis, polyneuritis, and coagulation disturbances. In the shoulder the treated pathologies were subacromial bursitis, supraspinatous tendinitis, subscapular tendinitis, and tendinitis of the long head of the brachial biceps. Relative side effects included severe forms of osteoarthritis, rotator cuff rupture, and tendinopathies arising from articular instability. In these cases ESWT can eliminate the pain temporarily but cannot modify the preexisting anatomical conditions. Occasionally we also observed small hemoatomas, small hemorrhagic petechinae, and temporarily increased pain.

8.3
Results

8.3.1
Nonunions

In 125 patients the final follow-up 6 months after the end of ESWT showed 84 cases (67.2%) of total fusion (Figs. 1, 2), 26 (20.2%) of partial fusion, and

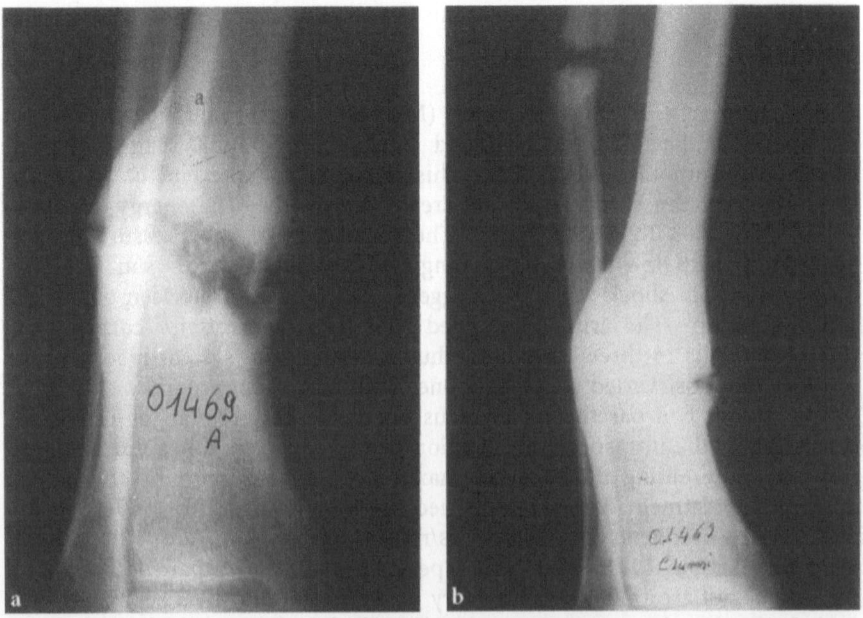

Fig. 1. a A 3-year-old nonunion of the distal one-third of a tibia in a 25-year-old man. **b** Total fusion after ESWT

Fig. 2. a A 2-year-old nonunion of the histmus of carpal scaphoid. **b** Total fusion 4 months after ESWT

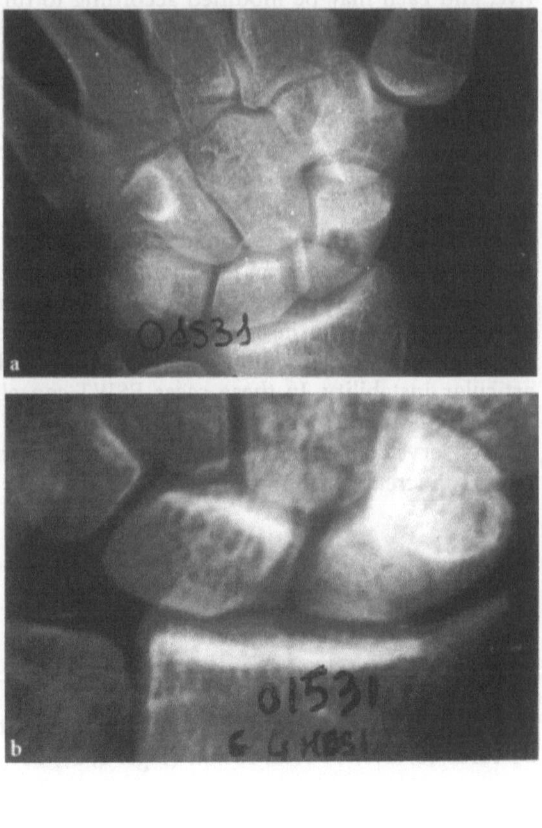

15 (12%) of no fusion. Specifically for carpal scaphoid nonunions there were 12 cases of distal pole and 29 of promial pole. In 13 scaphoides the pretreatment MRI showed prenecrosis. In cases of carpral scaphoid the 45-day follow-up at showed total fusion in 19 patients, partial fusion in 29, and no fusion in 16. At the second follow-up (45+45 days) after another treatment phase there was total fusion in 30, partial fusion in 22, and no fusion in 12. The final follow-up at 6 months showed no change in these results. In the other bones we observed after ESWT total fusion in 54, partial fusion in 4, and fusion in 3.

8.3.2
Soft Tissue Pathologies

The course of pain is very suggestive. The pain decreases substantially during the first 2–3 h following ESWT; thereafter it increases again, only to decrease again over the next few days. If the treatment is repeated when the lowest point is reached, the curve follows the same course as before and reaches an even lower level. This course of the pain results from two types of effects of shock waves: the immediate and the subsequent. The former account for the temporary disappearance of pain immediately after treatment but not for the absence of pain observed at a later date. Examples of these effects include an inhibition of pain receptors, in situ release of endorphines, and a change in pain-transmitting cortices by medullar inhibition according to the gate control theory. The later absence of pain is due to the increase in local vascularization and the local change in metabolism resulting finally in reduction in inflammation.

Our results were: in 83% cases good or very good (≥70% pain reduction; Fig. 3), in 11% satisfactory (40%–70% pain reduction), and in only 6% of cases poor (≤_40% pain reduction). It is difficult to compare these results to those obtained by other workers because of the paucity of such reports in the literature, and those that have reported are generally based upon different techniques.

8.4
Conclusions

Due to both its good results and its minimal invasiveness ESWT offers a very attractive technique for treating nonunion. Nevertheless, the therapeutic approach and the set of indications can be further improved. The present studies show that ESWT is not indicated in cases of congenital nonunion, and that results are better in hypertropic nonunions than in atropic forms. Careful measurement of the pretreatment signal by MRI can represent an important prognostic factor and thus identify patients with a greatly marked vascular crisis, such as in some case of atropic nonunion or scaphoid promial pole nonunion. In these cases the probability of recovery with high-energy ESWT is very low, and there is no indication to the treatment.

Regarding the mechanism of action on bone tissue, a number of biological effects together form a mosaic that explains the beneficial role of ESWT in resolving the pathology:

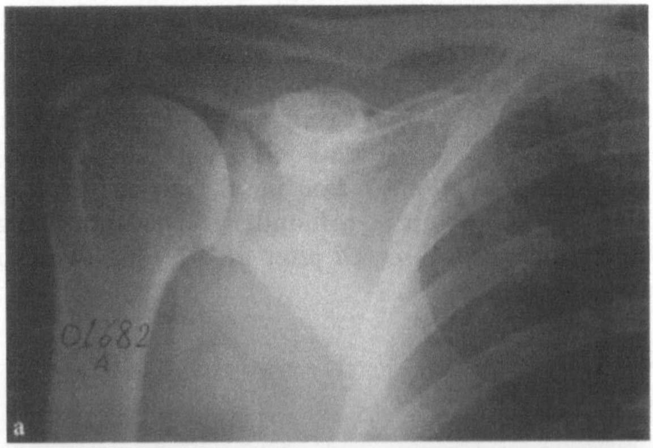

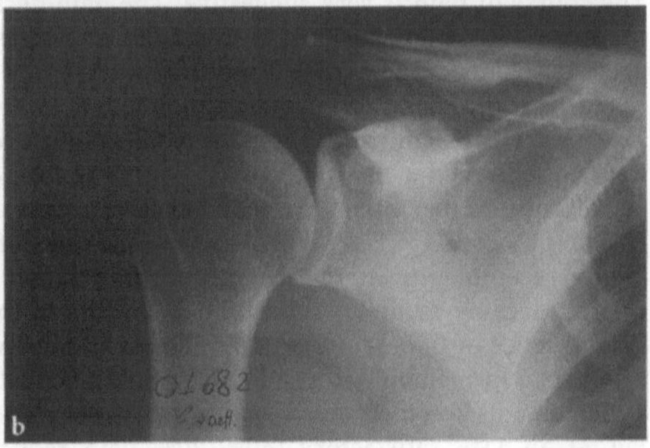

Fig. 3. a Calcifying tendinitis in the right should of a 50-year-old woman with a pain history of 12 months.
b Complete disintegration of calcification 4 weeks after ESWT

- Micronization of the osteogenic aggregation nuclei. The tricalcic phosphate crystal fragmentation frees microcrystals that behave as a calcic aggregation nuclei [2], as macrophages in recent fractures.
- Activation of stimulating osteogenic factors (e.g., bone morphogenetic protein, osteonectin).
- Increase in regional blood flow by temporary sympathetic paralysis induced by shock waves [14, 15].
- An interendothelial disjunction at the capillary level with fragmentation of the basal membrane. Migration of endothelial cells into the interstitial space with formation of new capillary beds follows [17].
- Activation caused by "capillary stress" of endothelial cell stimulating angiogenetic factor produced by endothelial and fibroblastic cells. This is the principal factor enhancing new capillary beds [1].

In the view of the encouraging results obtained with ESWT in treating soft tissue inflammations it must asked whether this mode of treatment is curative or adjuvant. Our own experience suggests that in posttraumatic disorders it is indeed curative. On the other hand, however, when used to treat secondary disease (e.g., due to muscular disequilibria, postural alterations, incorrect execution of athletics), where the shock waves have an anti-inflammatory effect, ESWT is an adjuvant therapy that is indispensable for treating the underlying causes of the disease.

References

1. Brown MD (1995) ESAF in relation to capillary growth. Int J Microcirc Clin Exp 15(3):111-115
2. Corrado EM, Russo S, Gigliotti S, De Durante C, Marinò D, Cozzolino F, Misasi N (1996) Le onde d'urto ad alta energia nel trattamento delle pseudoartrosi. Giornale Italiano OT 22(2):485-490
3. Dahmen GP, Meiss L, Nam V, Cruodis B (1992) Extrakorporale Stoßwellentherapie im knochennahen Weichteilbereich an der Schulter. Extracts Orthop 15:25-27
4. Delius M (1994) Medical applications and bioeffects of extracorporeal shock waves. Shock Waves 4:55-72
5. Graff J, Richter KD, Pastor J (1988) Effect of high energy shock waves on bony tissue. Urol Res 16:212
6. Haist J, Steeger D, Witzsch U, Burger RA, Haist U (1992) The extra-corporal shock wave therapy in the treatment of the disturbed bone union. 7th International Conference on Biomeical engineering, Singapore, December, pp 222–224
7. Haist J, von Keitz-Steeger D (1995) Shock wave therapy in the treatment of acute and chronic tendopathies in amateur and professional athletes. 34th Congress of German Specialists in Sport Medicine, 19-22 October
8. Haupt J, Haupt A, Senge T (1993) Die Behandlung von Knochen mit extrakorporalen Stoßwellen-Entwicklung einer neuen Therapie. Stoßwellenlithotripsie, Aspekte und Prognosen. Attempto, pp 120-126
9. Johannes EJ, Kaulesar Sukul DMKS, Matura E (1994) High energy shock waves for the treatment of non unions: an experiment on dogs. J Surg Res 57:246-252
10. Kaulesar Sukul DMKS, Johannes EJ, Pierik EGJM, Van Eijck GJWM, Kristelijn MJE (1993) The effect of high energy shock waves focused on cortical bone: an in vitro study. J Surg Res 54:46-51
11. Loew M, Jurgowski W, Mau HC, Thomsen M (1995) Treatment of calcifying tendinitis of rotator cuff by extracorporeal shock waves: a preliminary report. J Shoulder Elbow Surg 4(2)101-105
12. Rompe JD, Rumler F, Hopf C, Nafe B, Heine J (1995) Extracorporal shock wave therapy for calcifying tendinitis of the shoulder. Clin Orthop Rel Res 321:196-201
13. Russo S, Briganti F, Corrado EM, Gigliotti S, de Durante C (1995) Treatment of scaphoid non union by lithotripsy. Fifth IFSSH Congress, Helsinki, 3–7 July
14. Russo S, Lanza F, Passaretti U, Corrado EM (1996) Diagnosis and early treatment of aseptic bone necroses with high energy shock waves. Hand Surgery Br 21(1):15
15. Russo S, Gigliotti S, de Durante C (1996) L'uso delle onde d'urto nelle patologie ortopediche. In: Atti dei Seminari di Patol Arto Sup. Naples, pp 129–134
16. Schleberger R, Senge T (1992) Non invasive treatment of long bone pseudoartrosis by shock waves. Arch Orthop Trauma Surg 111:224-227
17. Seidl M, Steibach P, Worle K, Ofstader F (1994) Induction of stress fibers and intercellular gaps in human vascular endothelium by shock waves. Ultrasonics 32(5):397-400
18. Valchanou VD, Michailov P (1991) High energy shock waves in the treatment of delayed and nonunion of fractures. Int Orthop 15:181-184
19. Wirsching RP, Wirtz F (1995) Extracorporeal shock wave therapy (ESWT) – shock waves can do more than simply crush stones! Allgemeinartz 18:2056-2061

PART III

The Application of Shock Wave Therapy in Tendopathies and Tendinosis Calcarea

CHAPTER 9

The Orthopaedic Shock Wave Therapy in the Treatment of Chronic Insertion Tendopathy and Tendinosis Calcarea

J. Haist · D. von Keitz-Steeger · G. Mohr · G. Schulze and F. Weber

9.1 Introduction and History

Extracorporeal shock wave lithotripsy is an established therapeutic procedure for treatment of kidney stone diatheses, millions of patients having been treated successfully. It revolutionized the treatment of stones due to its extraordinarily successful outcomes with a minimally invasive procedure. Due to lithotripsy, surgical methods have been restricted to a few indications. Shock wave lithotripsy has thus become an established and acclaimed therapy worldwide.

In analogy to the disintegration model in the kidney, shock wave therapy has also been applied in the destruction of gallstones and salivary calculi. For various reasons, however, it has not achieved the ubiquitous success and the range of indications as in urology.

Since the mid-1980s, extracorporeal shock wave therapy has been implemented in experimental research in the treatment of pseudo-arthroses in only a few centres. Due to the obviously positive results, further hospitals soon resorted to this application. As an aside, the users note a pronounced analgesia in the focused area. This phenomenon was not only observed in the high-energy ranges used in the treatment of pseudo-arthroses, but was also reproducible at low-energy levels.

Considering that this phenomenon could be put to therapeutic use, Dahmen in Hamburg and Haist in Mainz began in early 1991 to implement extracorporeal shock wave therapy in the treatment of soft-tissue pain.

The first site of predilection was the shoulder; other localities were soon added, especially mentioning the elbow here.

Within the framework of the disintegration model, Loew in Heidelberg began treatment of tendinosis calcarea of the shoulder.

The individual orthopaedic work groups met under the auspices of the German Society for Shock Wave Lithotripsy for a consensus meeting at Schloß Weitenburg. Here, the foremost result was the definition of ranges of indications which, due to the clinically experimental advances in the individual groups with statistically significant proof of efficacy, could also be recommended for general use.

Notwithstanding the clinically impressive results, it is still not possible to postulate a definitive mode of action of extracorporeal shock wave therapy (ESWT) in soft-tissue pain near bones.

An extraordinary variety of lithotriptors have been used in orthopaedic shock wave therapy. At first, stationary large-size apparatuses common in urology were used. The localization of the site of action was carried out with both integrated X-ray devices and exterior sonographic devices. The energy range available was between 0.12 mJ/mm^2 and 1.2 mJ/mm^2.

Due to the demands of users, especially those treating pseudo-arthroses, experimental apparatuses with higher energy levels and better localization efficiency were made available.

The experimental apparatuses are clearly superior as concerns energy levels than those used in urology. Furthermore, localization was considerably enhanced due to the integrated mobile X-ray units (mostly as c-arches). The experimental apparatuses provide energy levels between 0.06 mJ/mm^2 and more than 2 mJ/mm^2.

In the therapy of soft-tissue pain near bones and tendinosis calcarea things moved in the opposite direction. The users wanted smaller mobile apparatuses, whose energy spectrum corresponded to the requirements of soft-tissue and calcification therapy. The localization unit was to be an exact in-line ultrasound generator, so as to do justice to radiological hygene. This lead to the development and sales of smaller apparatuses for use in orthopaedics. The enrgy range of these lies between 0.06 mJ/mm^2 and 0.4 mJ/mm^2.

9.2 Materials and Methods

In the framework of a multicentre study, patients with soft-tissue pain near bones were treated.

The indication was, on the one hand, prior treatment by a specialist during at least 3 months, in which, as a baseline, a sufficient number of infiltrations with peak value application of corticoids, cryo- and electrotherapeutic measures, physiotherapeutic exercises and an adequate provision of insoles in the case of heel spur disorder had been carried out.

If prior surgery had been carried out, this should date back at least 3 months.

It was fundamental that the adult patient had given consent.

Contra-indications for the orthopaedic shock wave treatment are systemic diseases, current pregnancy, malignant primary diseases and blood coagulation disease.

Furthermore, gross arthrotic changes or soft-tissue damage and, in the case of the shoulder, gross mechanical or instability impingement was to be ruled out.

9.3 Description of the Apparatuses

Therapy was undertaken with two different apparatuses.

One was a stationary large-size apparatus commonly used in urology, modified for orthopaedic use. This was a Lithostar plus manufactured by Siemens with a hanging module. It uses an electromagnetic shock wave generator, and localization is effected by means of an integrated inline sector scanner with a 3.5-MHz transducer. In addition, it is possible to carry out additional localization by means of a 7.5-MHz linear handscanner. The shock wave emitter is a flat coil. Steepening of the shock wave is effected via the run time and focusing is achieved by means of an acoustic lense. As mentioned above, this apparatus was originally intended for urological use and has a module hanging from the ceiling, thereby allowing total freedom of movement below the apparatus. However, the current version requires a lot of floor room for the water preparation and the processing and control units. Its energy range is between 0.08 mJ/mm^2 and 0.42 mJ/mm^2.

The other was the Minilith manufactured by Storz, a mobile apparatus especially conceived for use in orthopaedics. It also generates the shock wave electromagnetically. Localization is effected analogously to the Lithostar via an inline sector sonography unit with a 7.5-MHz transducer. In contrast to kidney stone lithotriptors, the apparatus has a considerably smaller therapy unit attached to a freely movable articulated arm which can be locked by means of brakes. The geometry of the shock wave is such that it guarantees a precisely defined focus zone of 2.5×25 mm with the coupling not putting putting too much strain on the tissue. The energy range is between 0.06 mJ/mm^2 and 0.27 mJ/mm^2, but can be optionally increased to 0.5 mJ/mm^2.

9.4 Treatment Modalities

In the entire range of indications, outpatient treatment is standard.

Treatment was repeated, depending on necessity, after 7–14 days. It was a monotherapy, i.e. further concomitant treatment was not carried out. An exception was painful limitation of the movability of the shoulder. In this case, concomitant physiotherapy was administered, so as to take advantage of the onset of painlessness for an increase in movability.

The region of interest was localized sonographically. Subsequently, rhomboidal application of 150 pulses each of 0.06–0.08 mJ/mm^2 to ten points was effected.

In the case of tendinosis calcarea, the calcification was localized sonographically and then 2000 pulses of 0.27mJ/mm^2 were applied. If necessary, therapy was repeated after 7–14 days.

9.5 Therapy Data

Over a period of 48 months ending on 1 April 1996 a total of 1842 patients underwent orthopaedic shock wave therapy. During this time, 5894 individual sessions were necessary to complete treatment, corresponding to an average of 3.19 sessions per patient.

The following range of indications was treated:

- epicondylitis radialis($N = 1002$)
- tendopathiae of the thoracic girdle ($N = 452$)
- epicondylitis ulnaris ($N = 251$)
- heel spur ($N = 62$)
- bursitis trochanterica ($N = 48$)

- achillodyniae ($N = 36$)
- others ($N = 31$)

9.6
Results

In the following, we have restricted ourselves to the results of the treatment of tendopathiae of the upper extremities, as these constitute the by far highest proportion of cases.

As concerns the results in the treatment of the lower extremities, publications by other work groups are available, e.g. Rompe in Mainz and Schleberger in Bochum, who report similar clinical results to those observed by us in the upper extremities. Our smaller numbers of cases in the lower extremities do, however, confirm these results.

Patients treated for tendopathia of the upper extremities up to 1 April 1996 underwent follow-up examination. This included both the radial and ulnar epicondylopathiae and tendopathiae of the thoracic girdle, as well as tendinosis calcarea. The patients had undergone extensive prior treatment. In nearly all cases, a sufficient number of injections and infiltrations, mostly of corticoids, as well as electrotherapeutic procedures and physiotherapy had been carried out. Nonsteroidal antirheumatic agents had been administered to at least half of the patients prior to treatment.

Due to the diagnoses, 50 patients had previously been treated surgically, of which 30 had been treated in the area of the epicondyles and 20 in the shoulder area.

A. Epicondylopathiae

Up to 1 April 1996 1253 patients had been diagnosed and treated for epicondylitis radialis or ulnaris. Of these, 917 were registered, whereby 731 had epicondylitis radialis and 186 had epicondylitis ulnaris. A total of 2659 sessions were held, which corresponds to an average of 2.9 sessions per patient.

So as to evaluate the success of the therapy, the patients were asked to individually assess the outcome on the basis of remaining symptoms:

- *Very good* (no complaints; they could go about their jobs and hobbies without restriction)
- *Good* (slight complaints; they could go about their jobs and hobbies without restriction)
- *Satisfactory* (tolerable remaining symptoms; overall considerably less pain; restrictions with regard to hobbies and jobs; continuation of conservative therapy necessary)
- *Unsatisfactory* (situation unchanged; pain profile unalterable)

Six months after therapy 31% considered the results of therapy as very good, 44.2% as good, 19.8% as satisfactory and 5% as unsatisfactory.

Furthermore, the patients were questioned according to the visual analog scale. Prior to treatment, pain was assessed as corresponding to 64.8 points, directly after therapy as 12.4 points, 3 months after treatment as 15.5 points,

6 months after therapy as 18.5 points and 12 months after treatment as 19.3 points.

B. Tendopathiae of the thoracic girdle

Up to 1 April 1996, 452 patients with various tendopathiae of the thoracic girdle underwent orthopaedic shock wave therapy. Most cases pertained to calcareous tendinosis syndrome ($N = 82$), followed by supraspinous tendon syndrome ($N = 71$) and infraspinous tendon syndrome ($N = 64$). Tendinosis calcarea was diagnosed in 68 cases. No exact topo-anatomical correlation could be found in 31 patients. A total of 793 sessions were necessary for conventional tendopathiae, corresponding to an average of 3.2 sessions per patient. In the cases of tendinosis calcarea, 170 sessions were held, corresponding to 2.5 sessions per patient. The overall average was 3.04 sessions per patient.

In analogy to the patients' assessment for the cases of epicondylopathiae, 33.3% judged the outcome as very good after 6 months post-treatment, 42.7% as good, 19.9% as satisfactory and 4.1% as unsatisfactory.

On evaluation according to the visual analogue scale, discomfort was valued as 71.3 points prior to therapy. Directly after treatment, the assessment of pain fell to 17.4 points, and rose slightly to 21.3 points 3 months after therapy. The values for 6 months and 12 months post-treatment were 19.7 and 16.3 points, respectively.

9.7 Conclusion

According to our observations, orthopaedic shock wave therapy is a minimally invasive and, with regard to radiation, safe method for the treatment of insertion tendopathiae and tendinosis calcarea. No side effects whatsoever were observed in the more than 5000 therapy sessions. However, due to the high expenditure of time and equipment, this therapy should be restricted to patients who do not experience considerable pain relief after a defined period of established conventional treatment. Nevertheless, shock wave therapy should be administered before resorting to surgical treatment.

CHAPTER 10

Ultrasound-guided Extracorporeal Shock Wave Therapy of Tendinosis Calcarea of the Shoulder, of Symptomatic Plantar Calcaneal Spur (Heel Spur) and of Epicondylopathia Radialis et Ulnaris

C. Jakobeit · L. Welp · B. Winiarski · R. Schuhmacher · T. Osenberg · T. Splittgerber · G. Spelsberg · W. Buntrock · U. Missulis · U. Kroll · A. Schmeiser · M. Beer · A. Watzlawik · G. Olschner and B. Winarski

10.1 Introduction

Extracorporeal shock wave therapy (ESWT) is a new alternative therapy for soft-tissue diseases near the bone. The German Society for Shock Wave Lithotripsy has classified ESWT as a therapy of equal value as surgery in the case of the following diagnoses:

1. Insertion tendinitis of the shoulder (with extraosseous calcium deposits)
2. Pseudo-arthroses
3. Epicondylitis humeri radialis/ulnaris
4. Plantar calcaneal spur

After more than 10 years of experimental and clinical shock wave application, we have since 1992 gained experience with more than 1000 patients with soft-tissue diseases near the bone, using purely sonographic localization. In the purely ultrasound-guided therapy we used lithotriptors manufactured by Dornier (experimental: MPL 9000/Compact; clinical: Doli). The use of a so-called inline transducer (coaxial to the shock wave axis) has proven especially advantageous. Subtile soft-tissue sonography has become our method of choice before (checking of the indication, localization), during (monitoring) and after (control) ESWT. The prerequisite for correct use is, however, ample experience with ultrasound diagnostics. Therapy was exclusively carried out by doctors with many years of experience in ultrasound diagnostics and shock wave application. It should be especially noted that the preselection of the patients in the so-called "soft-tissue consultation", the ESWT and follow-up examinations carried out solely by doctors mean a considerable expense in manpower and organization.

In the following, we will report on our experience with ultrasound-guided ESWT.

10.2
Ultrasound-guided ESWT of the Symptomatic Plantar Calcaneal Spur (Heel Spur) – Comparison of High-Energy (HE) and Low-Energy (LE) Therapy

The aim of our study was to check the efficacy of the purely sonographically guided ESWT in symptomatic plantar calcaneal spur and the comparison of HE and LE therapy.

Table 1. Inclusion and exclusion criteria for ESWT

Inclusion criteria	– radiologically and sonographically established and symptomatic calcaneal spur – prior (unsuccessful) conservative therapy
Exclusion criteria	– additional complaints in the area of the ankle joint or knee joint – rheumatic diseases, pregnancy

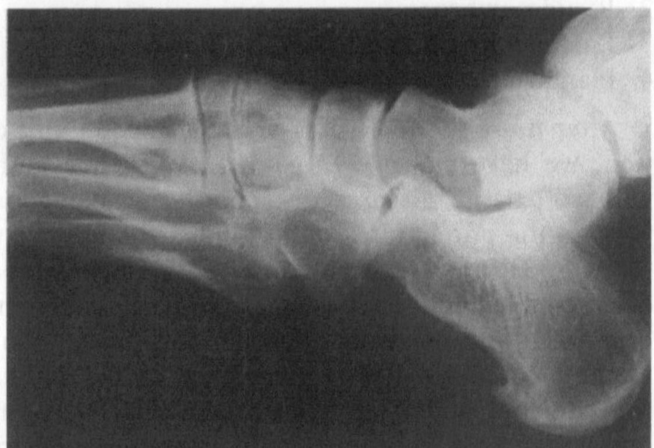

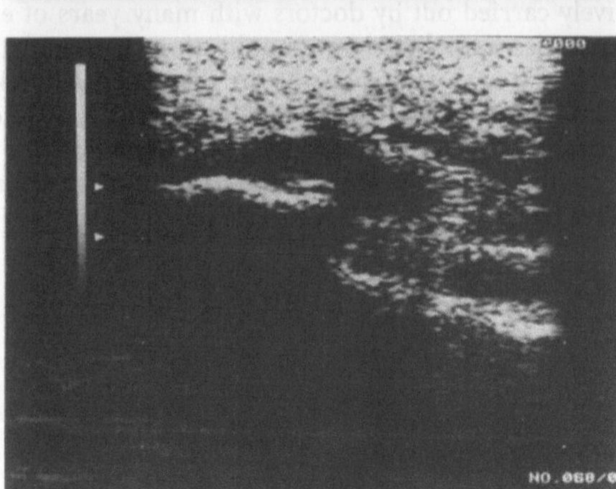

Figs. 1 and 2. Radiograph and ultrasound scan of a calcaneal spur

10.2.1 Patients and Methods

Over the course of 1 year, we applied ESWT to a total of 192 patients (118 females and 74 males) with therapy-resistant, painful plantar calcaneal spur. The average age of the female patients was 58.7 years, that of the males was 60.04 years.

The patients were randomly assigned to two (LE and HE) therapy groups. The number of sessions depended on the remaining complaints, with the aim of achieving total freedom of pain. All patients underwent follow-up examination after 3 months.

The inclusion criteria were the following (Table 1). In each patient, a calcaneal spur had been established both radiologically and sonographically (Figs. 1 and 2). All prior conservative treatment, such as orthotic devices, injection therapy with local anaesthetics or corticosteroids, X-ray stimulation, etc. had been unsuccessful.

Table 2. The following table is based on an estimation corresponding to several measurements with PVDF needle hydrophones (according to Coleman, 1989)

Level	EMSE 220 with inline transducer			Low-energy concept			High-energy concept			
	E_{eff}	E_{01}/mJ	E_{03}/mJ	Pulses S_z	E_{eff} $*S_z$	$E_{01}*S_z$	S_z	$E_{eff}*S_z$	$E_{01}*S_z$	$E_{03}*S_z$
10%	9	0.3	–	500	4500	150	100	900	30	–
20%	11	2	–	500	5500	1000	100	1100	200	–
30%	13	5	–	600	7800	3000	100	1300	500	–
40%	15	9	–				100	1500	900	–
50%	18	13	–				100	1800	1300	–
60%	21	16.6	0.9				100	2100	1660	90
70%	28	22	2				1000	28000	22000	2000
80%	35	35	4							
90%	42	50	8							
100%	50	84	13							
			Total:	1600 Pulses	17800 mJ	4150 mJ	1600 Pulses	36700 mJ	26590 mJ	2090 mJ

E_{eff} = effective acoustic energy in the focus plane, within an area of 12 mm diameter
E_{01} = effective acoustic energy in the focus plane, within an area in which a energy flux density of 0.1 mJ/mm^2 is exceeded
E_{03} = effective acoustic energy in the focus plane, within an area in which a energy flux density of 0.3 mJ/mm^2 is exceeded
– = threshold value was not reached at any point in the focus plane
Conclusion: in high-energy therapy, double the acoustic energy, namely 36700 mJ, is applied to an area with 12 mm diameter than in low-energy therapy, namely 17800 mJ = 17.8J
If one considers the energy E_{01}, i.e. the amount of energy at which the threshold of 0.1 mJ/mm^2 was exceeded (corresponds to an area of <1 mm to 3 mm in the case of the DOLI apparatus),the total "effective" energy applied is 26590 mJ = 26.6 J in the case of a high-energy strategy and 4150 mJ = 4.15 J in the case of a low-energy strategy
Thus, one requires between 2 and 6 low-energy treatments to apply the same amount of acoustic energy as in one high-energy treatment

Patients without definite plantar calcaneal spur symptoms or additional pain in the ankle joint or knee joint, as well as rheumatic diseases, were excluded from the study. Pregnancy was also an exclusion criterion.

The apparatus used was a Doli lithotriptor manufactured by Dornier. The shock wave is generated electromagnetically and covers both the LE and HE ranges. The energy density applied in the focus (in mJ/mm^2) in relation to the energy level (in %) is given in table 2. The LE range was defined as 10–30%. The HE therapy employed up to a maximum energy level of 70–80%.

Localization was carried out during therapy exclusively by ultrasound via an inline 5-MHz scanner (with continuous monitoring).

The group treated with high energy comprised a total of 113 patients, of which 62 were female and 51 were male (Table 3). In this group, all patients received 1600 shock waves in each sessions. Therapy was begun at an energy level of 10%, and every 100 shock waves the level was increased by 10%. After 600 shock waves, the maximum energy level of 70% had been reached. Due to the pain induced by the HE therapy analgesics [50 mg Pethidin-HCL (Dolantin®)] and sedation with Midazolam-HCL (Dormicum®) were administered intravenously, if necessary.

The group treated with low energy comprised 79 patients (56 females, 23 males). In this group also, 1600 shock waves were applied in each session.

Table 3. Distribution of patients in the treatment groups

Sex	Total	HE	LE
Female	118 (61%)	62 (55%)	56 (71%)
Male	74 (39%)	51 (45%)	23 (29%)
Total patients	192 (100%)	113 (100%)	79 (100%)

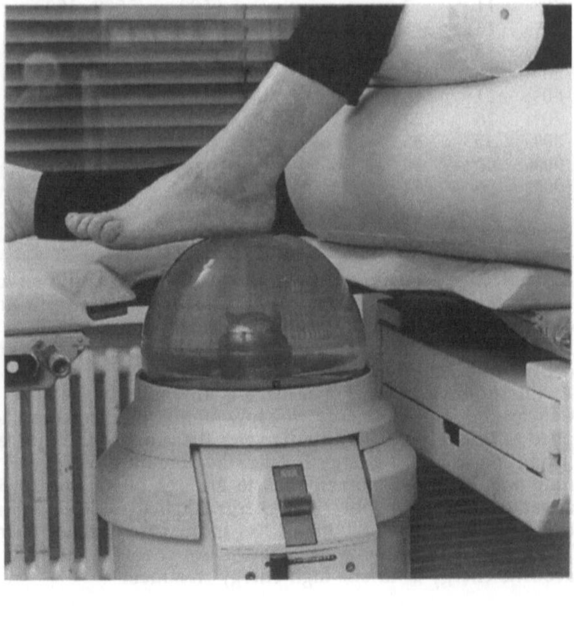

Fig. 3. Positioning of the patient during therapy

However, the maximum energy level applied was only 30%. The initial energy level of 10% was increased to 20% after 500 shock waves, and after 1000 shock waves increased to the maximum of 30%. Due to the low pain intensity, sedation and analgesics were not required.

The course of therapy was the same in both groups. Before each session, the calcaneal spur was localized sonographically and checked by palpation to confirm that the point of maximum tenderness corresponded to the location. The HE group then received the above-mentioned analgesia. In both groups, local anaesthesia in the area of the heel was foregone. The patients were positioned for treatment with the lithotriptor shown in Fig. 3.

During therapy, the person carrying out treatment established the optimal area of treatment in the region of the calcaneal spur by means of continuous ultrasound control. After each session, 50 g of Diclofenac was administered orally twice a day for 5 days. A new therapy session was performed at the earliest after 4 weeks.

The HE patients had to be monitored for about 2 h in hospital due to the sedation and analgesia administered. All patients were examined directly after treatment and the result of treatment checked the next day and after 1 week.

The success of treatment was checked according to the following parameters: the patient was required to state the intensity of pain according to a pain scale of 1–10 points (0 points meant maximum pain, 10 points meant complete freedom of pain) before the first session and before each subsequent session and follow-up examination.

Furthermore, in the evaluation, the criteria tenderness in the area of the calcaneal spur, pain at rest, starting pain after prolonged inactivity (e.g. in the morning after getting up), as well as the interval of painless walking, were taken into account. Each patient received a subsequent follow-up examination.

The evaluation was carried out for four complaint groups (Table 4).

Table 4. Criteria for allocation to group

Group	Criteria
Group 1: completely free of complaints	• no pain on weight-bearing • no tenderness • no starting pain
Group 2: few remaining complaints	• practically beneath the heel on weight-bearing • discrete local tenderness • no starting pain in the morning
Group 3: slight improvement	• pain beneath the heel on weight-bearing still present • tenderness in the region of the calcaneal spur • starting pain in the morning still present
Group 4: no change after therapy	• pain unchanged after therapy

10.2.2
Results

Painlessness or pain relief after ESWT was achieved in 187 patients. This corresponds to 97%. Only 5 patients did not experience improvement. In no case did a deterioration of the situation occur.

These results were independent of the form of therapy (LE or HE).

In the HE therapy group, 110 (97%) of the 113 patients profited from therapy. Only 3 patients (3%) did not show improvement.

In the LE therapy group, 77 patients (97%) showed positive response to therapy and only 2 patients (3%) experienced no improvement (Table 5).

Furthermore, the patients were assigned to the groups described before. The distribution was as follows (Table 6).

Groups 1 and 2 thus comprise 82.3% of the patients.

If one differentiates these patients according to the form of therapy (HE or LE), there are several differences (Table 7). Approximately 80% of the patients (HE: 84.1%; LE: 79.8%) in both of the forms of treatment are distributed over Groups 1 and 2.

In the case of the HE-treated patients, about 54.9% are in Group 1, whereas only 20.3% of the LE-treated patients are in this group. In Group 2,

Table 5. Improvement of complaints after ESWT

Improvement	Total	HE		LE	
		female	male	female	male
Yes	187 (97%)	60 (53%)	50 (44%)	54 (68%)	23 (29%)
No	5 (3%)	2 (2%)	1 (1%)	2 (3%)	–

Table 6. Results of treatment according to the individual groups

Group	Female	Male	Total
1	43	35	78 (40.6%)
2	52	28	80 (41.7%)
3	19	10	29 (15.1%)
4	4	1	5 (2.6%)

Table 7. Distribution of the patients after ESWT according to complaint group, differentiated by HE and LE

Group	HE			LE		
	female	male	total	female	male	total
1	30	32	62 (54.9%)	13	3	16 (20.3%)
2	21	12	33 (29.2%)	31	16	47 (59.5%)
3	9	6	15 (513.3%)	10	4	14 (17.7%)
4	2	1	3 (2.7%)	2	0	2 (2.5%)

Table 8. Number of patients completely free of complaints after one or two sessions

Number of sessions	Total (192 patients)		HE (113 patients)		LE (79 patients)	
	female	male	female	male	female	male
1	23 (12%)	14 (7.3%)	17 (15.0%)	11 (9.7%)	6 (7.6%)	3 (3.8%)
2	15 (7.8%)	12 (6.3%)	10 (8.8%)	12 (10.6%)	5 (6.3%)	–

there is an opposite relation. In the Groups 3 and 4, there are no great differences between the two forms of therapy.

We also investigated how many patients of the HE and LE groups were free of complaints after one or two sessions.

In the HE-treated group. 24.8% of the patients were completely free of pain after one session. In the LE-treated group, only 11.4% of the patients had no more complaints after one session. A total of 19.3% of the patients achieved complete freedom of pain after the first session.

Similar results were achieved as concerns freedom of pain after two sessions. In the HE group, it was 19.5% of the patients and in the LE group it was 6.3% (Table 8).

No complications (e.g. damage to nerves) or other side effects of therapy were detectable in any of the patients.

10.2.3 Discussion

The aim of this study was to check the success rate of purely ultrasound-guided ESWT in cases of painful calcaneal spur and the comparison of LE and HE therapy.

The results presented here show success in 97% of the patients treated. In 82% of the patients, complete painlessness or minimal remaining complaints was achieved. A comparison of our results with the data of other work groups [1–6], who mostly used radiological localization, shows similar success rates.

In studies by Rompe et al. [7] and Dahmen [8] on ESWT in the treatment of calcaneal spurs, using solely radiological localization, success rates of 75.8% (painlessness or considerable pain relief) are reported.

The advantages of ultrasound-guided therapy is the avoidance of radiation and the continuous exact localization of the area of application, the latter especially in cases of fidgety patients.

A comparison of LE and HE therapy showed that, in the former, patients had to be treated more often to achieve painlessness. The advantage of the former form of therapy is the much lower pain intensity in treatment, doing without sedation and analgesia, and therefore better tolerance on the part of the patient.

In the HE group, considerably more patients achieved freedom of complaints. Furthermore, we found that patients in this group achieved painlessesness more rapidly, often after only one session.

10.2.4 Conclusion

Ultrasound-guided ESWT is an effective and low-risk method of therapy for painful calcaneal spurs. The data of this study show good comparison of ultrasound-guided therapy with radiologically guided treatment.

HE therapy leads to quick success, whereas NE treatment is better tolerated by the patients. In view of the results currently available, ESWT could become the therapy of choice in cases of therapy-resistant calcaneal spur. So as to be able to comment on the long-term results of both forms of therapy, further studies should be carried out.

References

1. Dahmen G, Franke R, et al. (1995) Die Behandlung knochennaher Weichteilschmerzen mit extrakorporaler Stoßwellentherapie (ESWT), Indikationen, Technik und bisherige Ergebnisse. In: Chaussy C (Ed) Die Stoßwelle. Forschung und Klinik. Attempto Verlag, Tübingen, pp 175–186
2. Haist J, Steeger D (1994) Die Stoßwellentherapie der Epicondylopathia radialis et ulnaris. Ein neues Behandlungskonzept knochennaher Weichteilschmerzen. Orthop Mitteil 3:173
3. Haupt G (1995) Bisherige Ergebnisse der extrakorporalen Stoßwellentherapie im orthopädischen Bereich. 2. Konsensus Workshop der Deutschen Gesellschaft für Stoßwellenlithotripsie, 26–28 Januar 1995, Schloß Weitenburg
4. Loew M, Jurgowski W, Thomsen M (1995) Die Wirkung extrakorporaler Stoßwellen auf die Tendinosis calcarea der Schulter. Urologe [A] 34:49–53
5. Rompe JD, Hopf C, Rumler F (1994) 2 Jahre extrakorporale Stoßwellentherapie (ESWT) in der Orthopädie – Indikationen und Resultate. Orthop Mitteil 3:174
6. Schleberger R, Senge T (1992) Non-invasive treatment of long-bone pseudo-arthrosis by shock waves (ESWL). Arch Orthop Trauma Surg 111:224–227
7. Rompe JD, Hopf C, et al. (1996) Low-energy extracorporeal shock wave therapy for painful heel: a prospective controlled single-blind study. Arch Orthop Trauma Surg 115:75–79
8. Dahm K (1996) Shock wave treatment of painful plantar heel spurs. User Letter Dornier Medtech 1: 14–16

10.3 Ultrasound-guided Extracorporeal Shock Wave Therapy of Tendinosis Calcarea of the Shoulder

10.3.1 Introduction

The aim of our study was to investigate a new therapy concept: solely ultrasound-guided high-energy extracorporeal shock wave therapy (ESWT) of symptomatic tendinosis calcarea of the rotator cuff (after unsuccessful conservative therapy).

10.3.2 Patients

In this prospective study, there were 78 patients (41 females, 37 males) in the age range 34–71 years (average age 53.3 years) with pronounced painful im-

Table 9. Shoulder afflicted

Diagnoses	Number of patients
Tendinosis calcarea left	31
Tendinosis calcarea right	47

Table 10. Inclusion and exclusion criteria concerning tendinosis calcarea

Inclusion criteria	• complaints for more than 12 months • long-term, unsuccessful medication and physiotherapy
Exclusion criteria	• higher level arthroses • unrelenting thrombopathy

Table 11. Pain intensity

Pain	Number of patients
Severe to unbearable	66 (84.62%)
Moderate	12 (15.38%)

Table 12. Shoulder complaints before ESWT

Pain	Number of patients
On movement	78 (100%)
On weight-bearing	74 (94.8%)
At rest	65 (83.3%)
At night	70 (89.7%)
Painful arcus	55 (70.5%)
Restriction of movement	
Abduction	56 (71.7%)
Abduction	39 (50%)
External rotation	68 (87.1%)
Internal rotation	43 (55.12%)

Table 13. Location of calcium deposit

Location of calcium deposit	Number of patients
Supraspinatus tendon	72
Infraspinatus tendon	1
Supra-infraspinatus tendon	5

pairment of shoulder function due to tendinosis calcarea. The distribution concerning the side of the affliction is given in Table 9. All patients had had unsuccessful conservative treatment over a period of at least 12 months.

The indication for ESWT, exclusion and inclusion criteria are given in Table 10.

In addition to anamnesis and auto-evaluation of the complaints, standard clinical examinations, ultrasound examination of the joint (Fig 4; with a 7.5-MHz linear transducer) and standard X-rays were carried out before and after treatment (Tables 11 and 12).

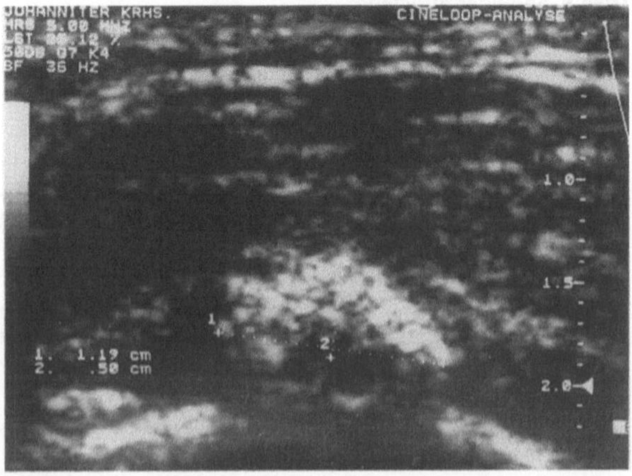

Fig. 4. Ultrasound scan of a calcium deposit in the area of the supraspinatus tendor

Table 14. Classification of the calcium deposits according to ultrasonographic and radiographic appearance

Group	Number of patients	Calcium type/diameter
I	9 (11.5%)	homogeneous >1 cm
II	16 (20.5%)	homogeneous >1 cm with amorphous portions
III	25 (32.1%)	amorphous >1 cm
IV	15 (19.2%)	homogeneous <1 cm
V	13 (16.6%)	amorphous <1 cm

The calcium deposits were topographically documented (Table 13) and classified in five groups according to radiological and ultrasonographical appearance and size (Table 14).

10.3.3
Methods

The apparatus used was a Doli lithotriptor (Dornier) with an 5.0-MHz inline scanner. Shock wave application was carried out with continuous ultrasound localization. The energy dose was increased each 100 pulses by 10% up to the maximum dose of 80%. The total number of pulses applied per session was 1800.

The best position for localization proved to be prone in retroversion and (as far as possible) abduction of the arm (Fig. 5).

The treatment was carried out with intervals of 4–6 weeks. Therapy was applied until the calcium deposit had entirely disappeared.

Follow-up examination was carried out at the earliest 1 month after the last lithotripsy, the longest interval being 13 months.

In 70 cases (89.7%), the patients suffered no more complaints or had experienced considerable improvement.

Therapy was unsatisfactory in 5 (6%) of the patients, 1 patient (1%) stated increase in complaint (in this case, pronounced calcification persisted).

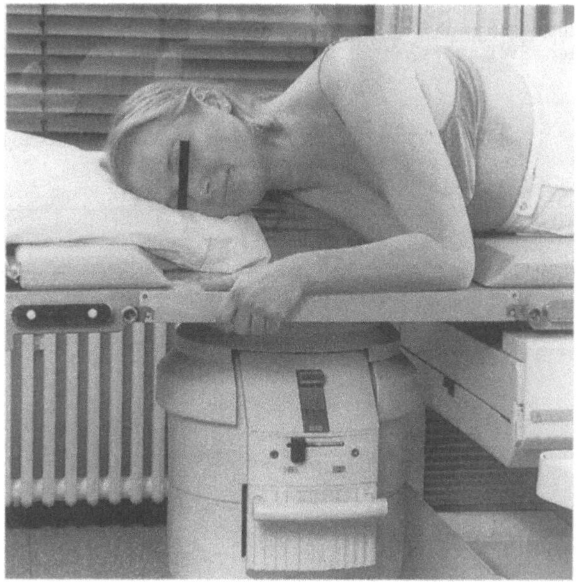

Fig. 5. Positioning of the patient during therapy

Table 15. Results after ESWT

Group	Number of patients	Subjective evaluation of patient
Free of complaints	59 (75.64%)	very good
Slight remaining complaints on weight-bearing	11 (14.1%)	good
Complaints considerably better (continued moderate restriction of movement)	2 (2.56%)	satisfactory
Insignificant improvement of the painful restriction of movement	5 (6.4%)	unsatisfactory
Increase in complaints	1 (1.28%)	worse

In 52 patients (66.6%), no more calcium was detected. In 16 patients (20.5%), the calcium deposit had considerably decreased. In 10 patients (12.9%), the calcium deposit was more or less unchanged (Table 16).

The results were unsatisfactory for the following patients (Table 17).

For all patients who were examined both by ultrasound and x-ray before and after ESWT, correspondence was established in the ultrasound and radiographic findings. All patients free of the calcium deposit were also free of complaints. Apart from the superficial bruises in the area of coupling (8 patients), no treatment-induced complications were observed sonographically. We found that constant modification of the angle of entry of the shock wave decreased the occurrence of bruises.

Table 16. Radiological and ultrasonographic findings after ESWT

Calcium deposits	Number of patients
Not detectable	52 (66.66%)
Considerably smaller and changed structure	16 (20.5%)
Slightly smaller and unchanged structure	9 (11.5%)
Larger	1 (1.28%)

Table 17. Unsatisfactory results of therapy

Results of therapy	Number of patients	Clinical course
Worse	1	Trauma – 1 month after last ESWT. Currently being neurologically treated. Increase in deposit size
Unsatisfactory	2	Complaints due to compression syndrome. Calcium remains in the therapeutic focus
	1	Surgery after first ESWT
	1	Recurrence of complaints 6 months after last ESWT. Calcium deposit exists
	1	Unessential betterment

Continuous ultrasound monitoring, in contrast to radiological localization, makes it possible to immediately identify possibilly occurring (early) complications in the soft-tissue area.

All patients felt that treatment under local anaesthesia (Novocain 2%) and, if required, in combination with an mild intravenous sedoanalgesia (Piritramid, Midazolam) was painful, but bearable.

10.3.4 Discussion and Conclusion

HE ESWT of tendinosis calcarea resistant to conservative therapy in the group of patients treated here is a low-risk, effective and non-invasive method. Our results clearly show that the desintegration of the calcium deposits leads to freedom from complaints. Therefore, the aim of therapy of tendinosis calcarea should be the total elimination of the calcium deposits.

This study substantiates that the results of purely ultrasound-guided ESWT are comparable with the good results of predominantly x-ray-guided therapy [1–4].

References

1. Loew M, Jurgowski W (1993) Erste Erfahrungen mit der extrakorporalen Stoßwellenlithotripsie in der Behandlung der Tendinosis calcarea der Schulter. Z Orthop 131:470
2. Dahmen GP, Meiss L, Nam VC, Skruodies B (1992) Extrakorporale Stoßwellen (ESWT) im knochennahen Weichteilbereich an der Schulter. Extr Orthop 11:25

3. Schleberger R (1995) Anwendung der extrakorporalen Stoßwellen am Stütz- und Bewegungsapparat im mittelenergetischen Bereich. In: Chaussy C (Ed) Die Stoßwelle, Forschung und Klinik. Attempto Verlag, Tübingen, 166–174
4. Rompe JD (1995) Bisherige Ergebnisse der Stoßwellentherapie bei der Behandlung chronischer Schmerzen an der Schulter und am Fuß. 2. Konsensus-Workshop der Deutschen Gesellschaft für Stoßwellenlithotripsie, 26–28 Januar 1995, Schloß Weitenburg

10.4 Ultrasound-guided ESWT of Refractory Epicondylopathia Radialis et Ulnaris – Experience with 170 Patients, using High-Energy Therapy

10.4.1 Introduction

The clinical problems concerning the so-called tennis/golfer's elbow are known: a multitude of conservative therapy concepts and many reports on surgical methods have as yet not been convincing. Due to the first optimistic data on the effect of extracorporeal shock wave therapy (ESWT) [1–4], we have carried out purely ultrasound-guided high-energy (HE) ESWT, using the electromagnetic apparatus Doli (Dornier) in 170 patients with therapy-resistant epicondylitis humeri radialis/ulnaris (calcarea and non-calcarea).

10.4.2 Patients and Methods

The following inclusion criteria applied to the 170 patients (Table 18) who formed the population of this study:

1. Therapy-resistant (more than 6 months) pain in the area of the epicondylus humeri radialis or ulnaris
2. At least 3 months of prior conservative (unsuccessful) therapy
3. At least two of the following tests had to be positive:
   a) Pressure pain above epicondylus humeri radialis (EHR)/epicondylus humeri ulnaris (EHU)
   b) Thompson test
   c) Middle finger extension test
   d) Chair test

Table 18. Patient population

	Total
Patients	170
females	68 (40%)
males	102 (60%)
Right arm affected (radialis/ulnaris)	134 (117/17) (79%)
Left arm affected (radialis/ulnaris)	36 (30/6) (21%)
Calcification observed in X-ray	47 (28%)
No calcification observed in X-ray	123 (72%)

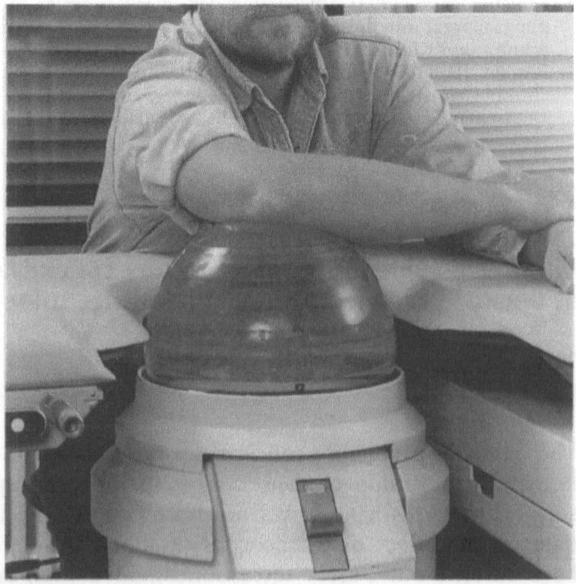

Fig. 6. Ultrasound-guided therapy of epicondylitis humeri ulnaris right

Exclusion criteria were local arthrosis/arthritis, primary chronic polyarthritis, pathological neurological or vascular findings, compression syndromes of the nervus radialis and unrelenting thrombopathy.

Before treatment, all patients were clinically, radiologically and sonographically (7.5-MHz transducer) examined.

Therapy was carried out with continuous ultrasound localization. The positioning of the patient is shown in Fig. 6.

Each patient received 1600 shock waves per session. Therapy began with an energy level of 10%, increasing by 10% after every 100 pulses up to the maximum energy level of 60%. During treatment, the point of maximum pain (trigger point) was focused under constant ultrasound visualization and, if necessary, corrected. The intervals between therapy sessions were 4 weeks until the patient was free of complaints. In the case of more severe complaints (during therapy), a mild intravenous sedoanalgesia (Midazolam/Piritramid) was administered.

All patients underwent clinical and ultrasonographic follow-up examinations directly after each session. The patients' assessments of pain were taken according to a visual analogue scale (VAS), whereby pain at night and provoked pain was taken into account.

10.4.3 Results

All patients tolerated treatment, no patient withdrew prematurely.

Of the patients, 89% reported improvement; in 11% of the patients no effect was established (Table 19).

Table 19. Improvement after ESWT

Improvement	151 (89%)
No improvement	19 (11%)

Table 20. Epicondylitis radialis et ulnaris

	Number of patients	Betterment
Epicondylitis ulnaris right		
Calcification	6	6 (100%)
No calcification	11	10 (91%)
Total	17	16 (94%)
Epicondylitis ulnaris left		
Calcification	2	1 (50%)
No calcification	4	4 (100%)
Total	6	5
Epicondylitis radialis right		
Calcification	29	25 (86%)
No calcification	88	76 (86%)
Total	117	101 (86%)
Epicondylitis radialis left		
Calcification	10	10 (100%)
No calcification	20	19 (95%)
Total	30	29 (97%)

There was no difference in the results for EHR and EHU, 73% of the patients stated no complaints or only minimal residual complaints (no impairment, only after greatest strain). These patients considered the success very good to good, 12% stated essential improvement (less than 50% residual complaints). Of the patients, 5% stated improvement of symptoms by 10–50% (in these cases, therapy was classified as unsatisfactory). If only patients with insertion calcifications are considered, success was very good or good (no complaints or minimal residual complaints only after greatest strain) in 86% (Table 20).

Early or late complications were observed neither clinically, sonographically or radiologically.

10.4.4 Discussion

Currently available studies concerning ESWT for epicondylitis clearly establish a considerable reduction of pain [1–4]. Rompe et al. [2] reported good results in 65% of the patients, using low energy levels.

Our study of HE therapy shows good results as concerns epicondylitis calcarea and non-calcarea. These good results may lead to HE therapy becoming the method of choice. Based on our experience to date, constant shock wave application to the point of maximum impulse of the pain (trigger point) is necessary for successful therapy of epicondylitis (non-calcarea).

In summary, the results presented here show that ultrasound-guided HE therapy of painful epicondylitis radialis et ulnaris is an effective and safe, side-effect-poor new alternative method in cases of patients who have undergone unsuccessful conservative therapy.

Further studies should be undertaken concerning the questions of whether results can be enhanced by means of greater modifications and which long-term results are achievable.

References

1. Dahmen GP, Meiss L, Nam VC, Skruodies B (1992) Extrakorporale Stoßwellen (ESWT) im knochennahen Weichteilbereich an der Schulter. Extr Orthop 11:25
2. Rompe JD, Hopf, et al. (1995) Extrakorporale Stoßwellenlithotripsie des therapieresistenten Ellenbogens – 1. Erste Ergebnisse von 150 Patienten. 2. Konsensus-Workshop der Deutschen Gesellschaft für Stoßwellenlithotripsie, 26–28 Januar 1995, Schloß Weitenburg
3. Haist J, Kreitz-Steeger D von (1995) Stoßwellentherapie knochennaher Weichteilschmerzen, ein neues Behandlungskonzept. 2. Konsensus-Workshop der Deutschen Gesellschaft für Stoßwellenlithotripsie, 26–28 Januar 1995, Schloß Weitenburg
4. Haupt G, Katzmeier P (1995) Anwendung der hochenergetischen extrakorporalen Stoßwellentherapie bei Pseudarthrosen, Tendinosis calcarea der Schulter und Ansatztendinosen (Fersensporn, Epicondylitis). In: Chaussy C (Ed) Die Stoßwelle, Forschung und Klinik. Attempto, Tübingen, pp 143–146

CHAPTER 11

Course Observations after Extracorporeal Shock Wave Therapy (ESWT) in Cases of Pain in the Locomotor System with Circumscribed Localization

Th. Wolf · J. Breitenfelder

Abstract. Extracorporeal shock wave therapy is an as yet not established method of treating chronic, local pain in soft-tissue near the bone; the therapy schema is not standardized or optimized. We have carried out a study in two small therapy groups with identical regime of treatment and present the results. In the mid-term we observed an improvement of the complaints. Patients with epicondylitis and pain due to calcaneal spur especially profited from treatment. Further studies are required to explore the mode of action of this method and to establish universally valid therapy methods.

11.1 Introduction

There are various causes of pain in the supportive and locomotor system. Pain is especially to be found in areas of special strain near joints. Here, articular capsule and ligament systems arranged spatially according to the requirements insert as passive structures, as opposed to inserting periarticular muscles and tendons belonging to the active control system.

The micro-architecture of these tendons and ligaments, as well as their collagen and elastic-fibre content and also the type of "rooting" of these structures in the periosteum and bones, are adapted to the local requirements and are therefore expected to display optimal function.

Natural aging processes slowly lead to impairment of the micro-architecture of the capsular ligament system by dehydration, changes in the ground substance, decrease in the proportion of elastic fibre and incorrect cross linkage of collagenic fibres. Overstrain or incorrect static strain by exceeding regenerative compensatory mechanisms can lead much more rapidly to structural damage and cause pain. Uhthoff [7] summarized this under the term *extrinsic* and *intrinsic tendinopathy*. Focal necroses, microruptures and granulations are the pathomorphological correlate, they lead to chronic and often refractory pain.

In addition to drug therapy, such as local infiltration of anaesthetics, also in combination with corticoids, and intake of analgesics and antiphlogistics, general strain relief and fixation therapy supported by physical and physiotherapeutic applications are administered. Deep X-ray therapy for pain relief, the effects and side effects of which is a matter of controversy, is often the last resort. Often one is liable to act polypragmatically due to the expectations of the patient. In the case of failure of conservative therapy, various surgical measures, depending on the location, can be undertaken.

Despite all endeavour, some of the patients experiencing pain are dissatisfied. The search for other forms of therapy is therefore justified.

Extracorporeal shock wave therapy (ESWT) is an established procedure in the treatment of lithiasis (kidney stones and gallstones).

For some years now, ESWT has also been used in several centres in the treatment of pseudo-arthroses and delayed bone union [6, 8].

The treatment of circumscribed soft-tissue pain near the bone or joint in tendinoses and tendopathies by ESWT has only been known since 1991, after work groups headed by GP. Dahmen (Hamburg) and J. Haist (Mainz) achieved first successful results. Further work groups have joined in and are endeavouring to widen the range of indications. There are indications that shock wave application in the painful tendinosis calcarea leads to quicker dissolution of the calcium deposits and more rapidly to pain relief [4].

11.2 Technical Remarks

ESWT is currently applied in two forms: higher energies are required for lithotripsy and the treatment of pseudo-arthroses, whereas both low- and high-energy pulses are recommended for pain therapy [8]. In the low-energy range of 0.08–0.12 mJ/mm^2, one hopes for less side effects and less pain for the patients. It is important to note that the threshold of high to low energy according to definition lies at 0.12 mJ/mm^2 and the transition is therefore fluid.

The range of indications for electrical shock wave therapy is as yet not exactly defined. This is also applicable to the therapy plan, which defines the number of pulses to be applied per session and the number of sessions daily or in with therapy-free intervals of several days. Furthermore, it is still the aim of studies to determine one (or more) optimally effective energy dosage(s) with which the point or area of pain can be treated.

Also, the machines available from various companies display generally different physical properties, of which the importance for therapy has yet to be determined.

All therapy forms have in common the transmission of differently generated impulses (piezoelectric, electromagnetic or hydraulic) bundled in in a shock wave to a limited area of pain via a coupling pillow.

In our study, we used a Minilith SL1 (Storz). The shock waves of this model are generated electromagnetically and focused via a parabolic reflector. The controllable focus pressure ranges from 10 to 40 MPa. The focus size is 2.4 × 25 mm, the focus distance is 40 mm. A 7.5-MHz sector scanner is integrated axially in the shock wave source. The machine is operated via normal line voltage. Impulses of energy settings 1–4 are applied with sonographic centering of the focus.

11.3
Theoretical Concepts of the Principle of Effect in ESWT

The analgesic effect of ESWT is as yet not known. There are various theoretical concepts, but they are a matter of controversy:

1.) The shock wave destroys the nerve ends. [3]
2.) The shock wave causes the nociceptor to emit a high frequency of nerve impulses whose transmission is prevented by "gate control" [3].
3.) The chemical medium surrounding the nociceptor is changed and disturbs the nerve function [3]. How far cavitation phenomena play a role in this, is the subject of further studies.
4.) A locally generated hyperaemia intensifies the degradation of inflammation mediators and induces a physiological healing process [5].

11.4
Side Effects of ESWT

In low-energy ESWT (below 0.12 mJ/mm^2), damage is quite unlikely [1]. However, when applying higher energy levels, haematoma in the cutis and subcutis, as well as in the deeper soft tissue have been reported. Animal experiments have shown subperiostal haematomas with consecutive callus formation and growth disturbance after application of shock waves to epiphyses [9, 2].

11.5
Contra-Indications for ESWT

With regard to the possible side effects, ESWT should not be applied in the following situations:

Blood coagulation diseases of various causes, open ephyses in the area to be treated pregnancy and masking of pain by neurological primary diseases.

We consider generalized pain syndromes, such as the fibromyalgia syndrome, as relative contra-indications.

In cases of considerable degenerative soft-tissue damage, such as ruptures of partial ruptures of the rotator cuff in the shoulder, we would rather prefer a cause-orientated therapy.

11.6
Materials and Methods

The aim of our study was to evaluate the results of ESWT in two groups of patients, (groups A and B), who were treated in the same way. It was a comparatively intensive therapy. 2000 pulses in the low-energy range were applied per session on five consecutive days. The duration of therapy was approximately 25 min.

Prerequisite was a long-term frustated drug and physical therapy with an average duration of 25 months.

Table 1. Diagnoses for the 17 patients to undergo ESWT in group A (19 therapies) and 12 patients in group B (13 therapies)

Diagnoses	Number of patients
Tendinosis of the supraspinatus	6
Epicondylitis humeri radialis	8
plantar calcaneal spur	10
Tendopathy of the greater trochanter	6
Z. n. Morbus Osgood Schlatter (with ossiculum)	2

Higher level degenerative defects were an exclusion criterion.

The patients had been informed of the study character of the therapy. Before beginning ESWT, the patients had to fill out a questionnaire, which, among other things, asked for information concerning the anamnesis, additional illnesses, therapeutic measures to date and a subjective evaluation of the complaints. The latter was determined according to the visual analogue scale (0 meant no pain and 100 meant maximum pain). The intensity of pain was assessed in both groups after completion of therapy and 3 months later. The patients of Group A were questioned again after 13 months posttherapy and those of Group B 6 months posttreatment. Only such patients who were not being treated locally or had undergone surgery in the meantime were considered.

Group A comprised 17 patients. Two patients were treated on both sides, giving 19 treatments. There were 7 females and 10 males. The average age was 51.5 years (25–68 years). Of the patients, 10 were still working and 6 were pensioners or had applied for pension. One patient was unemployed. The level of pain before begin of therapy was assessed as on average as 60 points.

Group B comprised 12 patients (13 treatments). The average age was 47.9 years (35–62 years). There were 9 females and 3 males. There were no pensioners in this group. The level of pain before therapy begin was assessed to be 76 points in average. The diagnoses are given in Table 1.

As the number of patients does not always correspond to the number of therapies, the percentage is given with regard to the number of therapies.

11.7
Results

ESWT was uncomfortable for all patients. Most of the patients intermittently required analgesics during the therapy cycle. No patient discontinued therapy.

- **Early results in Group A (13 therapies with 13 patients)**

After 5 days of therapy, 6 patients stated improvement of pain (46.1%). No patient was free of pain. Two patients reported an increase in pain since the begin of therapy and in 5 the level of pain remained unchanged. At discharge, an average pain intensity of 44 points on the visual analogue scale was registered.

Table 2. Comparison of the results in Group A (16 therapies with 14 patients) after 3 months and after 13 months (13 therapies with 12 Patienten) with regard to the diagnosis

after 3 months		after 13 months
1 × Epi. hum. rad. 1 × plantar calcaneal spur 1 × Tendopathy of greater trochanter.	pain-free	3 × plantar calcaneal spur
3 × Epi. hum. rad. 2 × calcaneal spur 2 × subacromial pain syndrome	better	3 × Epi. hum. rad
2 × Tendopathy of greater trochanter. 2 × subacromial pain syndrome 2 × Morbus Osgood Schlatter	no improvement	1 × Tendopathy of greater trochanter. 3 × subacromial pain syndrome 2 × Z.n. Morbus Osgood Schlatter 1 × plantar calcaneal spur

Out of all the questionnaires for interim results, 13 could be used for evaluation.

- **Results of Group A after 3 months (16 therapies with 14 patients)**

In 3 cases (18.7%), the pain had disappeared (0 points on the analogue scale). In 7 cases (43.7%), there were still complaints, but they were improved, and in 6 cases (37.5%), no improvement had occurred. Now the average level of pain according to the visual analogue scale was 47 points (Table 2).

- **Results after 13 months of Group A (13 therapies with 12 patients)**

Of the therapies, 6 had experienced improvement, of which 3 patients with plantar calcaneal spur were pain-free (23.7%). 53.8% showed no improvement. The level of pain was now at 37.5 points. Two patients had undergone surgery in the meantime.

- **Early results in Group B (13 therapies with 12 patients)**

None of the patients were free of complaints. In 5 therapies (38.4%), pain relief occurred. In 8 therapies (61.5%), no improvement was experienced. The level of pain was given on avergae as 53 points.

- **Results of Group B after 3 months (11 therapies with 10 patients)**

In 4 therapies (36.3%), no improvement was achieved. One patient with calcaneal spur was pain-free (9.1%). Five patients with 6 therapies (54.5%) showed considerable improvement (Table 3).

The level of pain was now 51.6 points.

- **Results of Group B after 6 months (11 therapies with 10 patients)**

Here, there was no essential change as compared to the results after 3 months. One patient with calcaneal spur stated increased pain. The average

Table 3. Comparison of the results of treatment for the patients in Group B after 3 and 6 months (10 patients, 11 therapies) with respect to the diagnoses

after 3 months		after 6 months
1 × plantar calcaneal spur	pain-free	1 × plantar calcaneal spur
2 × Epi. hum. rad. 2 × plantar calcaneal spur 2 × tendopathy of the greater trochanter	better	2 × Epi. hum. rad. 2 × plantar calcaneal spur 2 × tendopathy of the greater trochanter
2 × Epi. hum. rad. 1 × plantar calcaneal spur 1 × subacromial pain syndrome	no improvement	2 × Epi. hum. rad. 1 × plantar calcaneal spur 1 × subacromial pain syndrome

level of pain had, however, decreased considerably and now was at 38.5 points (Table 3).

11.8 Discussion

ESWT is a new form of therapy for somatic pain stellt. It is a local measure, as it is limited to the focus of the apparatus used. Correspondingly, only exactly localizable focuses of pain can be treated with this method.

The aim of this study was to investigate whether a therapeutic effect could be established with the chosen mode of therapy and whether a positive effect was still detectable after 6 months to 1 year.

The therapeutic procedure was identical in both groups: low-energy pulses on five consecutive days. The quality pain was assessed according to the visual analogue scale (Fig. 1) directly after and 3 months after treatment. Group A was additionally questioned after 13 months, Group B after 6 months.

Both groups had in common an anamnesis of more than 2 years on average. In both groups, to a large extent, the same locations of pain were treated (Table 1). The average age in Group A (51.5 years) was slightly higher in Group B (47.9 years). A total of 16 males and 13 females were treated. In Group A, the proportion of males was greater, in Group B the proportion of females was greater. It is notable that the patients in Group B stated a higher intensity of pain before therapy than those in Group A (76 points vs 60 points).

As the number of cases was small and there was no control group, only a descriptive view of the results of therapy is possible. The percentages do not pertain to the number of patients, but to the number of treatments.

In Groups A and B, 2 and 3 patients, respectively, stated a temporary local increase in pain during a session in the therapy cycle. In no case did a longer term detereoration occur after termination of therapy. The average level of pain in Group A decreased from 60 to 44 points and in Group B from 76 to 53 points. None of the patients in Groups A or B was immediately pain free after therapy.

0________________ 50________________ 100 points
no pain maximum pain

Fig. 1 Visual analogue scale for quantification of pain intensity

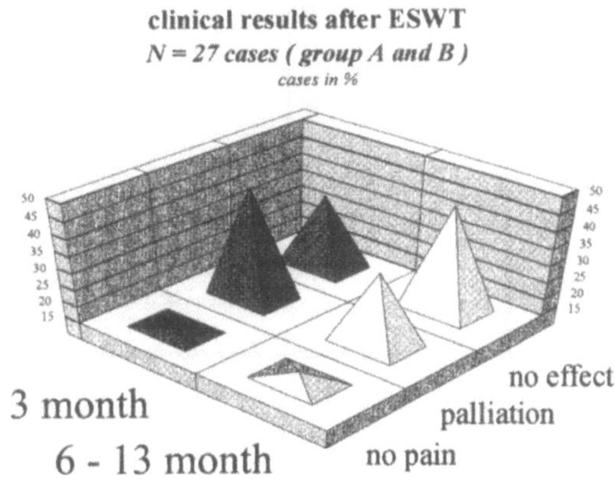

Fig. 2. Only a small proportion of the patients is really complaint-free after 3 and. 6–13 months. The proportion of cases showing no improvement is considerable in both groups

After 3 months only 4 cases of total pain relief in the 27 therapies (groups A and B) were found. This corresponds to a rate of 14.8%. Improvement occurred in 13 cases (48.1%), whereas no improvement occurred in 10 cases (37%).

If one considers the results with regard to the diagnoses, then some locations of pain appear to react better to therapy than others. Of the 7 cases of calcaneal spur (groups A and B), 6 showed improvement or freedom of pain. In the 8 cases of epicondylitis, 6 showed improvement. Of the 5 cases of tendopathy of the greater trochanter, 3 experienced improvement, and only 2 of 5 cases of tendinosis of the supraspinatus were satisfied with the result.

If we summarize the results of groups A and B (24 therapies) after 6 and 13 months only 4 cases achieved painlessness (16.6%). These were all cases of plantar calcaneal spur. Improvement was achieved in 9 cases (37.5%), whereby there were 5 epicondylitis humeri radialis and 2 calcaneal spurs. No improvement was achieved in 11 cases (45.8%), of which 4 were tendinosis of the supraspinatus (Fig. 2).

Despite the small number of cases, we conclude the following from our results:

- Low-energy ESWT appears to a large extent not to be dangerous, even in intensified therapy strategies. We registered no injuries.
- No long-term results can be expected after 3 months. There were no essential quantitive changes in the groups "pain-free", "better" and "no change", even if the patients later state a qualitative decrease in pain intensity (Fig. 3).
- Especially the painful plantar calcaneal spur and epicondylitis humeri radialis showed satisfactory results.
- Only a small percentage of the patients were subsequently free of pain.

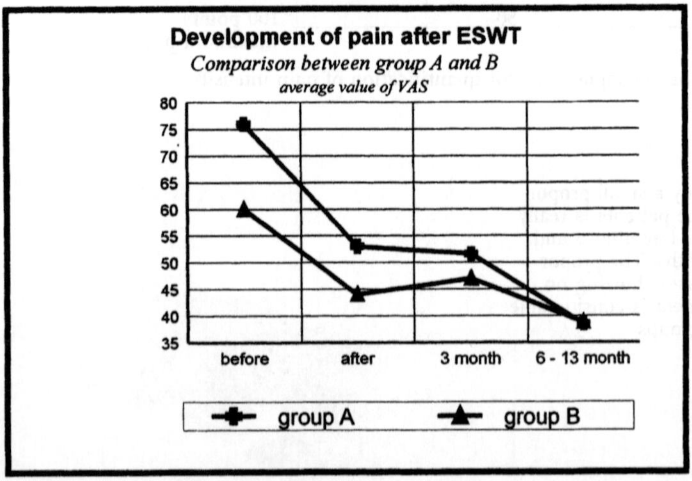

Fig. 3. The average pain intensity directly after therapy is considerably lower than before treatment. It does, however, decrease further in the following months

- The observed success of therapy justifies further controlled studies to achieve uniform standards in procedure and to clarify the biological effect of ESWT in more detail.

References

1. Dahmen GP, Meiss L, Nam V, Cruodis B (1992) Extrakorporale Stoßwellentherapie im knochennahen Weichteilbereich an der Schulter. Extr Orthop 15:25–27
2. Graff J (1989) Wirkung hochenergetischer Stoßwellen auf Knochen und Weichteilgewebe. Habilitationsschrift, Ruhr – Universität Bochum
3. Haist J, Steger von Keitz D (1995) Einsatzmöglichkeiten der analgetisch wirksamen ESWT an der Schulter. Kurzreferat auf der 43. Jahrestagung der Vereinigung Süddeutscher Orthopäden e.V., Baden – Baden, Germany
4. Loew M, Jurgowski W (1993) Erste Erfahrungen mit der extrakorporalen Stoßwellentherapie in der Behandlung der Tendinosis calcarea der Schulter. Z Orthop 131:470–473
5. Richter D, Ekkernkamp A, Muhr G (1995) Die extrakorporale Stoßwellentherapie – ein alternatives Konzept zur Behandlung der Epicondylitis humeri radialis? Orthopäde 24:303–306
6. Schleberger R, Senge T (1992) Non-invasive treatment of long- bone pseudarthrosis by shock waves (ESWL). Arch Orthop Trauma Surg 111:224–227
7. Uhthoff HK, Saker K (1995) Anatomie und Pathologie der Rotatorenmanschette. Orthopäde 24:468–474
8. Valchanou V, Michailov P (1991) High-energy shock waves in the treatment of delayed and nonunion of fractures. Int. Orthop 153:181–184
9. Yeaman LD, Christopher PJ, McCullough DL (1989) Effects of shock waves on the structure and growth of the immature rat epiphysis. J Urol 141:670–674

CHAPTER 12

The German Extracorporeal Shock Wave Society

R. Thiele

12.1 Introduction

The therapeutic application of extracorporeal shock waves (ESWT) in orthopedic and traumatological medicine developed from urological lithotripsy after initiation of the latter 1989 by Eckernkamp and Graaf.

The first orthopedic disorder considered to be an indication for ESWT was pseudarthrosis. The fracture/pseudarthrosis was consolidated through the application of ESWT. Further studies and clinical experiments have expanded the spectrum of indications to tendinitis calcarea of the shoulder, epicondylitis ulnaris/radialis, and calcaneal spur. For the first time in medical history it thus became possible to treat the cause of calcareous tendinosis without surgery. Since 1994 ambulatory shock wave therapy has been used increasingly by orthopedic physicians and surgeons in private practice. The successful application of this revolutionary therapeutic method has been expanding at a unforeseen extent.

The Berlin Society for Extracorporeal Shock Wave Therapy was founded in September 1995 to supervise the use of this promising method and to prevent its application for inappropriate diseases by untrained or profit-seeking physicians. A number of physicians from the Berlin/Brandenburg area defined quality-control and safety measures, and in this they enjoyed the full encouragement of the medical service and insurance companies. Support from throughout the country was given the efforts to develop these standards, overcome official and bureaucratic hurdles, and encourage and coordinate scientific advances. This led to the founding of the German Extracorporeal Shock Wave Society (DGST) in 1995. This independent, nonprofit society works to ensure quality, oversee certification, and promote scientific institutes conducting research aimed at improving ESWT therapy. Since 1996 the DGST has been conducting educational seminars. Upon completion of a seminar participants receive certification qualifying them to apply ESWT in the case of orthopedic disorders according to the recommendations and quality standards of the DGST.

12.2
Low-, Middle-, and High-Energy ESWT for Pseudarthrosis, Tendinosis Calcarea of the Shoulder, and Insertion Tendinosis: Results from the Berlin Center for Shock Wave Therapy

12.2.1
Introduction

Since 1994 two orthopedic practices and one surgical practice have joined the Berlin Center for Shock Wave Therapy to treat ambulatory patients suffering from pseudarthrosis, calcareous shoulder joints, tennis and golf elbow, calcaneal spur, and insertion tendinosis of the trochanter in accordance with DGST regulations. Between November 1994 and April 1997 a total of 1016 patients were treated in a total of 1610 sittings (Table 1). Further indications included chronic enthesopathies of the noncalcareous shoulder, chronic achillodynia, tendinosis of the trochanter major, cement-free endoprosthesis loosening, and delayed fracture healing.

ESWT was carried out only in cases of therapy resistance for over 3–4 months despite conservative therapy (local injections, physiotherapy, immobilization in cast or tape bandage, radiological therapy, antiphlogistica, insole therapy). In each case the application of shock wave therapy was authorized and covered by the patient's health insurance company. Patients with pseudarthrosis of larger bones were treated under regional anesthesia, and those with pseudarthrosis of smaller bones, shoulder, elbow, or heel were treated under local or conduction anesthesia.

Two Ossatron 120 systems (from HMT) were used to treat patients. This system produces an underwater shock wave by electrode induction and focus in a semiellipsoid. An image converter or a Sonoline 400 ultrasound system (both from Siemens) were used to visualize the pseudarthrosis region, i.e., calcareous deposits. The patients were treated in accordance to DGST recommendations (Table 2).

Patients with soft tissue disorders were examined 4 weeks after ESWT. At this clinical follow-up we decided whether further treatment was necessary (maximum 3×). Patients with tendinosis calcarea were subjected to radiological control 2 months after ESWT. Follow-up for the latter includes, according to the DGST, motoric ability status, subjective pain evaluation, and X-ray analysis. In the case of epicondylitis and calcaneal spur this includes subjective pain evaluation.

Table 1. Patients receiving ESWT

	No. of treated patients	No. of sittings per patient
Pseudarthrosis	23	1
Tendinosis calcarea	560	1.58
Epicondylitis radialis	242	1.6
Epicondylitis ulnaris	56	1.8
Calcaneal spur	106	1.53

Table 2. ESWT parameters

	Shock waves	kV	No. of treatments
Pseudarthrosis	2000–4000	24–28	1
Tendinosis calcarea	800–1000	16–18	1-3
Epicondylitis	800–900	14–16	1-3
Calcaneal spur	800–1000	14–16	1-3
Trochanter	800–1000	14–16	1-3

12.2.2 Results

The present study analyzed results in 127 patients with tendinosis calcarea, 50 with epicondylitis radialis or ulnaris, 28 with calcaneal spur, and 3 with insertion tendinosis of the trochanter. Three criteria were used in the examination: subjectivce pain, motoric ability status, and X-ray analysis in comparison to a constant score. In terms of subjective pain evaluation (n=127) the results showed that 58 (46%) were pain free, 15 (40%) had improved symptoms, and 18 (14%) experienced showed no change. This yields a success rate of 86%. Patients with a pain improvement of 50% (constant score) were considered a positive result.

As regards motoric ability status after 6 months 75 (59%) patients with tendinosus calcarea had unrestricted motoric ability, 37 (29%) were improved, and 15 (12%) were unchanged (Table 3). This means a success rate of 88%. Upon radiological analysis directly after ESWT (n=59) 20 (34%) patients were completely free of calcareous deposits, 23 (39%) showed notable disintegration, and 16 (27%) were unchanged. The success rate was thus 73%.

Patients with epicondylitis disorders (n=50) were evaluated for subjective pain. Of these 16 (32%) were pain free, 22 (44%) were notably improved, and 12 (24%) were unchanged. The success rate here was 76%. The subjective pain evaluation for calcaneal spur (n=28) showed 6 (21%) pain free, 17 (61%) notably improved, and 5 (18%) no change. The success rate was thus 82%.

The observed complications of ESWT include the following:

Table 3. ESWT success rates

	Complete success		Partial success		No success	
	n	%	n	%	n	%
Motility, tendinosis calcarea (n=127)	75	59	37	29	15	12
Calcareous deposits, tendinosis calcarea (n=59)	20	34	23	39	16	27
Subjective pain, epicondylitis (n=50)	16	32	22	44	12	24
Subjective pain, calcaneal spur (n=28)	6	21	17	61	5	18

- Tendinitis calcarea: local hematoma, temporary dysesthesia, acute arthritis (1×, in a patient who already suffered from primary chronic polyarthritis), deterioration within 10 weeks (2×), disorder recurrence after 3–5 months in patients who were treated once (2×)
- Epicondylitis: deterioration within 6 weeks (2×), disorder recurrence after 3 months (7×)
- Calcaneal spur: deterioration (1×), disorder recurrence after 5 months (2×)

12.3 Conclusion

Our success rates for the various indications of ESWT were between 73% and 88%. These results are in keeping with those from other ESWT centers, for example, those in Heidelberg and Kassel.

In the near future the following disorders may be considered as indications for ESWT, which would thus replace surgical treatment for them: material loosening, especially cement-free endoprosthesis loosening, delayed fracture healing, and aseptic bone necrosis. Furthermore, it may also become feasible to apply ESWT as a pain therapy to chronic noncalcareous enthesopathies of the shoulder, chronic achillodynias, and tendinosis disorders.

DGST - Protocol for Quality Control

Shoulder

Last name:...................................... **First name:**........................**birth date:**...............☐ m ☐ f..

Occupation:....................................Sports:...

Diagnosis:..☐ right ☐ left

Anamnesis:

disorder since:..

under medical treatment since:....................................sick leave

since:...

athletic ability:...in need of therapy:...............................

previous examination X-rays date:
result:..

stage:........size:........mm2

☐ Ultrasoundl date:
☐ CT/MRT date:

Previous treatment: ☐ medication ☐ physiotherapy.....times
☐ injections.....times ☐ radiological therapy.....times
☐ surgery.....times

Examination date: :

anteversion		abduction/elevation	
0- 30°	0	0- 30°	0
31- 60°	2	31- 60°	2
61- 90°	4	61- 90°	4
91-120°	6	91-120°	6
121-150°	8	121-150°	8
151-180°	10	151-180°	10
inner rotation/retroversion		**outer rotation**	
not possible	0	hand to back of neck, elbow forwards	2
back of hand to thigh	2	hand to back of neck, elbow sideways	2
to gluteal region	4	hand on head, elbow forwards	2
sacral region	6	hand on head, elbow sideways	2
lumbar region	8	hand over head	2
interscapular region	10		

pain													
during day	☺	0	1	2	3	4	5	6	7	8	9	10	☹
		10	9	8	7	6	5	4	3	2	1	0	
at night	☺	0	1	2	3	4	5	6	7	8	9	10	☹
		5	4	4	3	3	2	2	1	1	0	0	

Restrictions in daily life													
	☺	0	1	2	3	4	5	6	7	8	9	10	☹
		20	18	16	14	12	10	8	6	4	2	0	

strength in comparison to other side (in percent)

	☺	100	90	80	70	60	50	40	30	20	10	0	☹	
		25	22.5	20	17.5	15	12.5	10	7.5	5	2.5	0		

ESW-therapy
date: : 1. 2. 3.

Examination after three months
date: :

anteversion		abduction/elevation	
0- 30°	0	0- 30°	0
31- 60°	2	31- 60°	2
61- 90°	4	61- 90°	4
91-120°	6	91-120°	6
121-150°	8	121-150°	8
151-180°	10	151-180°	10
inner rotation/retroversion		**outer rotation**	
not possible	0	hand to back of neck, elbow forwards	2
back of hand to thigh	2	hand to back of neck, elbow sideways	2
to gluteal region	4	hand on head, elbow forwards	2
sacral region	6	hand on head, elbow sideways	2
lumbar region	8	hand over head	2
interscapular region	10		

pain													
during day	☺	0	1	2	3	4	5	6	7	8	9	10	☹
		10	9	8	7	6	5	4	3	2	1	0	
at night	☺	0	1	2	3	4	5	6	7	8	9	10	☹
		5	4	4	3	3	2	2	1	1	0	0	

Restrictions in daily life													
	☺	0	1	2	3	4	5	6	7	8	9	10	☹
		20	18	16	14	12	10	8	6	4	2	0	

strength in comparison to other side (in percent)														
	☺	100	90	80	70	60	50	40	30	20	10	0	☹	
		25	22.5	20	17.5	15	12.5	10	7.5	5	2.5	0		

X-ray on result .... stage ...... size ...... mm²

Examination after six months
date:

anteversion		abduction/elevation	
0- 30°	0	0- 30°	0
31- 60°	2	31- 60°	2
61- 90°	4	61- 90°	4
91-120°	6	91-120°	6
121-150°	8	121-150°	8
151-180°	10	151-180°	10
inner rotation/retroversion		**outer rotation**	
not possible	0	hand to back of neck, elbow forwards	2
back of hand to thigh	2	hand to back of neck, elbow sideways	2
to gluteal region	4	hand on head, elbow forwards	2
sacral region	6	hand on head, elbow sideways	2
lumbar region	8	hand over head	2
interscapular region	10		

pain													
during day	☺	0	1	2	3	4	5	6	7	8	9	10	☹
		10	9	8	7	6	5	4	3	2	1	0	
at night	☺	0	1	2	3	4	5	6	7	8	9	10	☹
		5	4	4	3	3	2	2	1	1	0	0	

Restrictions in daily life													
	☺	0	1	2	3	4	5	6	7	8	9	10	☹
		20	18	16	14	12	10	8	6	4	2	0	

strength in comparison to other side (in percent)														
	☺	100	90	80	70	60	50	40	30	20	10	0	☹	
		25	22.5	20	17.5	15	12.5	10	7.5	5	2.5	0		

X-ray on result .... stage ...... size ...... mm²

DGST - Protocol for Quality Control

Heel

Last name:..First name:...................................birth date.:...........

Height:...Weight:...☐ m ☐ f

Diagnosis:.. ....☐ right ☐ left

Anamnesis:

Disorder since:..

under medical treatment since:...................................sick leave since.....................................

Previous examinations: ☐ X-rays date:
☐ ultrasound date:
☐ CT/MRT date:

Previous treatment: ☐ medication ☐ physiotherapy.....times
☐ injections.....times ☐ insoles
☐ surgery.....times

Examination date:

Pain													
pain free walking range										0 m		0	
										< 100 m		15	
										< 1000 m		30	
										> 1000 m		45	
warming up pain												5	
pain on pressure	☺	0	1	2	3	4	5	6	7	8	9	10	☹
		20	18	16	14	12	10	8	6	4	2	0	

Restrictions in daily life													
at work	☺	0	1	2	3	4	5	6	7	8	9	10	☹
		10	9	8	7	6	5	4	3	2	1	0	
leisure time/sports	☺	0	1	2	3	4	5	6	7	8	9	10	☹
		10	9	8	7	6	5	4	3	2	1	0	
during sleep	☺	0	1	2	3	4	5	6	7	8	9	10	☹
		10	9	8	7	6	5	4	3	2	1	0	

ESW-therapy date: **1.** **2.** **3.**

Examination after three months
date:

Pain													
pain free walking range											0 m		0
											< 100 m		15
											< 1000 m		30
											> 1000 m		45
warming up pain													5
pain on pressure	☺	0	1	2	3	4	5	6	7	8	9	10	☹
		20	18	16	14	12	10	8	6	4	2	0	

Restrictions in daily life													
at work	☺	0	1	2	3	4	5	6	7	8	9	10	☹
		10	9	8	7	6	5	4	3	2	1	0	
leisure time/sports	☺	0	1	2	3	4	5	6	7	8	9	10	☹
		10	9	8	7	6	5	4	3	2	1	0	
during sleep	☺	0	1	2	3	4	5	6	7	8	9	10	☹
		10	9	8	7	6	5	4	3	2	1	0	

Examination after six months
date:

Pain													
pain free walking range											0 m		0
											< 100 m		15
											< 1000 m		30
											> 1000 m		45
warming up pain													5
pain on pressure	☺	0	1	2	3	4	5	6	7	8	9	10	☹
		20	18	16	14	12	10	8	6	4	2	0	

Restrictions in daily life													
at work	☺	0	1	2	3	4	5	6	7	8	9	10	☹
		10	9	8	7	6	5	4	3	2	1	0	
leisure time/sports	☺	0	1	2	3	4	5	6	7	8	9	10	☹
		10	9	8	7	6	5	4	3	2	1	0	
during sleep	☺	0	1	2	3	4	5	6	7	8	9	10	☹
		10	9	8	7	6	5	4	3	2	1	0	

DGST - Protocol for Quality Control

Elbow

Last name:..First name:......................................birth date.:.............

Height:...Weight:..☐ m ☐ f

Diagnosis:...☐ right ☐ left

Anamnesis:

Disorder since:..

under medical treatment since:...................................sick leave since....................................

Previous examinations:	☐ X-rays	date:
	☐ ultrasound	date:
	☐ CT/MRT	date:

Previous treatment:	☐ medication	☐ physiotherapy.....times
	☐ injections.....times	☐ insoles
	☐ surgery.....times	

Examination date:

Movement													
	☺	10	9	8	7	6	5	4	3	2	1	0	☹
		10	9	8	7	6	5	4	3	2	1	0	

Pain													
resting pain	☺	0	1	2	3	4	5	6	7	8	9	10	☹
		10	9	8	7	6	5	4	3	2	1	0	
stretching pain	☺	0	1	2	3	4	5	6	7	8	9	10	☹
		10	9	8	7	6	5	4	3	2	1	0	
pain on pressure	☺	0	1	2	3	4	5	6	7	8	9	10	☹
		10	9	8	7	6	5	4	3	2	1	0	
Chair-test (1kg)	☺	0	1	2	3	4	5	6	7	8	9	10	☹
		10	9	8	7	6	5	4	3	2	1	0	

Restrictions in daily life													
at work	☺	0	1	2	3	4	5	6	7	8	9	10	☹
		10	9	8	7	6	5	4	3	2	1	0	
leisure time/sports	☺	0	1	2	3	4	5	6	7	8	9	10	☹
		10	9	8	7	6	5	4	3	2	1	0	
during sleep	☺	0	1	2	3	4	5	6	7	8	9	10	☹
		10	9	8	7	6	5	4	3	2	1	0	

Strength in comparison to other side (in percent)													
fist formation	☺	100	90	80	70	60	50	40	30	20	10	0	☹
		10	9	8	7	6	5	4	3	2	1	0	
extension/flexion in wrist	☺	100	90	80	70	60	50	40	30	20	10	0	☹
		10	9	8	7	6	5	4	3	2	1	0	

ESW-therapy
date: **1.** **2.** **3.**

Examination after three months
date:

Movement													
	☺	10	9	8	7	6	5	4	3	2	1	0	☹
		10	9	8	7	6	5	4	3	2	1	0	

Pain													
resting pain	☺	0	1	2	3	4	5	6	7	8	9	10	☹
		10	9	8	7	6	5	4	3	2	1	0	
stretching pain	☺	0	1	2	3	4	5	6	7	8	9	10	☹
		10	9	8	7	6	5	4	3	2	1	0	
pain on pressure	☺	0	1	2	3	4	5	6	7	8	9	10	☹
		10	9	8	7	6	5	4	3	2	1	0	
Chair-test (1kg)	☺	0	1	2	3	4	5	6	7	8	9	10	☹
		10	9	8	7	6	5	4	3	2	1	0	

Restrictions in daily life													
at work	☺	0	1	2	3	4	5	6	7	8	9	10	☹
		10	9	8	7	6	5	4	3	2	1	0	
leisure time/sports	☺	0	1	2	3	4	5	6	7	8	9	10	☹
		10	9	8	7	6	5	4	3	2	1	0	
during sleep	☺	0	1	2	3	4	5	6	7	8	9	10	☹
		10	9	8	7	6	5	4	3	2	1	0	

Strength in comparison to other side (in percent)													
fist formation	☺	100	90	80	70	60	50	40	30	20	10	0	☹
		10	9	8	7	6	5	4	3	2	1	0	
extension/flexion in wrist	☺	100	90	80	70	60	50	40	30	20	10	0	☹
		10	9	8	7	6	5	4	3	2	1	0	

Examination after six months
date:

Movement													
	☺	10	9	8	7	6	5	4	3	2	1	0	☹
		10	9	8	7	6	5	4	3	2	1	0	

Pain													
resting pain	☺	0	1	2	3	4	5	6	7	8	9	10	☹
		10	9	8	7	6	5	4	3	2	1	0	
stretching pain	☺	0	1	2	3	4	5	6	7	8	9	10	☹
		10	9	8	7	6	5	4	3	2	1	0	
pain on pressure	☺	0	1	2	3	4	5	6	7	8	9	10	☹
		10	9	8	7	6	5	4	3	2	1	0	
Chair-test (1kg)	☺	0	1	2	3	4	5	6	7	8	9	10	☹
		10	9	8	7	6	5	4	3	2	1	0	

Restrictions in daily life													
at work	☺	0	1	2	3	4	5	6	7	8	9	10	☹
		10	9	8	7	6	5	4	3	2	1	0	
leisure time/sports	☺	0	1	2	3	4	5	6	7	8	9	10	☹
		10	9	8	7	6	5	4	3	2	1	0	
during sleep	☺	0	1	2	3	4	5	6	7	8	9	10	☹
		10	9	8	7	6	5	4	3	2	1	0	

Strength in comparison to other side (in percent)													
fist formation	☺	100	90	80	70	60	50	40	30	20	10	0	☹
		10	9	8	7	6	5	4	3	2	1	0	
extension/flexion in wrist	☺	100	90	80	70	60	50	40	30	20	10	0	☹
		10	9	8	7	6	5	4	3	2	1	0	

DGST - Protocol for Quality Control

Achillodynia

Last name:..First name:....................................birth date.:...........

Height:...Weight:...☐ m ☐ f

Diagnosis:..☐ right ☐ left

Anamnesis:

Disorder since:...

under medical treatment since:..................................sick leave since...................................

Previous examinations:	☐ X-rays	date:
	☐ ultrasound	date:
	☐ CT/MRT	date:

Previous treatment:	☐ medication	☐ physiotherapy.....times
	☐ injections.....times	☐ insoles
	☐ surgery.....times	

Examination date:

Movement													
	☺	10	9	8	7	6	5	4	3	2	1	10	☹
		20	18	16	14	12	10	8	6	4	2	0	

Pain		
painfree walking range	0 m	0
	< 100 m	5
	< 1000 m	10
	> 1000 m	15
warming up pain		5

pain on pressure	☺	0	1	2	3	4	5	6	7	8	9	10	☹
		10	9	8	7	6	5	4	3	2	1	0	

Restrictions in daily life													
at work	☺	0	1	2	3	4	5	6	7	8	9	10	☹
		10	9	8	7	6	5	4	3	2	1	0	
leisure time/sports	☺	0	1	2	3	4	5	6	7	8	9	10	☹
		10	9	8	7	6	5	4	3	2	1	0	
during sleep	☺	0	1	2	3	4	5	6	7	8	9	10	☹
		10	9	8	7	6	5	4	3	2	1	0	

Strength in comparison to other side (in percent)													
plantar flexion	☺	100	90	80	70	60	50	40	30	20	10	0	☹
		20	18	16	14	12	10	8	6	4	2	0	

ESW-therapy date: **1.** **2.** **3.**

Examination after three months
date:

Movement													
	☺	10	9	8	7	6	5	4	3	2	1	10	☹
		20	18	16	14	12	10	8	6	4	2	0	

Pain													
painfree walking range									0 m			0	
									< 100 m			5	
									< 1000 m			10	
									> 1000 m			15	
warming up pain												5	
pain on pressure	☺	0	1	2	3	4	5	6	7	8	9	10	☹
		10	9	8	7	6	5	4	3	2	1	0	

Restrictions in daily life													
at work	☺	0	1	2	3	4	5	6	7	8	9	10	☹
		10	9	8	7	6	5	4	3	2	1	0	
leisure time/sports	☺	0	1	2	3	4	5	6	7	8	9	10	☹
		10	9	8	7	6	5	4	3	2	1	0	
during sleep	☺	0	1	2	3	4	5	6	7	8	9	10	☹
		10	9	8	7	6	5	4	3	2	1	0	

Strength in comparison to other side (in percent)													
plantar flexion	☺	100	90	80	70	60	50	40	30	20	10	0	☹
		20	18	16	14	12	10	8	6	4	2	0	

Examination after six months
date:

Movement													
	☺	10	9	8	7	6	5	4	3	2	1	10	☹
		20	18	16	14	12	10	8	6	4	2	0	

Pain													
painfree walking range									0 m			0	
									< 100 m			5	
									< 1000 m			10	
									> 1000 m			15	
warming up pain												5	
pain on pressure	☺	0	1	2	3	4	5	6	7	8	9	10	☹
		10	9	8	7	6	5	4	3	2	1	0	

Restrictions in daily life													
at work	☺	0	1	2	3	4	5	6	7	8	9	10	☹
		10	9	8	7	6	5	4	3	2	1	0	
leisure time/sports	☺	0	1	2	3	4	5	6	7	8	9	10	☹
		10	9	8	7	6	5	4	3	2	1	0	
during sleep	☺	0	1	2	3	4	5	6	7	8	9	10	☹
		10	9	8	7	6	5	4	3	2	1	0	

Strength in comparison to other side (in percent)													
plantar flexion	☺	100	90	80	70	60	50	40	30	20	10	0	☹
		20	18	16	14	12	10	8	6	4	2	0	

CHAPTER 13

Therapy-Resistant Insertion Tendinosis: Indication for Extracorporal Shock Wave Therapy or Surgery?

C. von Hasselbach

13.1 Introduction

Since 1990 the Center for Shock Wave Therapy at the Orthopädische Universitätsklinik, Bochum, in Josef's Hospital has been treating patients with insertion tendinosis disorders. These patients had previously been subjected to surgical therapy - often more than one operation - without success. The surprisingly high rate of success with extracorporal shock wave therapy (ESWT) and the increasing number of positive reports in the literature [4, 5, 16, 19, 22, 30–33, 41] led us to compare results of ESWT to those of surgical therapy in a prospective study.

13.2 Material and Methods

13.2.1 Patients, Therapy Standards

From December 1995 until July 1996 we treated 191 patients with therapy-resistant insertion tendinosis, of whom 70.2% (n=134) belonged to the main indication groups: epicondylitis humeri radialis and supraspinatus and biceps tendon syndrome/tendinosis calcarea. Table 1 presents the complete list of indications. Inclusion criteria were:

- Pain anamnesis for more than 1 year
- Prior conservative therapy for at least 6 months
- Pathognomonic differential diagnosis with description of pain on palpation, monocausal dysfunction, and positive provocation tests

We used a standardized protocol to document the preliminary examination (Fig. 1). Exclusion criteria were:

- Age under 18 years
- Pregnancy
- Coagulopathy
- Infections
- Tumor disorders
- Overlapping vertebral disorder symptoms
- Entrapment neuropathy
- Arthrosis/arthritis in shoulder and/or elbow joint
- Rheumatoid arthritis

I. Patient

Last name, first name : .... Birth date: ....

Health insurance : .... Tel. : ....

II. Diagnosis

AD	OD	Right
AS	PA	Left
EHR	PTS	Both sides
EHU	SS- / BTS / TC	
BS / FP	Other	

III. History

Occupation	....	Sport activities		Date of accident	....
Years	....	Months	....	SL total	....
Occupational change		change of sport		Professional sports	
Number of prior therapists	....	IP / CD		Prior surgeries	

IV. Prior Therapy

NSAP Local	Corticoids Local	Immobilization
Oral	Oral	Physical therapy
Electrotherapy	Cryotherapy	Externa
Radiological therapy	Acupuncture	Laser
Orthesis	Ultrasound	Other

During the past 6 months:

NSAP Local	Corticoids Local	Immobilization
Oral	Oral	Physical therapy
Electrotherapy	Cryotherapy	Externa
Radiological therapy	Acupuncture	Laser

Intended surgical procedure

- Wilhelm's surgery
- Subacromial decompression
- Osteotomy
- Tenotomy
- Other

V. Clinical Findings

Continuous pain	Pain during rest	Pain on pressure
Point of maximum pain	PO	Impingement
Extension / flexion	Abduction / adduction	IR / OR ....
DD UL / UA cm	DD LL / LA cm	MA other cm ....
Middle finger stretch test	Finger snap test	Chair test
Neck grip	Apron grip	Strength reduction
Instability	Rotator cuff disorder	Other

AD	= achillodynia	BS	= bony spur of the heel	PMP	= point of maximal pain
SL	= invalid / unemployable	PTS	= patella tendon syndrome	PO	= polytope ossification
AS	= adductor sprain	FP	= fasciitis plantaris syndrome	SS	= supraspinatuss.-
BTS	= biceps tendon syndrome	CD	= % certified disability	TC	= tendinosis calcarea
IP	= invalidity pension	IR/OR	= inner / outer rotation	DD	= diameter deficit
EHR	= epicondylitis humeri radialis	NSAP	= nonsteroid antiphlogistics		
EHU	= epicondylitis humeri ulnaris	PA	= pseudarthrosis		
UL	= upper leg	UA	= upper arm		
LL	= lower leg	LA	= lower arm		

Fig. 1. ESWT documentation questionnaire

Table 1. Indications for ESWT (n=191)

	n	%
Epicondylitis humeri radialis	72	37.7
Supraspinatus, biceps tendon syndrome, tendinosis cascara	62	32.5
Achilles tendon	19	9.9
Fasciitis plantaris/bony spur	12	6.3
Epicondylitis humeri ulnaris	10	5.2
Adductor sprain	6	3.1
Peroneus tendon	6	3.1
Patella tendon	4	2.1

Table 2. Data on patients and treatment for epicondylitis humeri radialis (EHR), supraspinatus, biceps tendon syndrome, tendinosis calcarea (SS/BTS/TC), Achilles tendon (AT), fasciitis plantaris/bony spur (FP/BS), and epicondylitis humeri ulnaris (EHU)

	EHR	SS/BTS/TC	AT	FP/BS	EHU
Number	72	62	19	12	10
Women	34 (47.2%)	30 (48.4%)	6 (31.6%)	6 (50%)	2 (20%)
Men	38 (52.8%)	32 (51.6%)	13 (68.4%)	6 (50%)	8 (80%)
Age (years)	52.2	53.4	36.2	50	51.4
Women	54.0	52.5	37.3	51.7	52.3
Men	50.5	54.2	35.7	48.3	51.2
Anamnesis (years)	2.5	2.6	2.6	1.5	2.5
Number of prior therapists	3	2.7	2.7	2	2
Energy flow density (mJ/mm^2)	0.05	0.07	0.04	0.06	0.05
Number of therapy sittings	2.4	3.4	–	3.7	2.8
Number of prior operations	9 (12.5%)	0	2.4	0	0

- Systemic neurological/vascular diseases
- Shoulder and/or elbow joint instability

A 2-week-long treatment free period was mandatory prior to the commencement of ESWT. The distribution of age and gender (Table 2) varied in the various indication groups. The mean age was 51 years among patients with physiological degeneration syndromes in the shoulder, elbow, and heel but only 32 years among those with dynamic chronic stress syndromes in the Achilles, peronaeus, and patellar tendons and adductor attachments (professional sports, ballet).

During treatment and for 6 weeks thereafter patients were advised to use the affected extremity in a normal manner but to avoid painful movements and maximal loading. As a treatment standard neither the intake of medication nor absence from work were prescribed during this period. No patient was given sick-leave certification.

13.2.2 Treatment Methods

ESWT was administered only by the author himself using a Minilith system (Storz, Kreuzlingen, Germany). The target point for the shock waves was lo-

Table 3. Results of treatment at follow-up – VAS improvement and subjective evaluation – for epicondylitis humeri radialis (EHR), supraspinatus, biceps tendon syndrome, tendinosis calcarea (SS/BTS/TC), Achilles tendon (AT), fasciitis plantaris/bony spur (FP/BS), and epicondylitis humeri ulnaris (EHU)

	6 months		13 months	
	n	%	*n*	%
EHR[a] (*n*)	70	97.2	58	80.6
VAS (initial value 7.8)	1.3	83.4	0.9	88.5
Subjective evaluation				
Very good	22	31.4	30	51.7
Good	38	54.2	20	34.5
Satisfactory	5	7.1	3	5-.2
Poor	5	7.1	5	8-.6
SS/BTS/TC[b] (*n*)	58	93.5	48	77.5
VAS (initial value 8.4)	2.3	72.6	1.6	80.5
Subjective evaluation				
Very good	19	32.8	24	50.0
Good	25	43.1	13	27.1
Satisfactory	5	8.6	2	4-.2
Poor	9	15.5	9	18.7
AT[c] (*n*)	18	94.7	13	68.4
VAS (initial value 7.3)	0.9	87.6	0.8	91.0
Subjective evaluation				
Very good	13	72.7	10	76.9
Good	3	16.6	1	7-.7
Satisfactory	2	11.1	2	15.4
Poor	0	–	–	–
FP/BS[d] (*n*)	10	83.3	8	66.7
VAS (initial value 6.9)	4.2	55.1	4.2	55.1
Subjective evaluation				
Very good/good	3	30	–	–
Poor	7	70	–	–
EHU[e] (*n*)	10	100	10	100
VAS (initial value 8.1)	1.9	76.5	1.6	80.2
Subjective evaluation				
Very good/good	8	80	–	–
Poor	2	20	–	–

[a] 2×Wilhelm's surgery 2 weeks after therapy begin; total effect after 3.9 weeks.
[b] 3×OP SAD after 2/3 weeks, 2×misdiagnosis (rot. dis.), 1×OP SAD after 7 months, 2×IP/CD; total effect after 5.3 weeks.
[c] 1×4 prior surgeries, 1×application for IP; total effect after 4.8 weeks.
[d] Total effect after 3.5 weeks.
[e] Total effect after 4.7 weeks

cated through the scanner which was integrated coaxially to the shock wave direction and through pain feedback from the patient who was continuously questioned during treatment. Divergence very seldom occurred between the anatomical target point and punctum maximum of pain during the first sitting and was always a reason to check the indication.

The energy flow density was modulated so that the patient was able to tolerate the pain. An increase in the applied energy was generally possible during the second sitting and sometimes during the third. To avoid any additive effects no local anesthesia or other analgetics were administered.

The patient was prone during treatment and remained in a comfortable and relaxed position through the use of suitable padding. The number of therapy sittings and energy flow density varied according to the indication groups (see Table 3). On average ESWT was administered in two or three sittings using 1500 impulses, a frequency of 120/min, and an energy flow density of 0.05–0.07 mJ/mm^2.

13.2.3 Evaluation

A standardized follow-up protocol was used to document the patient's status during treatment and any changes versus the initial examination and prior sittings (Fig. 2). Further follow-up examinations were conducted 4 weeks and 6 and 13 months after the last therapy sitting. During each follow-up the patients were asked to quantify their pain according to a visual analog scale (VAS) ranging from 0 to 10 points (0=no pain, 10=unbearable pain). The following criteria were examined: intensity of pain on pressure, a possible shift in the punctum maximum of pain, functional changes, and the pathognomic provocation test. In the 6- and 13-month follow-up examinations the patients were asked to evaluate their pain status according to the following pain categories proposed by Roles and Maudsley [29]:

- 1, very good: no pain, uninhibited capacity of movement and activity
- 2, good: occasional pain, uninhibited capacity of movement and activity
- 3, satisfactory: pain during rest after exertion/loading
- 4, poor: daily activities are inhibited through pain

Patients treated unsuccessfully in this study, i.e., did not complete the treatment series or received surgery after treatment, received given category 4.

At 6-month follow-up 184 (96.3%) patients reported and at the 13-month follow-up 147 (77%). In addition to those lost to follow-up, 35 pain-free patients (18.3%) refused the personal examination. Their results were therefore obtained only via telephone and were not included in the data on the 13-month follow-up.

The first control examinations during the 3- to 6-week period after treatment were not conducted systematically, and these data are therefore not included in the evaluation. We did notice, however, that many patients who were initially disappointed in the immediate results after treatment later suddenly became pain free. Therefore the exact date at which the patient was completely free of discomfort was included in the 6-month follow-up protocol.

13.3 Results

The results are given Table 4 for the respective indication groups. VAS results were correlated with subjective pain evaluation in each of the groups.

VI. Development

No. of sittin g	Date	Time from-to	No. impulse	Impulse energy	Frequenc y	Positive immediate effect	Initial pain increase	Duration IS days	Transfer PMP	New PMP localizatio n	Subjective change +/- 0-10	Functional change +/- 0-10	Radiologica l change +/- 0-10	Notes
1														
2														
3														
4														
5														
6														

VII. Follow up

Final examination	Subjective change total +/- 0-10	Functional change total +/- 0-10	Radiological change total +/- 0-10	Mobility	Movement deficit	Finger-snap test	Chair test	Middle finger stretch test	Neck grip	Apron grip	Notes
3 months											
6 months											
1 year											
2 years											
3 years											

Fig. 2. Follow-up documentation protocol ESWT

Table 4. Evaluation of further indications (n=16, 6 months; n=13, 13 months)

	n	Success rate (%)	Energy flow density (mJ/mm^2)
Adductors	6	95	3×0.07
Peroneus tendon	6	93	3.5×0.05
Patella tendon	4	95	3×0.06

In the groups with epicondylitis humeri radialis the improvement in VAS was 83.4%, and subjective pain evaluation was good or very good in 86.2% of cases. In the shoulder group VAS improvement was 72.6%, and subjective pain evaluation was good or very good in 77.1%. The values were almost identical in the achillodynia group: VAS improvement 87.6% and 84.6% good or very good results in terms of subjective pain evaluation; this reflects the high success rate in this indication category.

The results for the fasciitis plantaris group (bony spur) were disappointing. Of the 12 patients 7 were complete failures. These poor results did not change over the course of 13 months. We believe the reasons for this failure to be: (a) an insufficient energy flow density of (0.06 mJ/mm^2), and (b) a high learning curve in this indication category for finding the exact focus target point. In the meantime we have adjusted the therapy regime for this indication group accordingly, i.e., using higher energy levels, and now have a similar success rate for fasciitis plantaris as for the other indication categories.

We found a surprisingly low rate of relapses after more than 1 year, although the literature [28] reports high relapse rates. We had only one notable relapse in the shoulder group: a woman was operated on al. loco 7 months after ESWT.

At the time of the second follow-up, 13 months after treatment, a tendency towards further improvement was observed. Figures for both VAS and subjective evaluation were improved, and there was also a significant shrift into a better evaluation group. For example, 14 patients of the epicondylitis group who were in the "very good" group at the time of the 13-month follow-up, had shown only "good" results 7 months earlier. In the shoulder group the values of 10 patients changed from "good" to "very good" and those of 3 patients from "satisfactory" to "good."

All results for the provocation tests and local pain on pressure were negative, with only one exception in the shoulder group and two in the epicondylitis group, and further listing was therefore deemed unnecessary. In addition, the fate of polyopter ossifications in the shoulder is not described because we found no correlation between shoulder pain and calcification. Among the shoulder patients 69% showed no radiologically positive calcifications. The lack of pain in the presence of concrements less than 1.5 cm in diameter is documented in the literature [2].

Analysis of our development protocols shows a characteristic pain curve in all indication categories, which can be divided into four phases (Fig. 3):

- Phase 1: immediate pain relief for up to 6 h after the first treatment
- Phase 2: notable deterioration in comparison to initial status during first to 3rd/4th day

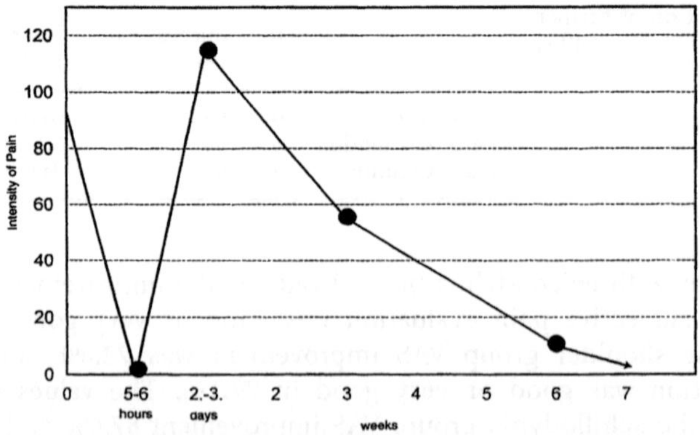

Fig. 3. Typical course of pain after ESWT

- Phase 3: 50%–60% gradual improvement during 4th/5th day until therapy is completed
- Phase 4: total effect completed during 4th–6th weeks after therapy

In this context the analysis of therapy failures is quite informative. Due to an initial deterioration in two patients in the epicondylitis group we decided to cancel further treatment after 2 weeks and conduct a denervation surgery (Wilhelm's). Similarly, in the shoulder group we canceled the therapy schemes for two patients after 2 weeks and for one patient after 3 weeks and conducted arthroscopic subacromial decompression procedures. Today we would no longer advise these patients to undergo surgery but would wait for the total effect to take place during the 4th–6th weeks after the last therapy sitting.

We noted that two patients showed a discrepancy between poor subjective evaluation and the negative provocation test. After inquiring into their social backgrounds it became clear that these patients' desires for early retirement had influenced the former. One patient had been unemployed for 14 months and had applied for disability employment; the other had applied for increased disability certification on the basis of disability. In future studies any current retirement application processes will be considered an indication for exclusion.

Two other therapy failures had been incorrectly diagnosed. In each case the correct diagnosis, rotator cuff rupture, was recognized later, and both patients were surgically treated. Despite these incorrect diagnoses, which we attribute to the learning curve of the first 6 months, we do not consider magnetic resonance imaging of the shoulder to be prerequisite for ESWT.

Since ESWT was introduced in our hospital the rate of surgery has been reduced dramatically. In 1995, 63 patients with epicondylitis received Wilhelm's surgery; in 1996 this number had declined to only 2. The number of arthroscopic subacromial decompressions with ligamental discission was reduced from 56 in 1995 to 9 in 1996. Our success rates with Wilhelm's surgery (77.6% good to very good results) and for subacromial decompression

(70.3% good to very good results) differ little from those reported in the literature [24, 26, 27, 40, 42].

13.4 Discussion

We examined the feasibility of ESWT in view of the contradictory results found in the literature on the success and mechanisms of ESWT on the musculoskeletal system [10, 16, 28, 32, 34, 35, 37, 41]. Is it genuinely represent a valuable addition to orthopedic medicine, or is it merely another type of superfluous medical machinery?

Despite the handicap of an unavoidable learning curve we were able successfully to treat 80%–85% of our patients who had suffered from their disorders for more than 2–3 years, except for the group of fasciitis plantaris group.

ESWT is not only much superior to conservative procedures for treating insertion tendinosis disorders but is also more effective than surgical methods. The number of denervation operations, decompression procedures, tenotomies, and osteotomies for treatment of insertion tendinosis in our clinic has been reduced by 90% since we began using ESWT.

Many authors, some with larger patient series, have reported similar successful results [3–5, 16, 30, 32]. To ensure personal therapeutic skill thorough control of results in follow-up examinations is necessary. We found the meticulous use of our follow-up protocol to be very helpful for monitoring progress. We were therefore very early able to discover the typical pain curves, with immediate pain for several hours, initial pain increase for 3–4 days, gradual improvement over 2–3 weeks, and finally a total effect 4–6 weeks after completion of therapy. The pain curve also offers evidence for the mechanisms of ESWT.

The initial pain-free period immediately after treatment can be accounted for by a temporary blockage of impulse transmission, according to the theory of gate control ([13, 14] and P. Steinbach, Regensburg, personal communication, 1996). The main effect is certainly based on the principle of therapy success through local disintegration. The well-measured local structural destruction triggers autonomic reparation processes, which also address the prevailing damage. This is apparent in the successful treatment of hypertrophic pseudarthrosis. ESWT resemble a surgical decortication: microfractures trigger the process of osteoneogenesis.

The same principle can be applied in bradytrophic collagenic tissue with an acidic oxygen milieu. Local tissue disintegration triggers the process of endothelic formation. This effect can be demonstrated with Doppler ultrasound ([34, 35] and P. Steinbach, Regensburg, personal communication, 1996). Shock wave application in animal models with delayed wound healing has led to significantly better rates of epithelization than conventional wound treatment [1, 18, 20, 34, 35, 39].

The reason for the delayed total effect which occurs 4–6 weeks after the last therapy sitting can be explained by the time required for complete healing of collagenic tissue. The improved vascularization evidently stabilizes a physiological metabolic milieu, and the results therefore not only remain steady but also improve, in this study over a period of 13 months.

Similarly to patients suffering from lumbar back pain, those aged over 50 years with shoulder and elbow disorders may also be influenced by socioeconomical problems due in part to their nearing retirement. It is therefore imperative to consider patients' social and economic conditions.

We could not answer the question of the dose-effect ratio. Other successful reports can be found in the literature in which similarly low impulse rates but higher energy densities were used [23, 33]. We are unable to determine the proportion of cases in which a single sitting using 1500 or 2000 impulses would have produced a successful result.

A further point of discussion is the set of qualifications necessary for approving ESWT. Requiring a patient to have been subjected to all current conservative therapy procedures, although these have proven useless [6–8, 11, 12, 15, 17, 21, 25, 38], before ESWT is allowed is a political consideration that is ethically unjustifiable. No patient would understand being required to undergo therapy procedures that may not only be useless but even harmful (corticoids!) before being treated with more effective methods. Nor would he understand why privately insured patients are able to take advantage of this therapy method, while nonprivate patients are forced to undergo an additional ordeal.

Of course not every painful symptom in the elbow, Achilles tendon, or shoulder should immediately receive ESWT because spontaneous healing often occurs. We believe that ESWT should be considered after a disorder has been chronic for more than 6 months, even if all possible conservative methods have not been tried.

References

1. Banner B, Ziesmer D, Collins LA (1991) Proliferative glomerulopathy following extracorporeal shock wave lithotripsy in the pig. J Urol 146:1425–1428
2. Bosworth BM (1941) Calcium deposits in the shoulder and subacrominal burdits: a survey of 12122 shoulders. JAMA 116:2477–2482
3. Dahmen GP, Meiss L, Nam VC, Skruodies B (1992) Extrakorporale Stoßwellentherapie (ESWT) im knochennahen Weichteilbereich an der Schulter. Extracta Orthopaedica 11:25
4. Dahmen GP, Meiss L, Nam VC, Francke R, Gonchars V (1993) Neue Wege der Schmerztherapie: Einsatz der Extrakorporalen Stoßwellentherapie (ESWT) zur Behandlung von knochennahen Schmerzen und Weichteilschmerzen. Orthopädie Mitteilungen 2:109
5. Dahmen GP, Francke. R, Gonchars V, Poppe K, Lentrodt S, Lichtenberger S, Jost S, Montigel J, Nam VC, Dahmen G (1995) Die Behandlung knochennaher Weichteilschmerzen mit Extrakorporaler Stoßwellentherapie (ESWT) Indikation, Technik und bisherige Ergebnisse. In: Chaussy C et al (eds) Die Stoßwelle. Attempo, Tübingen, pp 175–186
6. Day BH, Govindasamy N, Patnaik R (1978) Corticosteroid injections in the treatment of tennis elbow. Practioner 220:459–465
7. Demmer PJ, Rettig H (1982) Degenerative Erkrankungen und Osteonekrosen. In: Witt AN, Rettig H, Schlegel KF (eds) Orthopädie in Praxis und Klinik, vol VII, part 2. Thieme, Stuttgart, pp 7–18
8. Ebenbichler G, Resch KL (1994) Kritische Überprüfung des therapeutischen Ultraschalls. Wien Med Wochenschr 144:51–53
9. Ekkernkamp A, Haupt G, Knopf HJ, Püllenberg P, Muhr, Senge T (1991) Effects of extracorporal shock waves on standardized fractures in shees. J Urol 145:257A

10. Ekkernkamp A (1991) Die Wirkung Extrakorporaler Stoßwellen auf die Frakturbehandlung. Thesis, Ruhr University, Bochum, Germany
11. Ernst E (1992) Conservative therapy for tennis elbow. Br J Clin Pract 46:8–10
12. Ernst E, Fialka V (1993) Low-dose Lasertherapie: eine kritische Prüfung der klinischen Wirksamkeit. Schweiz Med Wochenschr 123:949–954
13. Folberth W, Köhler G, Rohwedder A, Matura E (1992) Pressure distribution and energy flow in the focal region of two different electromagnetic shock wave sources. J Stone Dis 4:1–6
14. Geisser ME, Robinson ME, Keefe FJ, Weiner ML (1994) Catastrophizing, depression and the sensory, affective and evaluative aspects of chronic pain. Pain 59:79–83
15. Grossi E, Monza GC, Pollavini S, Bona L (1986) NSAID ionisation in the management of softtissue rheumatism: role played by the drug, electrical stimulation and suggestion. Clin Exp Rheumatol 4:265–267
16. Haist J, von Keitz-Steeger D (1995) Stoßwellentherapie knochennaher Weichteilschmerzen – ein neues Behandlungskonzept. In: Chaussy C et al (eds) Die Stoßwelle. Attempo, *Tübingen*, pp 162–165
17. Haker E, Lundeberg T (1991) Is low energy laser treatment effective in lateral epicondyalgia? J Pain Symptom Manage 6:241–245
18. Haupt G, Chvapil M (1990) Effect of shock waves on the healing of partial-thickness wounds in piglets. J Surg Res 49:45–48
19. Haupt G, Katzmeier P (1995) Anwendung der hochenergetischen extrakorporalen Stoßwellentherapie bei Pseudarthrosen, Tendinosis calcarea der Schulter und Ansatztendinosen (Fersensporn, Epicondylitis). In: Chaussy C et al (eds) Die Stoßwelle. Attempo *Tübingen*, pp 143–146
20. Kaulesar JEJ, Sukul DM, Bijma AM, Mulder PG (1994) Effects of high energy shockwaves on normal human fibroblasts in suspension. J Surg Res 57: 677–681
21. Labelle H, Guibert R, Newman N, Fallah M, Rivard CH (1992) Lack of scientific evidence for the treatment of lateral epicondylitis of the elbow. J Bone Joint Surg Br 74:646–651
22. Loew M, Jurgowski W (1993) Extracorporale Stoßwellen-Lithotripsie bei Tendinosis calcarea. Z Orthop 131:470–473
23. Loew M, Jurgowski W, Mau H, Perlick L, Kuszniercak D (1995) Die Wirkung extrakorporal erzeugter hochenergetischer Stoßwellen auf den klinischen, röntgenologischen und histologischen Verlauf der Tendinosis calcarea der Schulter – eine prospektive Studie. In: Chaussy C et al (eds) Die Stoßwelle. Attempo, Tübingen, pp 153–156
24. Meine J, Eicher E (1981) Ergebnisse der Denervierungsoperation bei Epicondylitis radialis et ulnaris humeri. Handchirurgie 13:254–259
25. Mucha C, Wannske M (1989) Ergebnisse einer kontrollierten Studie zur physikalischen Therapie der Epicondylopathia humeri. Physikalische Therapie 10:564–573
26. Nelen G, Martens M, Burssens A (1989) Surgical treatment of chronic Achilles tendinitis, Am J Sports Med 17(6):754–759
27. Neuhaus P, Gabriel T, Maurer W (1983) Adduktoreninsertionstenopathie, operative Therapie und Resultate. Helv Akta Chir 49(5):667–670
28. Richter, D. et al (1995) Die Extracorporale Stoßwellentherapie – ein alternatives Konzept zur Behandlung der Epicondylitis radialis? Orthopädie 24:303–306
29. Roles, Maudsley (1972)
30. Rompe J-D, Hopf C, Eysel E, Heine, J. Witzsch U, Nafe B (1995) Extracorporale Stoßwellentherapie des therapieresistenten Ellenbogens – erste Ergebnisse von 150 Patienten. Presented at the 2. Konsensus-Workshop der Deutschen Gesellschaft für Stoßwellenlithotripsie, Schloß Weitenburg, 26–28 January
31. Rompe J-D et al (1996) Hoch-, mittel- und niederenergetische Stoßwellentherapie (ESWT) in der Orthopädie – eine Standortbestimmung. Presented at the annual meeting of the Süddeutschen Orthopädenvereinigung, Baden-Baden
32. Rompe J-D, Hopf D, Eysel P, Heine J, Witzsch U, Nafe B (1995) Extrakorporale Stoßwellentherapie des therapieresistenten Tennisellenbogens – erste Ergebnisse von 150 Patienten. In: Chaussy C et al (eds) Die Stoßwelle. Attempo, *Tübingen*, pp 147–152
33. Schleberger R (1995) Anwendung der extrakorporalen Stoßwelle am Stütz- und Bewegungsapparat im mittelenergetischen Bereich. In: Chaussy C et al (eds) Die Stoßwelle. Attempo, Tübingen, pp 166–174
34. Seidl M, Steinbach P, Hofstaedter F (1994) Shock wave induced endothelial damage – in situ analysis by confocal laser scanning microscopy. Ultrasound Med Biol 20:571–578

35. Seidl M, Steinbach P, Woerle K, Hofstaedter F (1994) Induction of stress fibres and intercellular gaps in human vascular endothelium by shock-waves. Ultrasonics 32:397–400
36. Steinbach P, Hofstaedter F, Nicolai H, Roessler W, Wieland W (1992) In vitro investigations on cellular damage induced by high energy shock waves. Ultrasound Med Biol 18:691–699
37. Steinbach P, Hoftstaedter F, Nicolai H, Roessler W, Wieland W (1993) Determination of the energy dependent extent of vascular damage caused by high-energy shock waves in an umbilical cord model. Urol Res 21:279–282
38. Stratford PW, Levy DR, Gauldie S, Miseferi D, Levy K (1989) The evaluation of phonophoresis and friction massage as treatments for extensor carpi radialis tendinitis: a randomized controlled trial. Physiotherapy Canada 41:93–99
39. Strohmaier WL, Bichler KH, Deetjen P, Kleinknecht S, Pedro M, Wilbert DM (1990) Damaging effects of high energy shock waves on cultured Madin Darby canine kidney (MDCK) cells. Urol Res 18:255–258
40. Wanivenhaus A, Widhalm R, Parzer R (1984) Insertionstendinose am Epicondylus unter Berücksichtung der Operation nach Gardern. Orthop Praxis 20:713–716
41. Wess O (1995) Speichelsteine, Schmerztherapie und die multifunktionale Nutzung von Lithotriphoren. In: Chaussy C et al (eds) Die Stoßwelle. Attempo, Tübingen, pp 226–231
42. Wittenberg R, Schaal S, Muhr G (1992) Surgical treatment of persistent elbow epicondylitis. Clin Orthop 278:73–80

Part IV

Further Fields of Application

CHAPTER 14

The Use of Extracorporeal Shock Wave Fronts for Treatment of Muscle Dysfunction of Various Etiologies: An Overview of First Results

H. Lohse-Busch · M. Kraemer and U. Reime

14.1 Introduction

Focused extracorporeal shock waves (ESW) are used to soothe local juxta-articular, ligamental and tendinal pain or to treat pseudarthrosis (2, 3, 7, 15). Discussions dealing with the mode of action of ESW generally distinguish between two different mechanisms (2, 4, 14, 16, 20): pressure and tractive forces when the impedance changes between two different mediums on the one hand and the phenomenon of cavitation on the other hand. Cavitation is characterized by nondirectional forces being set free as a result of the adiabatic deformation and change in volume of gas bubbles. These forces lead to microstructural changes of membranes and mitochondria.

Initial studies into the side effects caused by the application of ESW basically concentrated on possible damage to the organ parenchyma as a result of lithotripsy. During the last few years, however, greater attention has been given to possible damage to other types of tissue. In a literature survey (2) dose dependent damage to cells and cell organelles is described. Depending on the number of impulses triggered and the energy density of ESW, damage starts with transient subcellular changes, followed by notable destruction of cellular structures and to the disintegration of bones (2).

Threshold values above which damage to different cells and cell organelles occurs have been determined on the basis of tests carried out with human umbilical cord specimen (18, 20) and with cell cultures of prostate or bladder carcinomas. The application of 2000 ESW waves (1/sec.) with an energy density of 0.21 mJ/mm^2 has led to the detachment of endothelium cells in human umbilical cords. Changes in membranes and other subcellular structures (cell nuclei, mitochondria) in prostate and bladder carcinomas spheroids occurred after the application of 200 ESW with an energy density of 0.12 mJ/mm^2. However, these changes in cell organelles decreased 10 minutes after the ESW treatment and had disappeared after no longer than 50 hours (20). No histological changes were found in the epidermis, subcutis, muscles, sciatic nerve or cartilage of bloodless swine sections after the application of ESW (2).

The ex vivo examinations described above were performed by applying focused shock waves on immobilized specimens. The shock waves were focused on the same cell aggregates throughout the entire duration of the treatment.

14.2 The Problem

Insertion enthesopathy is generally treated with the aim to improve muscular dysfunction This dysfunction causes sensomotor disorders (6), thus leading to local pain and restriction of motion characterized by muscular dysbalances and increased viscoelasticity of the myofascial structures. Provided that such dysfunction can be successfully treated by means of physiotherapy, physical medicine, injections and pharmacotherapy, the pain and, consequently, the pain paresis disappears.

If, however, the above mentioned treatment methods prove ineffective, then ESW can be applied. The mode of action of extracorporeal shock waves is explained by dealing with the disintegration of possible calcareous deposits in the peritendinous connective tissue (2, 3, 7) on the one hand and by discussing the "sympathoplegic" (15) and analgetic effect of ESW on the other hand. ESW treatments have proved successful in most cases (2, 3, 7), even in the absence of peritendinous calcareous deposits.

As we have observed the treatment of insertion tendopathies with ESW improved the local muscular dysfunction immediately. The question is, however, whether the therapeutic effect can be entirely attributed to the focusing of the ESW or whether the improvement of the muscular function also derives from the shock wave fronts that disperse and diverge outside and away from the focus area. The question is also whether unfocused, planar ESW cause damage to muscle cells in man (study I).

Infantile cerebral palsy is accompanied by peripheral muscular dysfunction (6,8), which, from a clinical point of view, in some aspects is similar to functional disorders of insertion tendinosis. Consequently, the present study deals with the manifold symptoms of infantile cerebral palsy (studies II and III) and with nonspecific low back pain (study IV) in order to clarify whether shock wave fronts are a priori able to improve components of muscular dysfunction. Individual cases of muscular dysfunction affecting patients suffering from arthrogryposis multiplex congenita, myopathy and Charcot-Marie-Tooth disease have also been taken into account in the course of this research project. The treatment of children was authorized by the Ethics commission.

14.3 Methods

The treatment was conducted with the "Minilith SL 1" from the Storz Medical Company in Kreuzlingen (Switzerland). The focus of the ESW was first adjusted 3,5 cm inside the coupling cushion by overfilling the therapy source i.e. outside the tissue that was to be treated. The apparatus was subsequently modified by the manufacturer so that an overfilling with water, which causes damage to the coupling membrane, was no longer necessary.

When the energy switch is set to "1" this modified apparatus emits dispersing shock wave fronts with a pressure of 4.1 MPA $\hat{=}$ 0.012 mJ/mm^2. The pressure values for the energy levels "2", "3" and "4" are 5.6 MPA $\hat{=}$ 0.02

mJ/mm^2, 7.1 MPA $\hat{=}$ 0.03 mJ/mm^2 and 8.6 MPA $\hat{=}$ 0.042 mJ/mm^2 respectively.

Owing to the planar spreading of the shock waves, it is possible to avoid an immobile and focused application of ESW, thus minimizing the risk of side effects. The spherically dispersing energy fronts are attenuated as a function of the square value of the distance from the internal focus. The energy is further reduced by reflection and absorption of the shock waves inside the tissue. Furthermore, minimal changes in the wave angle of the shock waves occur due to respiratory and slight muscle activity of the patient.

The persons tested in the course of study I were exposed to a total of 2000 ESW ranging from energy level "1" to "4". 500 ESW were targeted on each of four different anatomical regions (muscle bellies of the flexors of the thigh and lower leg) at a frequency of 2 ESW/sec.

The children tested in the course of study II were exposed to ESW from energy level "1" to "3". 400 shock waves were targeted on each of the four different anatomical regions mentioned for study I at a frequency of 2 ESW/sec.

The children tested in the course of study III were treated for two weeks and exposed to ESW twice a week. In this case, the energy levels used were limited to levels "1" and "2". 400 shock waves were targeted on each of the four different anatomical regions (see studies I and II). In the course of this therapy, no physiotherapy was performed.

The adults tested in the course of study IV were exposed to ESW of energy level "1"-"4" on one or several sittings. 500 shock waves were targeted on each of the two to three different muscular regions of maximum pain. In this case, the treatment was accompanied by physiotherapy.

Consequently, the target areas were exposed to 400–500 low energy shock wave fronts which correspond to about 2% to 5% of the threshold value above which focused shock waves have been found to cause cellular damage (18, 20) and to 33% to 50% (children) and a maximum of 87.5% (adults) of the threshold value above which transient subcellular changes were detected from other authors (see above).

No control group was formed for study I as placebo effects could be ruled out almost entirely owing to the specific test set-up.

A double-blind test was carried out by Baumann and colleagues (1) by inserting an unnoticeable neoprene plate between the therapy source and the body of the children tested in the course of study II. The results of this test are published in this book.

No control group was formed for study III either as only a small number of children was examined to determine general tendencies. Similar conditions applied to study IV.

14.4
Study I. Biochemical Parameters

14.4.1
Objective

The muscle bellies of the ischiocrural groups and the gastrocnemius of 20 adults not exhibiting any disorders were each subjected to 500 ESW of energy level 1-4 (a total of 2000 shock waves).

The CPK, CK-MB, HBDH, LHD, aP and GPT values of the serum were examined just before treatment was started and three hours after completion of the treatment and, in individual cases, again 16 hours later.

14.4.2
Results

The changes in the biochemical parameters before and after the treatment with ESW were limited to a maximum of 2% and thus remained within the error range of the examination method. After treatment the parameter values tended even to be slightly lower, which possibly may be due to biorhythmical fluctuations. It can be concluded, that this type of application does not seem to cause damage of muscle cells.

14.5
Study II. ICP Symptoms

Some of the results obtained in the course of this randomized prospective study were discussed in earlier publications (12, 13).

14.5.1
Patients

So far, we have performed ESW therapy on a total of 360 children exhibiting motor disorders. After choosing the according values for energy levels, impulse frequency, tolerability and effect duration, we randomly chose 35 patients for standardized treatment.

These patients comprised 32 children and adolescents suffering from tetraspastic disorders due to infantile cerebral palsy (ICP), one female patient suffering from spastic tetraparesis as a result of cerebral trauma, one female patient suffering from arthrogryposis multiplex congenita and one female patient suffering affected by spastic athetosis as a result of nuclear icterus.

The 33 tetraspastic patients comprised 19 boys of an average age of 8.9 years, including one particularly reasonable young man aged 26, and 14 girls of an average age of 9.7 years, including one particularly reasonable dispastic young woman of 23 years. Among the boys, the youngest was 4 years old and the oldest was 15 years of age. Among the girls, the youngest was 4 years old and the oldest was 18 years of age.

All patients showed signs of flexion contractures of the lower extremities and had undergone Bobath or Vojta physiotherapy for several years and some of them used according aid devices and/or orthesesis. After having received intensive treatment for two to three weeks, comprising musculo sceletal medicine (manipulations of joints, myofascial release technique etc.), intensified physiotherapy, detonic and proprioceptive massage as well as exercises in a thermal bath, the potential of biomechanical and sensorimotor improvement seemed to be exhausted.

The patients examined included children with pronounced muscular hypertonia of the extremities and poorly innervated hypotonic erector spinae system, children with changing tonus conditions and three children with a pronounced hypotonic muscular system and minor spasticity but with contractures.

14.5.2 Methods

Treatment was performed on those muscles that are mostly responsible for the formation of contractures, i.e. the bellies of the biceps femoris muscle, semitendinous and semimebranosusus muscle and triceps surae muscle. These muscles were each exposed to 400 ESW from energy level 1 to 2. Additionally, the dorsal portion of the knee joint capsule and ankle joint capsule of 3 adult patients were treated. The epiphyseal lines of the children were always outside the ESW range.

Goniometric measurements were performed in prone position after the passive redressing of the hip, knee and ankle joints up to the "structural contracture" or up to the physiological "end feeling of the joint play" (6). The measured values were recorded applying the neutral zero method.

In the case of some patients, ultrasound images were continuously recorded in order to evaluate them by means of a computerized grey-tone analysis.

14.5.3 Results

The following data (Table 1) were obtained after completion of a single extracorporeal shock wave treatment.

Table 1. Improvement in the passive mobility of the joints of lower extremities after ESWT

	Hip		Hip		Knee		Knee		Ankle joint		Ankle joint	
n=33	right	p	left	p	right	p	left	p	right	p	left	p
Ext.	12,0°	0,001	12,3°	0,001	6,8°	0,001	9,8°	0,001	0,5°	0,005	3,9°	0,005
Flex.	5,3°	0,009	4,4°	0,008	5,3°	0,004	2,8°	0,07	7,7°	0,002	2,2°	0,048
Total	17,3°		16,7°		12,1°		12,6°			8,2°		6,1°

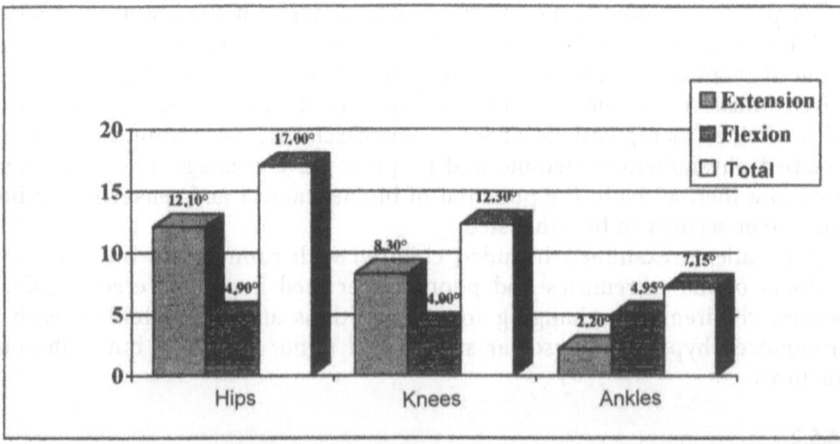

Fig. 1. The statistical evaluation of the measured values shows the changes produced by ESW with respect to the range of motion (measured in angular degrees) of the hip, knee and ankle joints of 33 children and adolescents suffering from spastic diparesis, spastic hemiparesis or spastic tetraparesis, generally accompanied by extrapyramidal disorders (dyskinesia, dystonia). The "p" value refers to the statistical relevance of the changes before and after the treatment

The table above shows the statistical evaluation on the basis of a two-factor variance analysis of all measured values. The improvement in the extension of the joints is quite significant from a statistical point of view. As far as typical spastic disorders are concerned, there was fewer and less severely disturbed flexion movement. Consequently, the improvement of such disorders was less pronounced.

The passive movement of the joints up to the hard-elastic resistance showed the following average improvement in the bilateral stretching deficit of the hip joints, knee joints and ankle joints of 12.1 °, 8.3 ° and 2.2 ° respectively. The overall mobility on both sides during the flexion/extension of the hip joints, knee joints and ankle joints increased by 17 °, 12.3 ° and 7.1 ° respectively (Fig. 1).

The treatment of the articular capsules in the case of three patients led to no further improvement in the mobility and was even considered unpleasant.

Furthermore, the effects produced on the muscular dysfunction occured independently in respect to the basic muscular tonus (hypertonia, hypotonia).

14.6 Casuistic Description of the ESW Effects on Various Neurological Diseases

14.6.1 Athetosis, Ataxia

Apart from the 18-year-old female patient suffering from athetosis as a result of nuclear icterus, 9 other children were treated who suffered not only from tetraspastic disorders of movement but who also exhibited pronounced dyskinetic and ataxic symptoms. All patients experienced a stabilization of their movement lasting for about three weeks and, according to the physiotherapists, a markedly improved posture.

14.6.2 Arthrogryposis Multiplex Congenita

The 13-year-old girl suffering from disorders of movement at her lower extremities experienced an improved redressing of her clubfeet lasting for two months and a stabilized gait pattern from a subjective point of view. The range of motion of the knee joints during extension/flexion could be improved from 0-0-25 to 0-0-35 during the same period. During the last 18 months, the girl had to be treated only every two months to maintain this improvement.

14.6.3 Duchenne-, Becker-Kiener-, Fukuyama Myopathy

In the case of children suffering from myopathy, it is crucial to delay the development of pes equinus in order to maintain the stability and ability to walk. ESW were administered on the flexors of the lower extremities in the described manner.

In the case of two boys aged 5 and 6 suffering from Duchenne myopathy, the range of motion of the ankle joints in dorsal extension/plantar flexion could be increased from 0/10/60 and 0/15/50 to 5/0/60 and 0/0/60 respectively after the ESW treatment. Regular stretching exercises at home and repeated ESW treatments at monthly intervals ensured that the results could be maintained for a period of over 16 months. According to their parents, the boys were less prone to fall and were able to do longer walks. The boys are still kept under observation.

Three brothers aged 9, 11 and 13 suffering from Becker-Kiener myopathy were submitted to ESW therapy described above for a period of 14 months. The individual treatments were performed at monthly intervals and resulted in a 10° improvement in the dorsal extension of the ankle joints. Again, these boys were less prone to fall after the treatment and were able to do longer walks. The boys are still kept under observation.

A 2-year-old boy suffering from Fukuyama myopathy exhibited flexion contractures of the hips of 40°. These contractures were reduced to 10° after the monthly treatment. However, the improvement lasts for only 10 days. The boy's condition did not worsen over a period of 14 months.

14.6.4 Charcot-Marie-Tooth I Disease

Three adults, one man and two women, were submitted to ESW therapy. The shock waves were targeted on the planta pedis and the gastrocnemii. All three patients exhibited an instantaneous improvement in the equilibrium reaction, a smoother gait and – even though this result is entirely subjective – improved strength.

14.6.5
General Clinical Observations Concerning the Disorders Discussed Above

There is the impression that regularly the intensity of the sonographic echo of the treated muscles decreased during the application of 400 ESW ranging from energy level 1 to 2. In some cases, the palpated viscoelasticity and rigidity diminished after only 200 to 300 ESW. However, it has to be mentioned that the slightest movement of the patients in the course of the treatment resulted in a considerable distortion of the sonographic images, thus preventing an evaluation of the grey tone values.

Goniometric measurements showed uniform results. The patients exhibited a reduction of the muscular rigidity and spastic co-contractures of the respective antagonists. The relaxation of the tonic muscles seemed to alleviate the pseudoparesis (9) of the phasic muscles.

There is every indication that ESW therapy has a particularly positive effect on the rigidity of the muscular system. The children submitted to ESW felt movement to be less strenuous. All patients experienced an increased proprioception, which was confirmed by an improved equilibrium reaction.

Despite the fact that only muscles of the lower extremities were treated, numerous patients experienced an improvement in the control of the upper extremities and erector spinae system. This seems to be due to a systemic effect of the therapy.

The physiotherapists of all patients declared that physiotherapy had been facilitated by the treatment and that the sensorimotor improvement had enabled the patients to learn motor patterns more easily and quickly.

In the case of children suffering from hypotonia and older children, the supporting spastic hypertonia of the muscles was found to have significantly decreased for two to three days, thus leading to a temporary deterioration in the static system. On the other hand, however, proprioception was found to have decisively improved, so that the patients still profit from ESW treatment.

In most cases, the biomechanical improvements seemed to increase in the course of the following two days. However, due to the necessary adaptation of the muscles, the improved abilities with respect to the patients' movement pattern could be seen two to three days after the first treatment.

Under regular physiotherapy the full extent of the improvement lasted for at least 18 days. Afterwards, the biomechanical improvements started to decrease, particularly when the range of passive movement was not fully utilized every day. It should be mentioned, however, that the movement patterns trained and continuously exercised were maintained.

Various parents declared that the treatment had instantaneously resulted in more vigilant reactions in their children. These reactions manifested themselves in the form of increased impetus and in general well-being with a cheerful inclination to talk. The children showed the inclination to dedicate themselves to independent occupations, a more skilful use of their hands, an improved power of concentration and reaction and unexpected questions or answers etc.. Adults, in particular, asked for repeated treatments "as they did so good".

14.7 Complications, Negative Effects

Some of the children found the apparatus and the noise it produced to be frightening. However, most of them hardly even felt the ESW or did not feel them at all. If anything, they perceived a slight impact which they got used to almost instantaneously.

About 50% of the patients suffering from tetraspastic disorders experienced an initial reduction in the postural tonicity, which, however, was compensated within a maximum of three days. Even patients who were kept under observation for several months (16 children were even observed for a period of 24 months) and submitted to repeated treatments did not exhibit any undesired effects.

14.8 Study III. Controlled Neuropsychological Pilot Study

14.8.1 Objective

It is a well-known fact that the reduction of motor disorders in the case of ICP children results in an improvement in the cognitive abilities (17). This is why we performed a controlled examination of neuropsychological parameters before and after having treated seven children suffering from moderate up to severe psychic retardation exclusively with ESW as a monotherapy for a period of two weeks.

14.8.2 Patients

Five children suffering from diparesis and two children affected by tetraparesis between 4.6 and 12.4 years of age (average age: 8.6 years) were selected at random.

14.8.3 Methods

These children were submitted to the aforementioned ESW therapy twice a week and examined about one to two days before and after this treatment. The examination methods applied were the ABC method (Kaufmann Assessment Battery for Children) and the TÜKI test (Tübingen Luria Christensen Neuropsychological Examinations for Children).

14.8.4 Results

Owing to the limited number of children examined (seven, of which five were submitted to the entire test series) and the differences in their age and degree of disability, the results obtained cannot be drawn upon for statistical evaluations.

Even if the tests could not be extended due to the limited resources available, the results are still sufficient to reflect tendencies.

The psychologist in charge of the examinations noted an increased vigilance in all children after completion of the treatment. The oral capabilities, in particular, improved considerably. The intellectual abilities, the cultural abilities, the intellectual equivalents and the sensorimotor integration improved by 15.1, 3.0, 5.5 and 18.5 T-values respectively. One child was no longer willing to cooperate during the follow-up examination, which resulted in a significant deterioration in the overall results of the entire group.

Some of the results obtained may be attributed to increased exercise. However, this is not plausible for the improvement of the oral praxy and sensorimotor integration.

14.9 Study IV. Nonspecific Low Back Pain

14.9.1 Objective

The objective of the pilot study was to test the effect of planar ESW on nonspecific and purely functional muscular disorders.

14.9.2 Patients

21 adults, 9 men and 12 women, of an average age of 48.7 who had been suffering from therapy-resistant lumbar pain over several months and had received in-patient rehabilitation treatment, were selected for treatment with ESW. All patients exhibited purely functional pain syndromes of different etiologies without detectable morphological alterations and had not experienced any relief of their nonspecific low back pain despite having undergone intensive and various forms of physiotherapy for two weeks.

14.9.3 Methods

In the course of the treatment, 500 ESW ranging from energy level 1 to 4 were targeted on each of the foci of maximum pain in the erector spinae complex on the pain side at the height of segments L4/L5 and mostly upon the erector spinae of the thoracolumbar transition zone. In 12 cases, ESW were also targeted on the gluteal complex.

14.9.4 Results

17 patients declared that they had experienced a pronounced pain relief immediately after completion of the ESW therapy. 15 patients were free from pain on the day following the treatment, and 3 patients declared that the sensation of pain had considerably diminished. Only three patients experienced no improvement of their condition. On the day following the treatment, the Schober index had increased by an average of 26 mm for all patients.
Three days after the treatment, only 11 patients were still free from pain and restricted mobility. Five patients stated that the pain was less intense. Five patients declared that their condition had not improved.

These results were unchanged on the 10th day. The five patients who had previously declared that the sensation of pain was less intense were submitted to manipulations of the dysfunctional segments, particularly of the ileosacral joints. After completion of this treatment, these patients were free from pain.

14.9.5 Interpretation

Particularly patients suffering from low back pain are considered to be frequently influenced by psychosomatic factors. Therefore a placebo effect may be possible. On the other hand, however, the results of our studies are comparable to those obtained by Eiden (5) who treated painful functional disorders of the ileosacral joints indirectly by means of reflexes of the cervical receptor field.

About 50% of the patients treated by Eiden exhibited dysfunctions that could be entirely attributed to muscular disorders. The treatment of these patients resulted in a complete disappearance of the sensation of pain. In cases in which the ileosacral joints were "blocked" by biomechanical factors, it was necessary to treat the joints by direct manipulations. About 25% of Eiden's patients showed persistent symptoms and turned out to be resistant to therapy, thus requiring a more complex treatment.

After the analgesic effect of ESW treatment had diminished, our patients had to be split up into three groups. The first group comprised patients who had primarily exhibited muscular disorders. The second group suffered from disorders caused by arthrogenic factors. The patients belonging to the third group could not be treated with physical therapy as they suffered probably from additional disorders, such as activated osteoarthritis, which had to be treated with more elaborated measures and time.

14.10 Discussion of Studies I to IV

The ESW applied in the course of study I did not produce any change in the biochemical parameters that are relevant for muscle cells. However, subcellular structures may have been affected. According to other authors, such changes disappear within a few days of the treatment (15). We surmise that ESW, as we administered, do not damage muscle cells.

In the case of spastic muscular dysfunction, not only the neurophysiological etiology but also secondary changes in the muscles themselves i.e. the increased viscoelasticity and rigidity of the contractile elements and connective tissue are to be examined (8). The same applies to myopathies and muscular atrophy (11). Regardless of their etiology some of the clinical symptoms of motor disorders and chronic pain (9) are to be classified as peripheral dysfunction. However, the functional symptoms vary for the individual diseases (11).

The observations we have made concerning the symptoms of low back pain confirm the positive effect of planar ESW. In fact, the application of ESW in the treatment of muscular dysfunctional low back pain has resulted in an measurable improvement in the patients' mobility and in a reduction in the sensation of pain.

The pathological consequence of muscular dysfunction both for ICP and nonspecific low back pain is muscular dysbalance, which, in its chronic form, may develop into Janda's pseudoparesis (9) and severely aggravate disorders and pain.

The objective of the study dealing with nonspecific low back pain is not to suggest the application of ESW for pure lack of discrimination. Instead we find the theoretical aspect in terms of muscular dysfunction per se to be important.

Regardless of the type of dysfunction treated, the use of planar ESW has resulted in an instantaneous biomechanical and thus sensorimotor improvement of the entire apparatus of movement after the first treatment. This improvement in the mechanical properties of individual muscles leads to a changed proprioception which influences the entire sensorimotor and psychosomatic system (17).

The benefits for patients suffering from spasticity are quite obvious. "Soft" (redressable) contractures caused exclusively by stiffness and increased viscoelasticity were greatly diminished. "Structural" (non redressable) contractures were reduced to a limited extent. Shortened muscular fascia became more flexible. Spastic cocontractions seemed to have been reduced.

An astonishingly positive effect has been achieved with respect to the rigidity of the muscles and the muscular hypertonia. The patients felt movement to be much easier. It has to be mentioned, however, that the supporting spastic tonicity of the lower extremities was weakened in many cases and that the paretic ICP component thus prevailed temporarily. Nevertheless, the improvement in the biomechanical abilities has still led to a substantial amelioration of proprioception.

After the treatment of motor dysfunction that are attributed to neurological factors, the instantaneous biomechanical effect lasts for an average of three weeks. The duration of the effect can be extended by performing repeated treatments. Throughout this period, physiotherapists can make use of their patients' biomechanical improvements and make them learn new motor patterns they will no longer unlearn.

Even if a control group had to be dispensed with, the effects discussed above can hardly be considered as placebo effects, all the more so as most of the patients treated were mentally handicapped, tetraspastic children and the effects lasted for several weeks. However, this question has to answered in further studies.

The cognitive-psychic development of children is closely linked with the development of their motor control. This close interrelationship is clearly reflected by the term "psychomotor" retardation. Developmental disorders of motion inevitably lead to disorders in the development of intellectual abilities. The intellectual potential of children is thus wasted away just like their potential abilities of movement if they are not continuously exercised and developed.

Even if only a limited number of controlled children affected by psychocognitive retardation has been examined, there is still an indication that the improvement in the biomechanical abilities as a result of ESW therapy also leads to considerable progress in the development of cultural, intellectual and sensorimotor abilities. These results were obtained after having carried out four treatments in two weeks, which is common practice in clinical routine.

Lasting improvements in the control system can obviously not be achieved if only a single treatment is performed. This applies to ICP symptoms in particular as they entail lasting cerebral disorders. Provided that ESW therapy is repeated at the aforementioned intervals, the effect will be felt for a prolonged period of time and lead to a lasting progress in the patients' development.

Low-energy planar ESW, such as the shock waves applied by means of the modified lithotripter "Minilith SL 1", have led to a step forward in the treatment of ICP symptoms. The System allows a pain free treatment suitable for children. Regardless of whether ESW therapy is performed to treat hypertonia or hypotonia, muscular dysbalances can be reduced.

Consequently, the approach that suggests a focused and thus strictly local ESW therapy (2,4,7), has to be reconsidered.

14.10.1
Possible Effect of ESW on Muscular Dysfunction

The phenomena and control mechanisms of biomechanical conditions that are typical of patients suffering from spasticity, muscular rigidity and increased viscoelasticity of the myofascial system have not been dealt with to a sufficient degree, and no universally valid definitions are available so far (21). The findings obtained to date can thus only be discussed from a clinical point of view.

Discussions dealing with the effects of ESW on the myofascial system are still purely hypothetical. The question whether the muscles as such or nervous structures are influenced by the physical process remains unanswered.

The indirect stimulation of nerves by extracorporeally induced shock waves has already been examined. This stimulation is attributed to cavitation (14, 16).

The arrangement of muscle fascicles, the closely innervated fascial structures (19), the different conditions of contraction within a fascicle, particularly in the case of muscular dysfunction, as well as their central blood vessels represent a variety of media with impedance surges (visible on the ultrasound image) in which shock waves can exert pressure and tractive forces.

It is conceivable that intracellular and extracellular cavitation processes occur within the muscle (2, 4, 14, 16). Furthermore, it is possible that these forces break the persistent actine-myosin chains that are considered to be responsible for muscular stiffness.

Secondary humoral effects are possible, too. A speculative approach might deal with the monoaminergic system which is of importance in the control of interneuronal connections of polysynaptic flexion and extension reflexes of the afferent nerves or neurones of groups II and III. Monoamine deficiency seems to be one of the main reasons for the disinhibiting reflex activity of persons affected by spasticity (10).

The mental and affective changes exhibited by some patients suggest that ESW have an effect on the endorphine/enkephaline balance.

14.10.2 Summarized Conclusions

Unfocused low energy ESW have no measurable disadvantage on the muscular system.

The treatment of painless muscular dysfunction is painless. The treatment of painful muscular dysfunction is painful, but has an analgetic effect.

The peripheral components of muscular dysfunction improve no matter what etiology underlies the disorder.

It is irrelevant whether a muscular dysbalance with pseudoparesis is caused on a hypotonically or hypertonically basis.

Muscular stiffness, increased viscoelasticity of myofascial structures, pseudoparesis due to muscular imbalance and spastic cocontractions are soothed by planar dispersing ESW.

Short term loss of supporting muscular tone is possible in spastic children until the altered proprioception is processed.

An increase in biomechanical possibilities after the ESW treatment leads to more vigilance and thus to improved psychocognitive abilities in children affected by cerebral palsy.

The immediate effect of ESW treatment is temporarily limited. Therefore ESW treatments are not suitable as a monotherapy. An intensive, synergetic physiotherapy as well as sensomotoric stimulation as a part of a comprehensive rehabilitation program will secure the results, which are limited by the underlying etiology.

14.10.3 Outlook

The results discussed above leave substantial scope for further research.

There is no reason why other neurological diseases that accompany muscular dysfunction should not be treated with ESW. We have also observed positive effects in the treatment of contracted and stiff muscles of professional athletes, adult hemiplegics and different myopathies. Based on our observations that proprioception is obviously improved through ESW treatment, we have also treated the soles of patients suffering from polyneuropathic symptoms. The results in terms of ataxic symptoms were in part surprisingly good. Similar results were produced for the ataxia of multiple sclerosis patients who received ESW to the foot soles, i. e. the very important m. quadratus plantae pedis. Dosage and sequence of treatments must still be defined for these diseases.

References

1. Baumann JU, Baumann JB (1997) Extracorporeal Shock Waves in Orthopaedics. Chapter 15, Springer Berlin Heidelberg New York
2. Chaussy C, Eisenberger F, Jocham D, Wilbert D (eds) (1995) Stoßwellenlithotripsie, Aspekte und Prognosen. Standortbestimmung der Arbeitsgruppe "Experimentelle ESWL" - Übersicht und Perspektiven. Attempto, Tübingen, 93-103
3. Dahmen GP, Meiss L, Nam VC, Skruodies B (1992) Extracorporale Stoßwellentherapie (ESWT) im knochennahen Weichteilbereich an der Schulter. Extracta Orthopaedica 11:25
4. Delius M (1994) Medical applications and bioeffects of extracorporal shock waves. Shock Waves 4:55-72
5. Eiden KJ (1990) Therapy of the atlas compared with traditional manipulation in sacroiliac dysfunction. in Paterson JK, Burn L (eds) Back pain, Kluwer Academic, Dordrecht, pp 404-409
6. Frisch H (1995) Programmierte Therapie am Bewegungsapparat: Chirotherapie. Springer, Berlin Heidelberg New York, pp 47-69
7. Haist J (1995) Einsatzmöglichkeiten der analgetisch wirksamen extracorporalen Stoßwellentherapie (ESWT) an der Schulter. Orthop Praxis 9(95):591-593
8. Hummelsheim H, Mauritz K (1993) Neurophysiological mechanisms of spasticity - modification by physiotherapy. In: Thilman AF, Burke DJ, Rymer WZ (eds.) Spasticity: mechanisms and management. Springer, Berlin Heidelberg New York, pp 426-438
9. Janda V (1988) Muscles and cervicogenic pain syndromes. In: Grant R (ed) Physical therapy of the cervical and thoracic spine. Churchill Livingstone, Edingburgh, pp 153-165
10. Jankowska E (1993) Monoaminergic inhibitory control of spinal interneurons. In: Thilman AF, Burke DJ, Rymer WZ (eds) Spasticity: mechanisms and management. Springer, Berlin Heidelberg New York, pp 222-232
11. Lohse-Busch H (1990) Symptomatische Verbesserung der Muskelfunktion bei neuromuskulären Erkrankungen der Reflexe der oberen HWS. Orthop Prax 12:775ä781
12. Lohse-Busch H, Kraemer M, Reime U (1996) A pilot investigation into the action of low-energy shock waves on impaired muscular dysfunction in children with cerebral palsy and low back pain in adults. MITAT 5 [Suppl. 1], p 87
13. Lohse-Busch H, Kraemer M, Reime U (1997) Pilotuntersuchung zur Wirkung von niedrigenergetischen, extracorporalen Stoßwellen auf Muskelfunktionsstörungen bei spastischen Bewegungsstörungen von Kindern. Schmerz 11:108–112
14. Mihran RT, Barnes FS, Wachtel H (1990) Temporally-specific modification of myelinated axon excitability in vitro following a single ultrasound pulse. Ultrasound Med Biol. 16(3):297-309
15. Russo S, Gigliotti S, De Durante C, Corrado B (1996) Diagnosis and early treatment of aseptic bone necrosis with high energy shock waves: preliminary notes. MITAT 5 [Suppl. 1]:p 87
16. Schelling G, Delius M, Gschwender M, Grafe P, Gambihler S (1994) Extracorporeal shock waves stimulate frog sciatic nerves indirectly via a cavitation-mediated mechanism. Biophys 66:133-140
17. Schlack HG (1996) Stimulation der Körperwahrnehmung - ein wichtiges Konzept in der Behandlung zerebralparetischer Kinder. Sozialpäd KiPra 18(5):274-276
18. Seitz R (1993) Analyse von stoßwelleninduzierten Zell- und Gewebeschäden. Thesis, Regensburg.
19. Staubesand J, Yi L (1996) Zum Feinbau der Fascia cruris mit besonderer Berücksichtigung epi- und intrafaszialer Nerven. Man Med 34:196-200

20. Steinbach P, Wörle K, Seidl M, Seitz R, Hofstädter F (1995) Effekte hochenergetischer Ultraschallstoßwellen auf Tumorzellen in vitro und humane Endothelzellen. In: Chaussy C, Eisenberger F, Jocham D, Wilbert D (eds) Stoßwellenlithotripsie, Aspekte und Prognosen. Attempto, Tübingen, pp 1995, 104-109
21. Thilmann AF (1993) Spasticity: definitions, and usage of the term. In Thilman AF, Burke DJ, Rymer WZ (eds) Spasticity: Mechanisms and Management. Springer, Berlin Heidelberg New York, pp 1-5

CHAPTER 15

Treatment of Neuromuscular Dysfunction in Children with Spastic Cerebral Palsy by Extracorporeal Unfocused Shock Waves

Jürg U. Baumann · Joyce B. Baumann

Summary. A study to assess the effects of non-focused extracorporeal shock waves (ESW) of low energy on spastic and contracted muscles of the lower extremities of 11 ambulatory children with cerebral palsy is reported. In the first part of the study, a single application of 400 impulses with a frequency of 2/s was applied to the shortened hamstring and calf musculature in a randomized sample of 5 children. The remaining 6 children received a fake treatment. Evaluation before and after treatment included subjective interrogation of patients and parents, clinical assessment of spasticity and muscle length, gait measurements and parts D and E of the Gross Motor Function Measure Testing (GMFM). In the second part of the study, all 11 subjects received three consecutive treatments with ESW before being examined for a third time, whereby each patient acted as her/his own control. In this pilot study, no statistically significant effects of treatment could be demonstrated, although there was a trend towards reduction in muscle tension and improvement in gait, calling for further tests with a greater number of subjects.

15.1 Introduction

In persons affected by spastic and dystonic cerebral palsy, "permanent" muscle shortness, i.e. muscle contractures, represent major obstacles to improved outcomes of treatment by exercise. Since the muscles mainly affected are those used most intensively for walking, their treatment is of importance and should aim at increasing muscle length, while maintaining strength, elasticity and contractility. The effect of the present non-surgical procedures, including stretching excercises and relaxation techniques, are insufficient.

Experience using focused extracorporeal shock waves (ESW) for treating musculo-skeletal and other disorders, including lithiasis of the urinary system, gall bladder and salivary glands, has accumulated over the last years [1]. With proper application and dosage, few side effects are reported [2]. In orthopaedic surgery, effective pain reduction following serial focused shock wave application has been observed in ulnar and radial epicondylitis of the elbow, plantar fasciitis, as well as in calcareous tendinosis of the shoulder [3, 4]. Promotion of the healing of pseudarthrosis has also been reported. There has been extensive research to explain the pain reducing effects by direct action on the peripheral nervous system or other mechanisms [3]. The same or different direct or indirect effects of low energy non-focused shock waves have been reported to induce muscle relaxation when applied to children and adults with muscle contractures due to spastic cerebral palsy and chronic low back pain [5, 6]. This pilot study involving 11 children attempted to determine the therapeutic potential of treatment by low energy shock waves taking into account the placebo effects.

15.2 Methods

15.2.1 Subjects

Five boys and 6 girls, aged between 4.2 and 12.4 years (average 8.9 years) took part in the study. All patients could walk without canes or crutches and were able to speak and express themselves with ease. The protocoll was divided into two parts: For the first part, the subjects were randomly divided into two groups. Four girls and 1 boy, average age 8 years 10 months, were treated by ESW. Three subjects had spastic tetraparesis and additional rigidity/dystonia, two had spastic diplegia. Of the 2 girls and 4 boys in the control group, average age 8 years 9 months, 2 were classified as spastic diplegia, 4 had spastic tetraparesis, of which one had additional athetosis and one ataxia with dystonia. The subjects were examined on the day before and 48 h after the single application. In the second part, all the subjects received three consecutive treatments with ESW before being examined for the third time, each child acting as its own control.

15.2.2 Treatment

In the first part of the study, 400 "flat" shock waves with a frequency of 2 Hz generated by a "Minilith" lithotripter (Storz Medical AG, Kreuzlingen, Switzerland) were applied to the test group. Each wave produced a front pressure between 4.1 MPa corresponding to an energy density of 0.012 mJ/mm^2 and 5.6 MPa corresponding to 0.02 mJ/mm^2. The focus of the ESW was kept 3 cm within the apparatus by overfilling of the coupling pillow with water. In the placebo-group, the wave generator produced the same pulsating sound effect but without shock wave generation. In the second part of the study, all patients received three consecutive treatments with shock waves as originally applied to the test group alone.

On the basis of the extensive literature on the biological effects of shock waves, the research plan was approved by the hospital ethics committee. All parents signed a form of informed consent.

15.2.3 Examinations

All assessments and evaluations were made without knowing whether the subject had received real or placebo treatment.

1. **Clinical assessment**, including parent interrogation for history, *expectations*, the evaluation and grading of distribution and degree of spasticity, rigidity/dystonia, ataxia and dyskinesia. In the measurement of the passive range of motion (ROM) of hip, knee and ankle joints, care was taken to avoid effects of neurogenic rigidity and spastic reflex activity.

2. **Gait evaluation.** The subjects who wore bathing suits walked back and forth at least twice over a 12-m walkway at their normal speed with SVHS video registration from front and back, and left and right by cameras on rails moving parallel with the child. Special spherical reflecting markers, at least three per segment, located over the pelvis, hip, knee, and ankle and optimized for video-assessment were employed. The exposure time was 1/500 s. Fifty half-images/s were recorded with two video recorders (Panasonic 7355AG) and stored on video tapes. Time-distance parameters were measured using a customized video time code and synchronisation of two cameras positioned at a right angle to each other and to the walkway as described previously [7]. Step length, stride length and walking distance were measured on the video images from distance calibrations on the walkway. Stride length and walking velocity were normalized to leg length. Stride and step length were averaged over four steps, velocity over five steps. Because of the short steps taken by most of the subjects, reliable force plate registration proved impossible for 10 of the 11 children with the force plate arrangement in use at the time of this study.

3. **Gross motor function measure (GMFM)**, parts D (Standing) with 13 tasks and E (walking, running, jumping, stair climbing) with 24 standard tasks were always evaluated by the same person [8, 9].

15.3 Results

For each subject, a total of 77 items before and after each of the two treatment series were recorded and evaluated.

15.3.1 Subjective Impressions of Patients and Parents

After randomized therapy, no effect was reported in the control group by any of the patients or parents in 4 of the 5 subjects. One 10-year-old boy said he could walk better, one 4-year-old was said to have shown particular endurance in walking after placebo treatment. Among the 5 treated persons, 3 with prevalent spasticity reported no change when moving, 2 with considerable dystonia/rigidity felt more relaxed for several hours, one walked faster, but, according to her parents, trailed her feet more following treatment.

Following three consecutive treatments in all patients, 10 of the 11 children felt improvement. Increased endurance was reported by 4, improved lifting of the foot when walking by 3, slower walking with improved balance and fewer falls by 4.

15.3.2
Passive Range of Motion

On repeated examination, a change, mainly improvement, either at the hip or knee level was found in all persons at least at one level and on one side of up to 10°. In 2 non-treated and 1 treated patient with mixed spastic and dystonic tetraparesis, differences of up to 25° were recorded. Improvements in

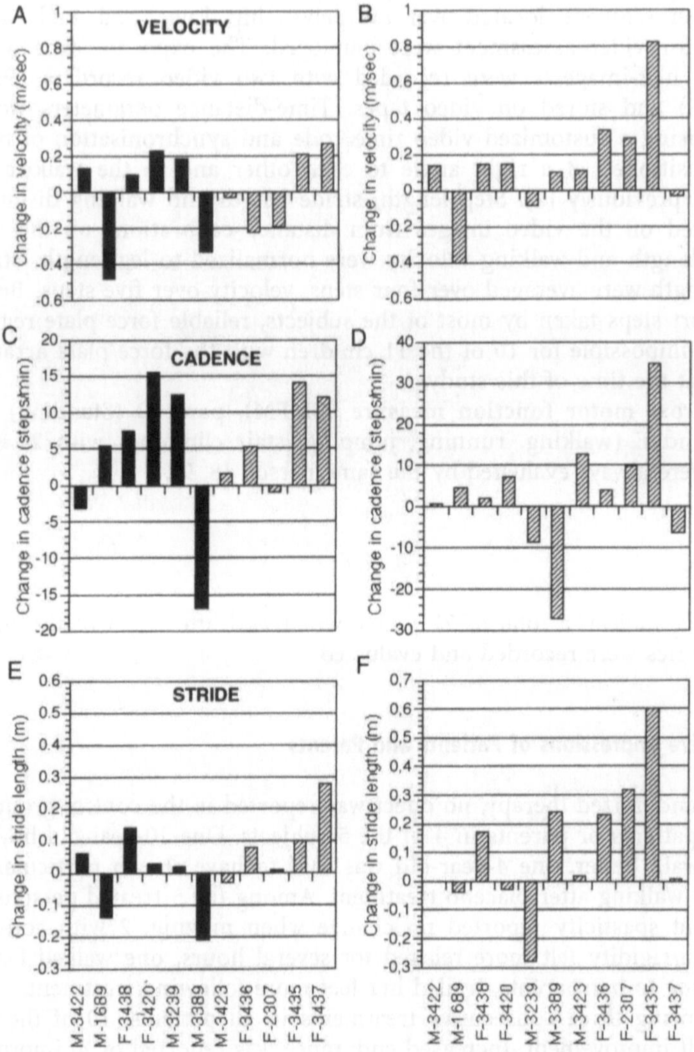

Fig. 1 a–f. The results of gait analysis in individual patients expressed as the difference between values before and after treatment. Graphs A (Velocity), C (Cadence) and E (Stride) represent the values after randomized treatment (*solid bars* = placebo treatment, *hatched bars* = real treatment) and graphs B, D and F the corresponding values after three further treatments of all patients

ankle dorsiflexion with the knee extended up to 10° were found in 1 patient with placebo and 2 patients following serial shock wave application. No change at the ankles was found in 8 of the 11 children. In summary, this

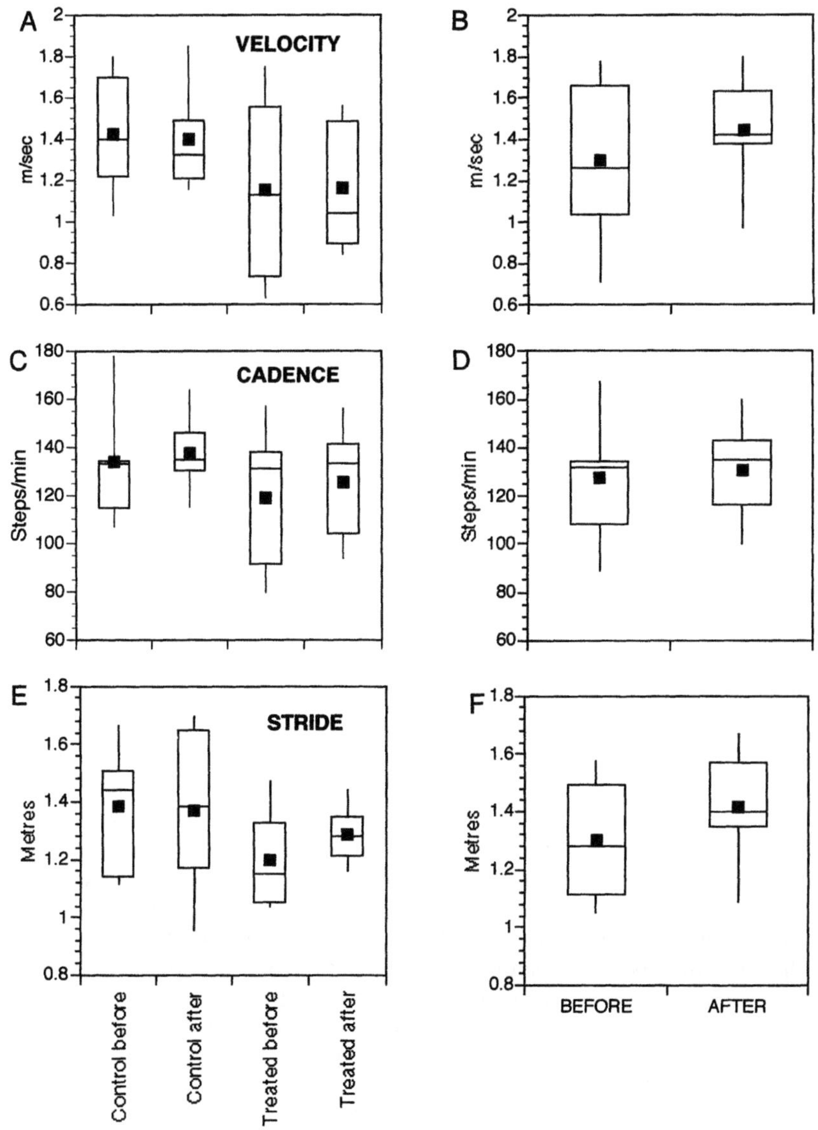

Fig. 2a–f. The results of gait analysis expressed as box plots, showing the variability of the results. The horizontal lines at the top, bottom and through the middle of the box correspond to the 75th, 25th and 50th percentile (median), respectively. The symbol shows the arithmetic mean. The whiskers extend from the 10th percentile (bottom) to the 90th percentile (top). A, C and E show the absolute values of the control and treated groups before and after apparent or real treatment. B, D and F show the values of all patients before and after three additional treatments

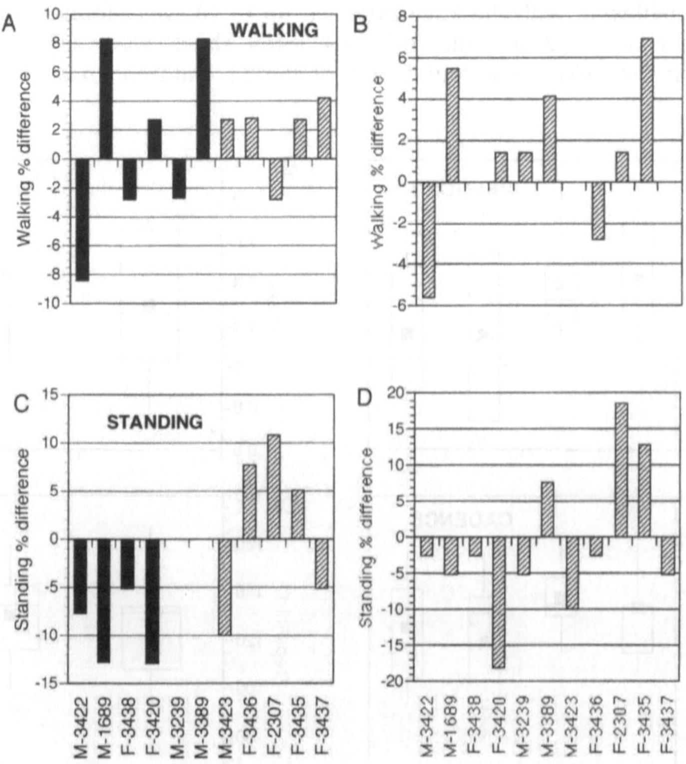

Fig. 3 a–d. The results of GMFM testing expressed as percentage difference from pretreatment values. Graphs A (Walking) and C (Standing) represent the values after randomized treatment (*solid bars* = placebo treatment, *hatched bars* = real treatment), graphs B and D the corresponding values after three further treatments of all subjects

measurement was found unreliable due to a multiplicity of factors in this group of patients. No trend for a change related to treatment was observed in the double-blind examination.

The results in the two groups after randomized therapy are presented as differences from pretreatment values in each individual in Fig. 1A, C, E and as corresponding box plots of actual values in Fig. 2A, C, E. After three further treatments of all subjects, differences from pretreatment values in each patient are represented in Fig. 1B, D, F, and the corresponding box plots of actual values in Fig. 2B, D, F. The results after GMFM testing are similarly represented as percentage differences in individual values in Fig. 3A-D and as box plots in Fig. 4A-D.

15.3.3
Spatio-temporal Parameters of Walking

On statistical evaluation, there were no significant differences, the P-values were >0.05 in all examinations.

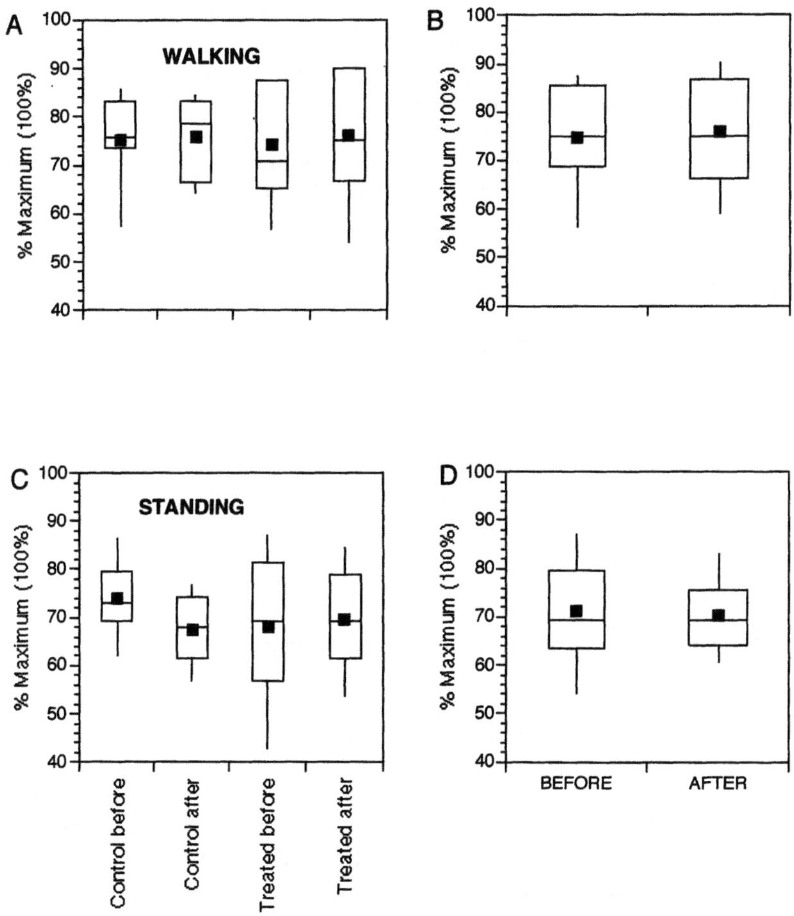

Fig. 4a–d. The results of GMFM testing expressed as box plots (see Fig. 2). A and C show the absolute values of the control and treated groups before and after apparent or real treatment. B and D show the values of all patients before and after three additional treatments

Walking velocity increased slightly in 3 and decreased in 2 of the persons treated by shock waves, but also increased in 4 of the untreated group (Fig. 1A). Differences of up to 18% were observed in the control group. In the treated group, 2 patients improved their speed of walking by over 30%.

After three further treatments of all patients, velocity increased slightly in 7 of the 11 patients and markedly in 1 (Fig. 1B).

Cadence increased in 4 of 5 treated patients, but also increased in 4 of 6 of the placebo group. Changes in both groups were <20% (Fig. 1C).

After the following three treatments, 8 patients showed improvement (Fig. 1D).

Stride length increased in 3, remained unchanged in 1 and dimished in 1 person treated, whereas it improved in 4 and became shorter in 2 under placebo management (Fig. 1E). The percentage changes, however, were minimal, except in one treated person whose stride length increased by 27%.

After further treatment, 5 improved considerably, 4 remained similar and 1 showed a somewhat poorer result (Fig. 1F).

The improvements after three consecutive treatments in all patients in both velocity and cadence are reflected in the increases in the average values as seen in the corresponding box plots (Fig. 2B and F).

15.3.4 GMFM Scores D and E

The score values for test groups D ("Standing") and E ("Walking") for the treatment and placebo groups are shown as individual values in Fig. 3A and B, with their distribution and mean values in Fig. 4A and B. No statistical difference was observed in either test between the treament and placebo groups, the percentage changes for both walking and standing being <15%.

After three further treatments of all patients, 6 showed some improvement in scores for "walking" (Fig. 3B), but not in "standing", where only 3 showed any improvement (Fig. 3D).

15.3.5 Correlation of Different Test Results Among Individuals

Evaluation of the total score of each individual in the six tests was interesting. Following shock wave treatment in the randomized part of the study, 1 patient improved in all six tests and a further 2 in five tests. In the placebo group, improvement was only observed in four of the tests by 2 subjects. Counting improvements and deteriorations among the functional test items (GMFM), there was 70% improvement in the treated group, but only 51% improvement in the placebo group.

15.4 Discussion

Reduction in muscle tension was the main aim of the shock wave application in this study. Lohse-Busch et al. [5, 6] have reported such effects following the application of non-focused serial shock waves to biarticular muscles of the lower extremities in patients with spastic cerebral palsy.

Analysis of results of treatment in children of different ages and with differing neurological symptoms, especially in such a small sample, is difficult, and a randomized study is mandatory. Apart from the heterogeneity of the patients, such factors as learning effects due to repeated examinations and the occupations of the children between treatments are also important variables. These and other factors are probably reflected in the marked differences in the individual results.

Assessment of treatment including patient interrogation combined with measurement of time-distance parameters of walking from video films and supplemented by gross motor function testing using a standardized protocol

[8, 9] revealed no difference between the treated and placebo groups in either part of the study. Statistically, there was no proof of a reduction in muscle tension and increased mobility, but the results showed a tendency towards slight improvement in the dynamic abilities, as well as in the GMFM scores in walking, both in the treated group of the randomized study and after three further treatments of all patients. In contrast, a tendency towards deterioration in more static components of the GMFM tests (standing) was observed. This can be interpreted as a sign of reduced muscle tension in the presence of muscular weakness, which can be compensated by spastic muscle overactivity [10]. However, double-blind studies with a larger number of subjects will be necessary to prove these trends.

No adverse functional effects were observed following shock wave treatment. Improvements observed by Lohse-Busch and co-workers [5, 6], as well as those reported by some of our patients, are similar to those after manipulative treatment and after specific applications of rhythmic mechanical neuromuscular stimulation. The effects of vibration are reported to depend equally on the frequency of stimulation and intensity. Unfocused serial shock waves can achieve deep penetration, but should be further optimized for frequency and intensity. The results reported here show that a similar randomized study with a much larger group of patients, after optimizing the treatment, is necessary before the effects of shock wave treatment can be further objectively analyzed.

Acknowledgements. Our thanks are due to the patients and their parents who volunteered for this study. Treatment was performed in the outpatient Department of the Institute for Manipulative Medicine of the Theresienklinik, Bad Krozingen, Germany (Dr. H. Lohse-Busch).

The Study was supported by the "Stiftung für Bewegungsstörungen, Basel" and the "Swiss Cerebral Palsy Foundation". The examinations were carried out at the Motion Analysis Laboratory of the Department of Pediatric Orthopaedic Surgery, University of Basel, Switzerland (Prof. F. Hefti). We would particularly like to thank Mrs. Doris Gassert for organizing the study as well as the engineer, Mr. Georg Meier-Hofmann.

References

1. Chaussy C, Eisenberger F, Jocham D, Wilbert D (Hrsg.) (1995) Die Stosswelle – Forschung und Klinik. Attempto Verlag, Tübingen, Germany
2. Dahmen G, Haupt G, Rompe J, Loew M, Haist J, Schleberger R (1995) Orthopädische Stosswellenbehandlungen. In: Die Stosswelle – Forschung und Klinik. Attempto Verlag, Tübingen, Germany
3. Rompe JD, Hopf C, Küllmer K, Heine J, Bürger R (1996) Analgesic effect of extracorporeal shock wave therapy on chronic tennis elbow. J Bone Joint Surg (Br) 78-B:233-237
4. Rompe JD, Rumler F, Hopf C, Nafe B, Heine J (1995) Extracorporeal shock wave therapy for calcifying tendinitis of the shoulder. Clin Orthop 321:196-201
5. Lohse-Busch H, Kraemer M, Reime U (1997) Pilotuntersuchungen zur Wirkung von niedrigenergetischen, extrakorporalen Stosswellen auf Muskelfunktionsstörungen bei spastischen Bewegungsstörungen von Kindern. In: Der Schmerz (in press)
6. Lohse-Busch H, Kraemer M, Reime U (1997) In: Extracorporeal Shock Waves in Orthopaedics, Chapter 14, Springer Berlin, Heidelberg, New York
7. Baumann JU, and Hänggi A (1977) A method of gait analysis for daily orthopaedic practice J Med Eng & Technol 1:86-91
8. Russell D, Rosenbaum P, Gowland C, Hardy S, Lane M, Plews N, McGavin H, Cadman D, Jarvis S (1993) GMFM Gross motor function measure manual. 2nd Edition. Easter

Seals Research Institute, Toronto/Ontario, Canada. Neurodevelopmental Research United, Ontario Ministry of Health, McMaster University, Hamilton, Ontario, Canada
9. Damiano DL, Abel MF (1996) Relation of gait analysis to gross motor function in cerebral palsy. Dev Med Child Neurol 38:389-396
10. Damiano DL, Vaughan CL, Abel MF (1995) Muscle response to heavy resistance exercise in children with spastic cerebral palsy. Dev Med Child Neurol 37:731-739

Subject Index

MIX
Papier aus verantwortungsvollen Quellen
Paper from responsible sources
FSC® C105338

If you have any concerns about our products,
you can contact us on
ProductSafety@springernature.com

In case Publisher is established outside the EU,
the EU authorized representative is:
Springer Nature Customer Service Center GmbH
Europaplatz 3, 69115 Heidelberg, Germany

Printed by Libri Plureos GmbH
in Hamburg, Germany